A CULTURAL HISTORY
OF MEDICINE

VOLUME 1

A Cultural History of Medicine

General Editor: Roger Cooter

Volume 1
A Cultural History of Medicine in Antiquity
Edited by Laurence Totelin

Volume 2
A Cultural History of Medicine in the Middle Ages
Edited by Iona McCleery

Volume 3
A Cultural History of Medicine in the Renaissance
Edited by Elaine Leong and Claudia Stein

Volume 4
A Cultural History of Medicine in the Enlightenment
Edited by Lisa Wynne Smith

Volume 5
A Cultural History of Medicine in the Age of Empire
Edited by Jonathan Reinarz

Volume 6
A Cultural History of Medicine in the Modern Age
Edited by Todd Meyers

A CULTURAL HISTORY
OF MEDICINE

IN ANTIQUITY

Edited by Laurence Totelin

BLOOMSBURY ACADEMIC

LONDON • NEW YORK • OXFORD • NEW DELHI • SYDNEY

BLOOMSBURY ACADEMIC
Bloomsbury Publishing Plc
50 Bedford Square, London, WC1B 3DP, UK
1385 Broadway, New York, NY 10018, USA
29 Earlsfort Terrace, Dublin 2, Ireland

BLOOMSBURY, BLOOMSBURY ACADEMIC and the Diana logo are trademarks of
Bloomsbury Publishing Plc

First published in Great Britain 2021
This paperback edition first published 2024

A catalogue record for this book is available from the British Library.

Library of Congress Cataloging-in-Publication Data
Names: Cooter, Roger, editor.
Title: A cultural history of medicine / general editor, Roger Cooter.
Description: London ; New York : Bloomsbury Academic, 2021. |
Series: The cultural histories series | Includes bibliographical references and index. |
Identifiers: LCCN 2020051490 | ISBN 9781472569936 (hardback)
Subjects: LCSH: Medicine–History.
Classification: LCC R131 .C78 2021 | DDC 610.9—dc23
LC record available at https://lccn.loc.gov/2020051490

ISBN: HB: 978-1-4725-6993-6
        Set: 978-1-4725-6987-5
        PB: 978-1-3504-5148-3
        Set: 978-1-3504-5164-3

Series: The Cultural Histories Series

Typeset by RefineCatch Limited, Bungay, Suffolk
Printed and bound in Great Britain

To find out more about our authors and books visit www.bloomsbury.com
and sign up for our newsletters.

CONTENTS

LIST OF ILLUSTRATIONS   vii

LIST OF TABLES   x

GENERAL EDITOR'S PREFACE   xi
Roger Cooter

NOTE ON ANCIENT MEDICAL TEXTS   xii

Introduction   1
Laurence Totelin

1   Environment   21
Ido Israelowich

2   Food   43
John Wilkins

3   Disease   69
Julie Laskaris

4   Animals   93
Chiara Thumiger

5   Objects   119
Patricia Baker

6   Experiences   143
Rebecca Flemming

7   Brain   165
    David Leith

8   Authority   189
    Laurence Totelin

SOURCES   211
BIBLIOGRAPHY   229
NOTES ON CONTRIBUTORS   251
INDEX   253

ILLUSTRATIONS

INTRODUCTION

0.1 Recipe for Mithradatium in the London Pharmacopoeia, 1746   2
0.2 Seven ancient authorities represented on one of the frontispieces
to the 'Vienna Dioscorides' manuscript, 512 CE   4
0.3 Italian terracotta drug jar for Mithradatium, sixteenth century   6
0.4 Carbonized figs from Herculaneum, 79 CE   8
0.5 Roman limestone stele of a female pharmacist, second century CE   13

CHAPTER 1

1.1 Three Roman terracotta votive offerings representing heads   23
1.2 The Roman military fort at Hardknott Pass, United Kingdom   28
1.3 Plaster and wood model of the Asclepeion of Epidaurus, Greece   34
1.4 The swimming pool at the Roman baths of Caerleon,
United Kingdom   35

CHAPTER 2

2.1 Galen's home city of Pergamum, view from the Asclepeion   44
2.2 The cereal plains of Turkey   45
2.3 The bottle gourd   55
2.4 Chickpeas   59
2.5 The myrtle   62

CHAPTER 3

3.1 Terracotta statuette of an emaciated woman, first century BCE 71
3.2 Representation of women weaving on a black-figure lekythos, *c.* 550–530 BCE 74
3.3 Mummy of a priest of Ammon affected with Pott's disease, *c.* 1000 BCE 81
3.4 Greek marble votive relief fragment of mother, nurse and infant, late fifth century BCE 85
3.5 Illustration of Greek or Roman instruments used to perform embryotomies 88

CHAPTER 4

4.1 Roman earthenware feeding bottle in the shape of a swan 96
4.2 Roman terracotta votive offering representing a nursing mother, 300–100 BCE 98
4.3 Frontispiece showing Galen dissecting a pig, 1565 107
4.4 Greek marble statue of Asclepius, 400–200 BCE 111

CHAPTER 5

5.1 Scan of the original receipt from the Park collection 120
5.2 The tools in the Park Collection 121
5.3 Roman bronze ligula 124
5.4 Reproductions of Roman medical implements from Pompeii 127
5.5 Roman scalpel, first–third centuries CE 128
5.6 Roman collyrium stamp decorated with a caduceus design, second–third century CE 136
5.7 Park Collection showing where samples were taken for the XRF study 138

CHAPTER 6

6.1 Marble tombstone of a physician from Athens named Jason, second century CE 144
6.2 Cast-bronze head of the emperor Marcus Aurelius, second century CE 148
6.3 Roman painted wood tablet showing woman on birthing stool, first–second century CE 161

CHAPTER 7

7.1 Medieval diagram of the brain and senses, fifteenth century   167
7.2 Roman terracotta votive representing a male torso   171
7.3 Detail of a woodcut depicting the Hellenistic physicians
     Herophilus and Erasistratus, 1532   175
7.4 Engraving representing Democritus laughing and
     Heraclitus weeping, seventeenth century   181

CHAPTER 8

8.1 Roman ivory medicine box, fifth century CE   190
8.2 The earliest preserved copy of the Hippocratic Oath, third
     century CE   192
8.3 Marble sarcophagus of a physician from Ostia (near Rome),
     early fourth century CE   195
8.4 Relief sculpture representing the surgeon Ulpius Amerimnus
     from Ostia (near Rome), mid second century CE   204

TABLES

5.1 XRF readings for the spoon   137
5.2 XRF readings for the stylus   139
5.3 XRF readings for the spatula probe   139
5.4 XRF readings for the handle   139
5.5 XRF readings for the small spoon probe   140
5.6 XRF readings for the disc probe   140

GENERAL EDITOR'S PREFACE

ROGER COOTER

The cultural history of medicine is all embracing. Virtually nothing can be excluded from it – the body in all its literary and other representations over time, ideas of civilization and humankind, and the sociology, anthropology and epistemology of health and welfare, not to mention the existential experiences of pain, disease, suffering and death and the way professionals have endeavoured to deal with them. To contain much of this vastness, the volumes in this Series focus on eight categories, all of contemporary relevance: Environment, Food, Disease, Animals, Objects, Experience, Mind/Brain and Authority. From the ancient through to the postmodern world these themes are pursued with critical breadth, depth and novelty by dedicated experts. Transnational perspectives are widely entertained. Above all these volumes attend to and illuminate what exactly is a *cultural* history of medicine, a category of investigation and an epistemological concept that has its emergence in the 1980s.

NOTE ON ANCIENT MEDICAL TEXTS

Greek and Roman medical texts can be difficult to navigate. Whenever possible, we have given references to editions and translations that are widely available, and in particular to the Loeb Classical Library editions. Some texts attributed to Hippocrates and Galen, however, are not available in modern editions. In such cases, we have given conventional references to the nineteenth-century editions by Émile Littré for the Hippocratic texts and Gottlieb Jacob Kühn for the Galenic texts. These references are given in the format 'K/L6.515', where 'K' refers to 'Kühn'; 'L' refers to 'Littré'; '6' refers to the volume number; and '515' refers to the page number.

Introduction

LAURENCE TOTELIN

In his fourteenth satire, the Roman poet Juvenal (late first–early second century CE) jokingly advised a father to take a prophylactic drug to protect himself against his son, who wished to inherit his wealth:

> Quickly look for [the physician] Archigenes; purchase the mixture which Mithradates
> Created; if you wish to pluck off one more fig,
> And handle other roses, you must have some medicine
> To swallow before food, when you are a father or a king.
>
> —Juvenal, *Satires* 14.252–5[1]

In the conventional language of fruits and flowers, the poet alluded to a long life filled with sexual exploits for the father, if he consulted the physician Archigenes (a common Greek name, but also that of a famous doctor active in the first century CE) and took the mixture of Mithradates before eating.[2] This medicine, often called Mithradatium or the Mithradatic antidote, was the antidote that the king of Pontus Mithradates VI (120–63 BCE) had invented.[3] It was one of the two most famous remedies of Western pre-modern medicine; the other was theriac, which the imperial physician to Nero, Andromachus the Elder, created by, among other alterations, adding viper flesh to Mithradatium (see e.g. Watson 1966; Stein 1997; Boudon-Millot 2010). These remedies allegedly protected their consumers against the threat of poisoning, as in the case of the father in Juvenal's satire, but they also proved helpful against numerous diseases. They were the main object of ancient treatises on antidotes, such as Galen's *On Antidotes*, and the pseudo-Galenic *On Theriac to Piso* and

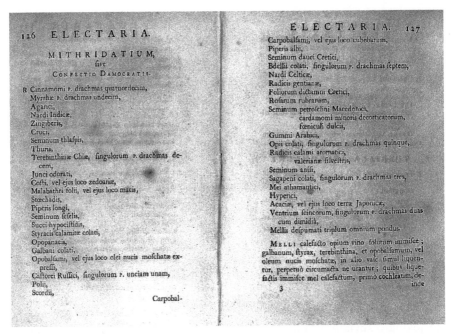

FIGURE 0.1: Recipe for 'Mithridatium sive confectio Damocratis' (Mithradatium or preparation of Damocrates) in the London Pharmacopoeia, 1746. Each ingredient is listed on a new line, thereby facilitating the reading of the recipe. Courtesy of the Wellcome Library.

On Theriac to Pamphilianus (on the question whether these two last treatises are authentic or not, see Nutton 1997; Leigh 2015; Boudon-Millot 2016: LII–LXXIV).[4] Mithradatium and theriac had an enduring success beyond antiquity, and their recipes were still included, for instance, in the official London Pharmacopoeia in the eighteenth century (see Figure 0.1; see Cowen 1985). Through the complex early history of Mithradatium, and with some references to the history of theriac, I will introduce the eight themes of this volume: environment, food, diseases, animals, objects, experience, mind/brain, and authority, as well as some prominent scholarly approaches.

ROYAL AUTHORITY, AUTHORSHIP AND EXPERIENCE

Much scholarship on ancient medicine focuses on two corpora, two large collections of texts. The first is the Hippocratic Corpus, a series of treatises attributed to Hippocrates of Cos, the physician active in the second half of the fifth and beginning of the fourth century BCE, although it is unclear whether Hippocrates himself wrote any of the texts preserved in this collection (for introductions, see Craik 2015; Pormann ed. 2018). The second is the Galenic

Corpus, the collection of texts written by or attributed to Galen of Pergamum (129–200/216 CE), the doctor from Asia Minor who served in Rome as physician to several emperors: Marcus Aurelius and his son Commodus, Septimius Severus and his son Caracalla (for introductions, see Hankinson ed. 2008; Boudon-Millot 2012; Nutton 2020). Galen's writings are also important because they are one of the main sources for our knowledge of medical texts written during the Hellenistic period (the period from the death of Alexander the Great, 323 BCE, to the battle of Actium, 31 BCE), which are for the most part lost. Thus, the medical treatises written during the reigns of Mithradates and the Hellenistic rulers are now only known through fragments quoted by Galen and other later authors, such as Oribasius (fourth century CE), Aetius of Amida (sixth century CE) and Paul of Aegina (seventh century CE).

The present volume acknowledges the significance of the Hippocratic and Galenic corpora while also considering an array of other sources, written and material, some of which (as in the case of Juvenal's verses quoted above) are not usually classified as medical (for this type of approach, see Nutton 2013). This volume also recognizes that most ancient sources relevant to a cultural history of medicine were produced by members – often male – of social elites, but it seeks to recover the voices of women, enslaved people and other less privileged social actors (on 'popular medicine', see Harris ed. 2016). Thus, the antidote of Mithradates was allegedly created by a king, but through its history, we get glimpses of the lives of criminals, market sellers, social climbers and sick women and children.

Mithradates was the king of Pontus, a kingdom bordering the Euxine Sea (the Black Sea). He was one of the fiercest enemies of Rome in the first century BCE: three Mithradatic Wars were waged against him, until he was defeated by the Roman general Pompey the Great and killed himself (for a biography, see Mayor 2010). Intellectuals, including medical authorities, gathered at his court where Greek served as the vernacular language. The king had a strong interest in medicine. Sources associate him with three reputed medical authorities of his time: Asclepiades of Bithynia, who apparently declined to visit Mithradates' court but sent treatises instead (Pliny, *Natural History* 25.6; see also 7.124);[5] Crateuas 'the root cuter' who named a plant '*mithridateia*' in his honour (Pliny, *Natural History* 25.62; see Figure 0.2); and the Empiricist physician Zopyrus of Alexandria (see below). The historian Plutarch (*How to Tell a Flatterer* 15) reported that the king himself 'posed as an amateur physician', to whom his courtiers flocked in flattery to be cut and cauterized.[6] It is pharmacology, however, that most fascinated the king. According to Galen (*On Antidotes* 1.1, K14.2), he 'eagerly sought experience (*empeiria*; see von Staden 1975) of almost all simple drugs', and this led him to develop his antidote. The Roman encyclopedist Pliny the Elder (*Natural History* 25.6), for his part, noted that Mithradates drank poison every day to immunize himself (a process still known in French as *mithridatisation*) and was the first to invent antidotes, one of which was remembered by his name. While one of Mithradates' doctors or reputed medical correspondents might in fact have carried out – or at least supervised – these pharmacological experiments, it is the king who was remembered as the authority behind the creation of antidotes. Who could be a better figurehead of antidotes than a king rumoured to have poisoned some of his relatives, and who was himself constantly under the threat of poisoning?

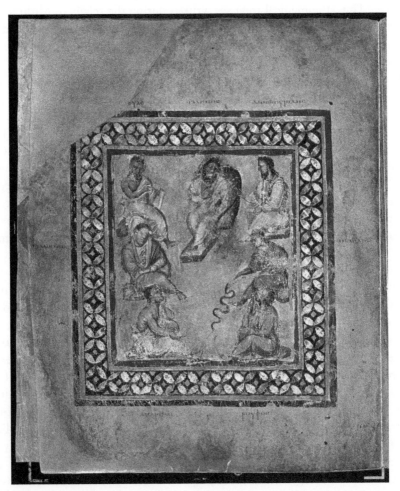

FIGURE 0.2: Seven ancient authorities represented on one of the frontispieces to the famous 'Vienna Dioscorides' manuscript, a copy of Dioscorides' pharmacological work *Materia Medica* produced in 512 CE. The authorities represented are, clockwise starting from the central top figure: Galen, Dioscorides, Nicander of Colophon, Rufus of Ephesus, Andreas of Carystus, Apollonius Mys and Crateuas. MS Vienna, Österreichische Nationalbibliothek medicus graecus 1, fol. 3v. © Österreichische Nationalbibliothek.

The ancient sources explicitly posited a link between Mithradates' political power and his pharmacological prowess. Pliny observed (*Natural History* 25.5–7) that the king gathered detailed information on medical substances directly from his subjects 'who constituted a great part of the world'. He was able to do so by addressing these people in their own languages, as he was fluent in twenty-two languages (or twenty-five according to Aulus Gellius, *Attic Nights* 17.17).[7] Mithradates the ethnographer, then, was keen to understand the environment and peoples of his kingdom literally down to their roots – empire and medicine are intimately linked (see Flemming 2003; Totelin 2012a). Still according to Pliny, Mithradates recorded his findings, together with specimens, in a series of treatises, which Pompey the Great seized and ordered his freedman Lenaeus to translate into Latin, ensuring that his victory be 'beneficial no less to life than to the state'. Pompey had understood the political ramifications of Mithradates' botanical and pharmacological interests, and keenly imported them into Roman culture, where they took roots of their own.

Political power was essential to Mithradates' discoveries in another way. According to Galen (*On Antidotes* 1.1, K14.2), the king tested the properties of pharmacological ingredients on 'evil men who were condemned to death'. Galen (*On Antidotes* 2.7, K14.150) also recounted the story of the physician Zopyrus who sent the king one of the antidotes he had devised (it is unclear whether the physician sent the actual physical remedy or its written recipe) to be tested on a condemned criminal. Zopyrus encouraged Mithradates to experiment by giving either the poison or the antidote first. The prisoner survived, we are told. It is because he was the ruler, the embodiment of the legal system, that Mithradates was able to procure these criminals on whom to experiment. Ancient physicians benefited from associations with rulers who had the right of life and death over their subjects, and they exonerated their patrons from moral guilt, as Galen did (*On the Powers of Simple Drugs* 10.1, K12.252): 'if, as kings, they try out drugs on people condemned to death, they do nothing terrible' (on morality and ancient science, see Lloyd [1985] 1991).[8] The author of *On Theriac to Piso* (chapter 2) made a similar claim, adding that, since he did not have the ability to test theriac (a necessity to detect whether the drug had been adulterated) on humans, he had to resort to trying it out on animals: a venomous beast was made to bite a wild cock who would survive if it had been given true theriac but die otherwise. One cannot escape the conclusion that ancient learned physicians profited from the torture of humans and animals, which at times took place in public in the form of 'spectacles' that were reminiscent of ancient circus games, where animals and dissenters (such as Christians) were killed for the 'entertainment' of the crowd (see Gleason 2009 for the comparison between ancient anatomy demonstrations, on the one hand, and games and public criminal interrogations, on the other).

While ancient rulers had the power of life and death over their subjects, no antidote could offer them eternal life, even though some antidotes were called 'immortality' (*athanasia* in Greek; for the recipe of an *athanasia* attributed to Mithradates, see Galen, *On Antidotes* 2.8, K14.148). The legend of Mithradates acknowledged that reality, as it included an anecdote about his failed suicide (see Harig 1977). Various versions of the story exist, the most dramatic of which is found in the pseudo-Galenic treatise *On Theriac to Piso* (16.20–2). Allegedly, when he had been defeated by the Roman general Pompey the Great, Mithradates chose to kill himself by drinking a poison. His daughters, who had taken the same drug, died quickly, but he remained alive, 'the poison being ineffective because he was used to consuming antidotes'. He then called his friend Bistocus and asked him to cut his throat 'to accomplish with the sword the work of the poison' (see Figure 0.3). Although Mithradates undoubtedly

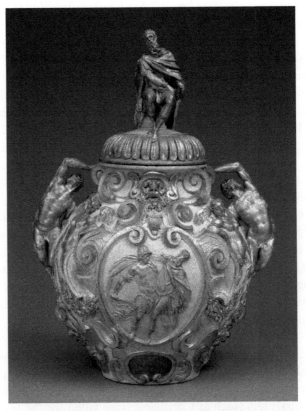

FIGURE 0.3: Terracotta drug jar for 'Mithridate' (Mithradatium), Italian, sixteenth century, attributed to Annibale Fontana. This side of the jar shows King Mithradates being killed by sword by a friend, after having failed to kill himself by poison. The Getty Museum, object number 90.SC.42.1. Courtesy of the Getty Museum.

took his life (a common act among defeated rulers in antiquity, see for instance Cleopatra's suicide after her defeat at Actium), it is possible that the story of his death was embellished shortly after his death to promote antidotes, which became fashionable at Rome in the first century CE.

Pliny the Elder (*Natural History* 23.149) claimed to transmit the original recipe of Mithradates' wonderful antidote, which Pompey had allegedly discovered in a notebook written in the king's own hand. It was composed of two dried nuts, two figs (see Figure 0.4), twenty leaves of rue, crushed together with a pinch of salt. Taken while fasting, it would protect against the threat of poisoning for the day. The poet Quintus Serenus (end of second–beginning of third century CE?), recast the information he found in Pliny's work into verse, adding a few sarcastic jabs:

> The Mithradatic antidote is reported
> To be composed of many ingredients; but Magnus [Pompey] in the king's desk
> When victorious, he seized it, discovered among the possessions,
> Such a trifling mixture of well-known ingredients that he laughed:
> Two times ten leaves of rue, a few grains of salt,
> Two walnuts, as many figs, crushed together.
> The king took a small amount of this every morning, mixed with wine,
> Fearing the goblets which his mother handed him.
>
> —Quintus Serenus, *Medical Book* 1061–8[9]

Serenus and Pliny both knew that this simple, hearty preparation composed of common household ingredients bore no resemblance to the Mithradatic antidote as it was prepared in Rome in the first centuries of the Common Era. The contrast was indeed risible, and it is likely that this short recipe was a spoof, similar in no way to the antidote a king like Mithradates would have invented. Pliny (*Natural History* 29.24) noted that the antidote with which he was familiar included fifty-four ingredients, some of which were prescribed in absurdly small quantities.[10] The encyclopedist objected to such compound remedies, which he considered to be dangerous Greek imports into Rome; he favoured a less complicated form of healing, based on few ingredients, preferably grown in Italy.

Pliny did not give the full recipe of the fifty-four-ingredient Mithradatium. Several recipes for the Mithradatic antidote, however, are preserved in the writings of medical authors active in the first and second centuries CE: Scribonius Largus (*Composite Remedies* 170), Celsus (*On Medicine* 5.23.2), Andromachus the Younger (preserved by Galen, *On Antidotes* 2.1, K14.107–8), Antipater and Cleophantus (preserved by Galen, *On Antidotes* 2.1, K14.108–9), Damocrates (preserved by Galen, *On Antidotes* 2.2, K14.115–19), and Xenocrates and

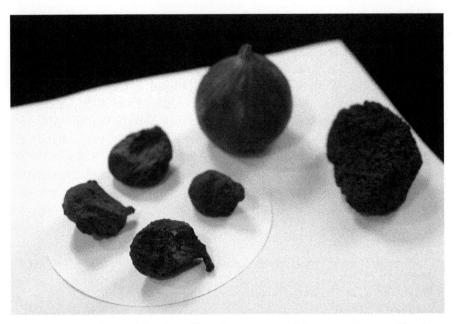

FIGURE 0.4: Carbonized figs from Herculaneum, one of the towns destroyed by the eruption of Vesuvius in 79 CE. Figs figured in a four-ingredient recipe which Pliny believed to be the original Mithradatic antidote. Stories also circulated about Livia feeding poisoned figs to her husband, the emperor Augustus. © Getty images.

Nicostratus (preserved by Galen, *On Antidotes* 2.10, K14.164–5).[11] Galen also transmitted several other recipes attributed to Mithradates, and in particular an antidote named 'with skink' (Galen, *On Antidotes* 2.9, K14.152–4), which included a type of lizard, an ingredient also found in other Mithradatium recipes (see below).

Every single one of these recipes is different from the next in the number of ingredients it contains and their quantities. Among this diversity, the original recipe of Mithradatium is unrecoverable (see Watson 1966: 44; Totelin 2004). The wish to find the authentic original recipe, however, is a modern one: ancient medical authors had no qualms in producing their own Mithradatic antidote and in using the name of the king as a form of advertisement for their own products. Damocrates, for his part, put his stylistic mark on the recipe by versifying it, a method which Galen (e.g. *On the Composition of Drugs according to Kind* 5.10, K13.820) praised as it made it easier to memorize complex recipes.[12] The attitude of ancient medical authors towards authorship and intellectual property, then, was very different from modern ones.

VEGETABLE, ANIMAL, MINERAL: NATURE
IN A DRUG

All the preserved recipes for Mithradatium (except for the four-ingredient recipe discussed above), while each was different from the next, have several points in common. Most obviously, they include a long list of ingredients, from thirty-eight to fifty-four.[13] They are polypharmaceutical (containing many ingredients) preparations, a type of remedy that was still relatively new at the time of Mithradates. According to Galen (*On the Composition of Drugs according to Kind* 2.1, K13.462), the Empiricist physician Mantias (second half of the second century BCE) was the first to write about such multi-ingredient drugs.[14] Before that time, pharmacological recipes had been much shorter, as is the case with the recipes preserved in the Hippocratic Corpus, which rarely contain more than five or six ingredients (see Totelin 2009: 259). Among the remedies attributed to Mantias by Galen (*On the Composition of Drugs according to Places* 8.3, K13.162–3) is a twelve-ingredient Attalic antidote, that is, a remedy bearing the name of another king: Attalus III of Pergamum (170–133 BCE).[15] Like Mithradates, Attalus was known for his botanical and medical interests (see Totelin 2012a), and he may have been a source of inspiration to the king of Pontus. The wording of Galen makes it unclear whether Mantias devised an antidote for the king or whether he recorded an antidote created by the king. In any case, we here have a link between a courtly setting and the development of multi-ingredient antidotes. These would have appealed to kings and other prominent political figures, not only because they promised protection against poisoning, but also because of their expensive and expansive nature: they could be conspicuously consumed as signs of the king's wealth, trading abilities and power over the natural world. Conversely, the conquests of huge territories by Alexander the Great and the subsequent creation of large kingdoms, the Hellenistic kingdoms, had created the conditions in which numerous 'new' substances could be traded from Asia into Europe, thereby contributing to the creation of polypharmaceutical remedies (see e.g. Nutton 1985).

Indeed, the recipes for Mithradatium read as long catalogues of costly ingredients, many of which came from beyond the boundaries of the Pontic Kingdom and even the much larger Roman Empire: from distant Arabia, India and further East. They include various types of pepper, cinnamon, cassia, cardamom, Troglodytic Arabian myrrh, Indian nard, frankincense and ginger.[16] The availability of these ingredients depended on the existence of trading routes, which could prove very unstable in antiquity. Galen (*On Antidotes* 1.1, K14.24), who constantly stressed the importance of selecting the best-quality ingredients for the preparation of Mithradatium, theriac and other multi-ingredient recipes, admitted that this was easier to do in a city such as Rome, the centre of the empire and its trading routes (on Roman eastern trade, see e.g. Young 2001). But even in trading hubs such as Alexandria and Rome, stocks

could easily become depleted. Thus, Galen lost in the great fire of Rome in 192
CE his stock of cinnamon, which was larger than those of all the city's shops put
together (*Avoiding Distress* 6).[17] He could still use the imperial reserves, but
even those were getting a little old, since the emperor Commodus had sold off
most of his father's, Marcus Aurelius', personal stock, leaving Galen to use
cinnamon dating to the rules of Trajan (98–117 CE) and Hadrian (117–138 CE)
(*On Antidotes* 1.13, K.14.65). In a context where ingredients could be very
hard to procure, merchants did not hesitate to adulterate ingredients. For
instance, they kneaded black pepper and added to it pyrethrum (a common
European flower) and mustard to mimic the shape and taste of another type of
pepper, the long pepper (pseudo-Galen, *On Theriac to Piso* 12.10).

Some of the exotic, oriental ingredients mentioned above were qualified
geographically: Indian nard and Troglodytic Arabian myrrh. Geographical
epithets, alluding to European and Near Eastern locations, were similarly
attached to other ingredients of the Mithradatic antidote: Cretan wild carrot,
Attic honey, Chian wine, Illyrian iris, Lemnian earth, Pontic castoreum,
Pontic *phou* (a wild nard) and Gallic nard. These geographically qualified
ingredients are what ancient historian Lin Foxhall (1998 and 2005), in her
study of archaic trade, has called 'local specialties'. She suggested that the
conspicuous and competitive consumption of such products contributed to the
identity definition of elites in the archaic period (roughly from 800 to 500 BCE).
Local specialties can be said to play a similar role in the much later period in
which Mithradatium was first developed and became fashionable. Reading
recipes for Mithradatium brought to mind the various locations named, giving
a sense that all trade routes led to the place where the antidote was prepared
and consumed.[18]

Mithradatium and other multi-ingredient antidotes can be said to the 'world
in a drug' (see Totelin 2016b), as they contained ingredients from all parts of
the world known to the inhabitants of Europe and the Near East at the time.
For a king, a general or an emperor to consume such a drug was a symbolically
charged act: it amounted to swallowing a macrocosmic representation of the
world every day.

At an even more fundamental level, Mithradatium was also 'Nature in a
drug', as all preserved recipes for the antidote included animal ingredients in
addition to vegetable ones; and some versions also included a mineral ingredient.
Thus, all versions included castoreum, a secretion which the ancients believed
to be found in the beaver's testicles (it is in fact found in the beaver's anal sac);
some contained skink, which according to Dioscorides (first century CE, *Materia
Medica* 2.66; see Figure 0.2), was a land crocodile from Egypt, India or
Mauretania; and some versions included the earth from Lemnos, a mineral
product that was stamped with the figure of the goddess Artemis as a proof of
authenticity (see Marganne 1997).[19] The Mithradatic antidote, then, harnessed

the power of all sections of nature, of the environment, to protect its user against poisons and diseases.

OBJECT OF DESIRE: ANTIDOTE CONSUMPTION AMONG ROMAN ELITES

Numerous material sources relevant to a cultural history of medicine have come down to us (for an overview, see Baker 2013), among which we can mention surgical instruments, osteo-archeological remains and archaeological structures. Pharmacological containers are a relatively common archaeological find; at times these containers state which preparation they held, as is the case for the small vessels for *lukion*, an expensive unguent (see Taborelli and Marengo 1998 and 2010). To this day, no ancient container for Mithradatium has been securely identified in the archaeological record. The archaeologist Marina Ciaraldi (2000), however, has suggested that the remains of a complex antidote like Mithradatium or theriac might have been discovered near Pompeii. These were found in the so-called Villa Vesuvio, in a *dolium* (a large container), which in addition to peaches and walnuts, had held a mixture of plant and animal ingredients used medicinally in antiquity. Other finds in Villa Vesuvio included a small cooker, which might have been used in the production of soap, dyes or medicines.

Ancient antidotes, then, have left few tangible traces. The history of these objects is mainly to be written through texts. It is nevertheless important always to remember that these medicines were material objects, which people in antiquity coveted and consumed in a conspicuous manner (on using the notions of 'consumption' and 'consumerism' in relation to antiquity, see Greene 2008). 'It is remarkable how the rich emulate the tastes of the emperors – or at least desire to be seen to emulate them': such was the damning opinion Galen had of wealthy Romans consuming theriac, Mithradatium and other antidotes (*On Antidotes* 1.4, K14.24). The physician reported that, under the rule of Marcus Aurelius, who took a daily dose of theriac, the Roman elites all wanted to purchase antidotes, but under that of his son Commodus, who had no interest in medicine, few continued to prepare them. Pseudo-Galen (*On Theriac to Piso* 2.9) further noted that these drugs came back in fashion under the joint rule of Septimius Severus and his son Caracalla, at which time its use became more general: 'indeed it is now possible for all of us liberally to use what we receive from them [the emperors] and ungrudgingly be cured, receiving the medicine one from another'.

The use of the word 'fashion' in relation to ancient medicine, and more generally in relation to the ancient economy, may appear anachronistic. Fashion is often thought to be a phenomenon restricted to post-industrial societies. In the last twenty years, however, historians have started to explore the notions of fashion and consumerism in pre-industrial societies. Lin Foxhall for instance, in her aforementioned study of archaic trade (2005), argued that 'need' in the absolute sense was not the main driving force in the growth of trade in the archaic period. Rather, desire for goods played an important role. She further suggested that this desire was analogous to the modern notion of 'fashion':

> This isn't as daft as it sounds. By 'fashion' I mean the widespread, relatively large-scale consumption of standardized goods with rapidly changing styles. Stylistic change in itself contributed to the cultural value of the item and is thus practically driven by the desires of the consumers.
>
> —Foxhall 2005: 241

While the concept of 'stylistic change' is not entirely applicable to antidotes, the changes many physicians made to the antidote's recipe are somewhat analogous. It is also possible that there were rapid stylistic changes in antidote containers, which as mentioned have unfortunately not been identified in the archaeological record.

According to Galen (*On Antidotes* 1.4, K14.24), the popularity of antidotes had some negative effects. Some doctors prepared them without including those ingredients that were difficult to find. Worse, beside the excellent physicians who prepared these drugs, people who were far less qualified sold sub-standard antidotes. Galen singled out the *muropōlai*, the unguent sellers (see Figure 0.5), for criticism: they all made mistakes, some more severe than others. Pseudo-Galen (*On Theriac to Piso* 2.5), for his part, deplored the fact that some dishonest people were in the antidote business entirely for monetary gain, peddling poor-quality preparations at the highest prices.

The voice of those *muropōlai* and other peddlers whom elite medical authors despised so much is lost. Many might have been illiterate or have limited literacy skills (for an interesting redefinition of literacy skills in the ancient context, see Woolf 2015). They have, however, left some traces in the epigraphical record (see Korpela 1995). Thus, we can read the funerary inscription in honour of a *thurarius* (an incense seller or maker) named Lucius Lutatius Paccius active in Rome perhaps during the rule of Augustus (*CIL* I^2 1334 = *ILS* 7612). This seller claimed to be 'from the family of King Mithradates'. The Latin *familia* covers much more than the nuclear family, and it can be assumed that Paccius was a freedman somehow attached to the entourage of a king named Mithradates. Whether the king in question was Mithradates VI, the inventor of Mithradatium, or a later king Mithradates (kings of the Bosporan Kingdom were thus named), is however unclear. One cannot but ask whether Paccius sold antidotes, and more particularly the Mithradatic antidote. Adrienne Mayor (2010: 243) suggested that Paccius might have known Mithradates' original recipe, and that he was related to

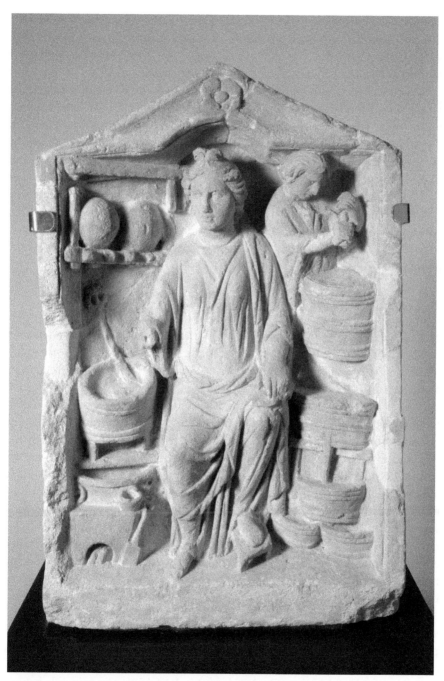

FIGURE 0.5: Limestone stele possibly representing a female pharmacist with her
attendant, Roman, second century CE. The central figure is depicted seated in the
middle of a workshop, with an assistant working in the background. Musée
Départemental d'Art Ancien et Contemporain, Épinal, France.

another pharmacologist named Paccius. That other Paccius is well attested in medical literature; he invented a remedy called *hiera* ('the sacred remedy'), which he bequeathed to the emperor Tiberius (14–37 CE), after having kept it a secret all his life (Scribonius Largus, *Composite Remedies* 97).

Whether Galen had people like the two Paccii in mind when he criticized the *muropōlai* who prepared antidotes, or people lower on the social scale, we do not know. In any case, the physician stressed that it was the rich who emulated the emperor and purchased poor-quality antidotes from quacks. While he mentioned the testing of antidotes on people condemned to death, he did not discuss the consumption of these drugs by ordinary people, who were neither rich nor poor. We simply do not know whether these people had access to – presumably simpler versions of – Mithradatium and other antidotes. This is an issue that is common in ancient history: sources tend to provide information on social elites and the people they enslaved but very little on the majority of the population.

DISEASES AND EFFICACY: IT'S ALL IN THE MIND

Mithradates had developed his antidote in the hope to protect himself against poison. By the first century CE, however, the medicine had many other uses beside that as a prophylactic. It was also used against the bites of all venomous animals, although against the bite of the viper it was considered less effective than theriac, which contained viper flesh – similar is a cure for similar (Galen, *On Antidotes* 2.1, K14.106). Finally, it was recommended in the treatment of other internal afflictions, ranging from simple indigestion (dyspepsia), to the very severe respiratory illness peripneumonia, and passing by stomach ailments, liver ailments, jaundice, spleen ailments, kidney ailments, sciatica, gout, affliction of the nerves, pleurisy, coughs, fevers, chills, tetanus and opisthotonos, urine retention and tired eyes. What exactly these disease labels referred to is very difficult to determine: even when the same words are used in ancient and modern medicine, as in the case for instance of dyspepsia and tetanus, the reality covered by the words might be different. That is, ancient and modern tetanus might not be the same disease, and scholars have pointed to the issues inherent in trying to retrospectively diagnose ancient patients (see e.g. Leven 2004).

The ailments listed so far affect all people, irrespective of their gender. The version of Mithradates' antidote called 'with skink', however, claimed to be particularly helpful in gynaecological treatments: its recipe stated that it 'helps conception; brings down the menses; brings down the dead foetus; and brings down the afterbirth' (Galen, *On Antidotes* 2.9, K14.152). The principle behind these four gynaecological applications, which at first sight might appear quite disparate, is the same: the antidote was supposed to regulate blood in the female body. The ancients conceived of health as a state of balance of humours. The body of a woman, because of its very texture, was thought to accumulate more blood than that of man in the process of digestion. If that blood was not evacuated on a regular basis through menstruation, or used up in pregnancy or lactation, it could cause ill health and infertility (see Dean-Jones 1994; King 1998). Regulating a woman's blood by means of drugs might at times have brought on abortions, willingly or not (see Riddle 1994).

While very much a multi-purpose drug, Mithradatium was not prescribed for maladies of the soul, for what we would call mental illnesses (on mental illnesses in antiquity, see e.g. Harris ed. 2013; Thumiger 2017). Theriac, on the other hand, according to Pseudo-Galen (*On Theriac to Piso* 15.26 and 16.18) could be effective against diseases of the soul caused by black bile (melancholy); more generally it sharpened the mind by clearing it of exhalations.

One can justifiably ask how ancient antidotes could be thought effective in so many different cases. Galen explained the efficacy of these medicines in the following way:

> If all unhealthy states could be treated by single remedies, there would be no need for any compound remedies, but that is far from the case . . . The need for compound drugs is greatest in diseases that require opposite powers at the same time: for instance, both repulsive and dispersing; or both purgative and laxative; both thickening and thinning of the humours. The most useful and best drugs have in themselves opposite powers, as we will show. The compounding of remedies is necessary when we want to have a single remedy effective against many venomous animals or deadly poisons. And it is that need that has led to the preparation of the antidote called 'theriac', and before that Mithradatium and many others.
>
> —Galen, *On the Composition of Drugs according to Kind* 1.3, K13.371 and 374

To Galen (whose reasoning seems somewhat circular) antidotes were particularly beneficial in complex cases, where they could be used as an all-encompassing form of treatment. From the point of view of modern medicine, Mithradatium, theriac and other antidotes appear to be complete frauds. Yet to the ancients, these drugs worked: Galen and many other physicians, whatever their sects, prescribed those remedies to their patients. Their positive judgement of antidotes was based on their experience, on their practice.

Modern readers might be tempted to attribute the efficacy of antidotes to some of its ingredients. Thus, most recipes for Mithradatium listed opium, which is a well-known analgesic (on opium in antiquity, see Scarborough 1995). Pseudo-Galen wrote extensively about opium in theriac (rather than Mithradatium), and explained how the emperor Marcus Aurelius altered the opium content of his antidote:

At first, preparing it for his own security, Marcus Aurelius took it every day in the amount of an Egyptian bean, either swallowing it without mixing it with water or wine, or mixed with those. But as he sometimes fell deeply asleep during his daily activities, he removed the poppy juice from the preparation. But then again, because of his previous habit, since he was of dry temperament by nature, and since he had been taking this drying remedy for a long time, he then spent most of the night wakeful. And because of this he was forced again to take the antidote that includes the opium juice, but this time somewhat matured. For, I have already said it often, when they mature, these types of drugs contain a gentler opium.

—Galen, *On Antidotes* 1.1, K14.4

Some scholars have taken this passage, together with a chapter from the historian Dio Cassius' *Roman History* (72.6.3–4), as a sign that Marcus Aurelius was addicted to opium (Africa 1961; Trancas et al 2008).[20] Others have rightfully dismissed this theory, stressing among other things, that the amount of opium contained in the antidote would have been too small to cause addiction (see e.g. Hadot 1984). Whatever one thinks of Marcus Aurelius' attitude to opium, it is historically problematic to reduce very complex polypharmaceutical preparations to one or a handful of ingredients. To fully understand Mithradatium or theriac, we must consider all their components, as well as the set of cultural connotations attached to them.

Perhaps a better way to approach the question of ancient antidotes' efficacy is to go back to first principles and reflect on the notion of efficacy and the way it meshes with expectations. In her fundamental work, the medical anthropologist Nina Etkin (1988: 302) stressed that efficacy 'might mean a number of things, ranging from full symptom remission to some physical sign (e.g., fever, salivation, emesis, etc) which is interpreted as a requisite *proximate* effect that indicates that the curing/healing *process* is under way'. That is, those who took Mithradatium might not have expected to recover from their ailments by taking the antidote, but rather were content with small changes, which could be attributable to the drug itself or to the powerful placebo effect. Those consumers might have been satisfied to take antidotes as tonics, in a way that is not dissimilar to the modern consumption of vitamin complexes.

ANTIDOTES AS FOOD; ANTIDOTES AS POISONS

Antidotes had originally been designed as prophylactics against poisons, which were often administered as part of dishes or drinks. Stories about poisoning and poisoning attempts at Hellenistic and Roman courts abound (see Winder 2017). For instance, Marc Antony apparently became so suspicious of his lover Cleopatra that he declined to eat anything she offered him unless it had been sampled by a food taster (Pliny, *Natural History* 21.12); Livia allegedly smeared with poison the figs growing in the imperial gardens in order to kill her husband Augustus (Dio Cassius, *Roman History* 56.30.2); and Agrippina the Younger famously served a dish of poisoned mushrooms to her husband, the emperor Claudius (Tacitus, *Annals* 12.67).[21] The fear of poisoning by food ingestion played an important role in the institution of the food tasters (Collins 2012), courtiers who risked their lives daily for their patron.

Against the threat, real or imagined, of poisoning by food, antidotes promised a simple, and even pleasant solution. The emperor Marcus Aurelius, we are told, thought of his theriac as a food. The historian Dio Cassius (*Roman History* 72.6.3–4) wrote that 'Marcus would not tend to eat during the day, unless it was some of the drug called theriac'; and pseudo-Galen (*On Theriac to Piso* 2.7) noted that 'the divine Marcus . . . used the remedy abundantly, as if it were some food'. To the sick emperor, who suffered from digestion issues, theriac was almost a meal replacement. Taking the drug might have been a relatively agreeable experience, as it contained many herbs and spices such as anise, rose, pepper and cardamom (for the use of these ingredients as food items, see Dalby 2003), taken as an electuary (a medicinal paste) in wine and honey. One should note that the English word 'treacle', which today mostly refers to a sticky confectionary syrup, derives from the old French *triacle*, itself derived from the late Latin *triaca* for *theriaca* (Oxford English Dictionary, s.v. treacle). Until the nineteenth century, the word 'treacle' was used to designate antidotal pharmacological preparations. A common baking ingredient, then, is the direct descendent of the antidote of choice of Roman emperors.

The question of where to locate the boundary between medicine and food, between pharmacology and dietetics was a vexed one in ancient medicine (this remains a complex question, and anthropologists talk of a continuum between food and medicine, see Etkin 2008; on food in the ancient world, see Wilkins and Nadeau eds 2015). Galen (*On Mixtures* 3.2; translation Singer 1997: 271) defined the difference as follows: 'Now those substances which are assimilated [by the body] are called foods; all others are called drugs'.[22] In other words, foods can be digested whereas drugs cannot; the body acts upon foods, whereas the body is acted upon by drugs. Galen acknowledged that some substances could fall in both categories, but he did not count antidotes among those food-drug substances. To ancient physicians, antidotes were drugs, *pharmaka*. As such they could have a deleterious effect on the body, and they were certainly not to be recommended to everyone. Pseudo-Galen (*On Theriac to Piso* 17.7) reported the sad story of a child who died because his father insisted on giving him theriac: the drug was too strong for the child's body, which could not digest it (see Gourevitch 2001). Antidotes themselves could turn poisonous. In fact, they were mild poisons (the Greek word *pharmakon*, and the Latin equivalent *venenum*, can refer both to a curative drug and to a poisoning one, see Samama 2002) that were taken against worse ones: poisoned foods, animal venoms and humours that had turned poisonous in the body.

CONCLUSION

This volume, like all others in the *Cultural History of Medicine* series, is organized around eight seemingly simple themes: environment, food, disease, animals, objects, experience, mind/brain and authority. In this introduction, through the case study of Mithradatium, I have started to unpack these notions, at times reading against the grain.

The phrase 'Hippocratic triangle' refers to the three main components of the medical art, as identified in the Hippocratic treatise *Epidemics* 1 (chapter 11): the patient, the disease and the physician.[23] Patients and physicians are deliberately excluded from the list of key themes in the *Cultural History of Medicine*, and the history of Mithradatium and other antidotes shows us why this might be the case. For who exactly are the meek patients and the powerful physicians in our story? Galen and Pseudo-Galen, while most knowledgeable on the topic of antidotes, do not appear as authoritative doctor figures here: rather they pander to the whims of their imperial patrons, wax lyrical about ancient kings who tortured prisoners for the sake of their experiments and look on in despair while merchants sell counterfeited goods. Meanwhile, the patients–consumers of antidotes dictate its composition and swallow them as if they were foods.

NOTES

1. This and all citations hereafter are from the Loeb Classical Library edition by Morton Braund (2004). Unless stated otherwise, all translations in this introduction are the author's own.
2. Archigenes is mentioned as a physician by Juvenal in his *Satires* 6.236 and 13.98. Information on the ancient physicians and other medical authorities mentioned in this introduction can be found in Keyser and Irby-Massie eds (2008).
3. Rather than the more familiar spelling 'Mithridates', I opt here for the more correct spelling 'Mithradates', as historian McGing (2012) does in his entry for the Oxford Classical Dictionary. For the sake of consistency, I will also refer to the 'Mithradatic antidote' and 'Mithradatium'.
4. This and all citations hereafter of *On Antidotes* are from the fourteenth volume of the Kühn's edition, thereafter abbreviated as 'K14'. This and all citations hereafter of *On Theriac to Piso* are from the Les Belles Lettres edition by Boudon-Millot (2016). This citation of *On Theriac to Pamphilianus* is from the fourteenth volume of Kühn's edition.
5. This and all citations hereafter of books 24 to 27 of Pliny's *Natural History* are from the Loeb Classical Library edition by Jones (1956).

6. This citation is from the Loeb Classical Library edition by Babbitt (1927).
7. This citation is from the Loeb Classical Library edition by Rolfe (1927).
8. This and all citations hereafter are from the eleventh and twelfth volumes of the Kühn's edition, thereafter abbreviated as 'K11' and 'K12' respectively.
9. This citation is from the Teubner edition by Vollmer (1916).
10. This citation is from the Loeb Classical Library edition by Jones (1963).
11. This citation of Scribonius Largus' *Composite Remedies* is from the Teubner edition by Sconocchia (1983). This citation of Celsus' *On Medicine* is from the Loeb Classical Library edition by Spencer (1935–38). Numerous recipes for the Mithradatic antidote are also preserved in later medical writings.
12. This citation is from the thirteenth volume of the Kühn's edition, thereafter abbreviated as 'K13'.
13. The recipe in Scribonius Largus' *Composite Remedies* only includes twenty-two ingredients, but the text is incomplete.
14. This and all citations hereafter are from the twelfth and thirteenth volumes of Kühn's edition, abbreviated as 'K12' and 'K13'.
15. This citation is from the thirteenth volume of Kühn's edition, abbreviated as 'K13'.
16. The identification of ingredients listed in ancient recipes can be difficult, but I will not dwell on this question.
17. This citation is from the Collection des Universités de France edition by Boudon-Millot and Jouanna (2010).
18. That is the case even if the produce often did not actually come from the location whose name was attached to it.
19. This citation is from the edition by Wellmann (1907).
20. This and all citations hereafter of Dio Cassius is from the Loeb Classical Library edition by Cary (1927).
21. This citation of Tacitus is from the Loeb Classical Library edition by Jackson (1937).
22. This citation of Galen's *On Mixtures* is from the Teubner edition by Helmreich (1904).
23. This citation is from the Loeb Classical Library edition by Jones (1923a).

CHAPTER ONE

Environment

IDO ISRAELOWICH

INTRODUCTION

It is meaningful to talk about the environment in a study of the cultural history of medicine in classical antiquity in two distinctive fashions. The first examines the impact of the environment on health and healthcare in the Graeco-Roman world. The second explores how contemporaries perceived the effect of the environment on the human constitution and how these views shaped healthcare. In addition, and in tune with some recent historiographical contributions, it must be borne in mind that the environment itself is not unchanging and that it has a history in itself. This non-human history, either man-induced or otherwise, also meant that the impact of the environment on health and healthcare was continuously changing. Thus, a volcano erupting, a famine, a flood or a plague could and should be seen as hereby relevant. Likewise, migration, urbanization, grand-scale building works and exploitation of natural resources had a profound effect on the environment, which, in turn, had health-related resonance. However, the changing nature of the environment was only seldom acknowledged by contemporaries, laypeople and medical authors alike. It is because of these reasons that this non-human history will take a marginal place in this chapter.

These distinctions, however, though illustrative and historically significant, are conceptual, not concrete. Soldiers under the command of Germanicus Caesar (15 BCE–19 CE), encamped across the Rhine in the maritime district of Germany, whom Pliny the Elder (23–79 CE) reported to have been struck by severe illnesses, which Roman doctors called '*stomacace*' and '*scelotyrbe*' and were treated by a plant named '*Britannica*' made no such distinctions (Pliny,

Natural History 25.20–1).[1] They became ill. Their knees and teeth were severely damaged. They were led to believe that drinking local water caused their ailments. They were cured by the healing power of a local plant. In turn, acquaintance with this illness and its cure became widespread throughout the Roman world. Hence, it is impossible to distinguish between the 'real' impact of the environment on the soldiers under the command of Germanicus Caesar and its perception by them. It is also impossible to discern real-time perceptions from their latter reformulation by Pliny, who was a scholar writing elsewhere and relying on post-factum reports. Though local drinking water might not have had actual poisonous attributes, the soldiers believed that the local drinking water caused their ailments, which, in turn, led to actual actions then and there, and to a dissemination and codification of knowledge throughout the Roman world. Likewise, a sick person such as Aelius Aristides, who followed the commands of his healthcare providers and travelling to convalesce in particular spas, a worshipper following a similar exhortation of a healing deity, and an architect planning a city were conscious of the impact of the environment on the human body. Aristides was a Greek scholar, living during the second century CE, who fell ill and consulted physicians, priests and deities in pursuit of cure (on Aelius Aristides' health, see Israelowich 2012). Both his doctors, as well as Asclepius, the god of medicine, sent him on various expeditions to salubrious places, such as rivers, seas, springs or spas (on Aristides' pilgrimages, see Petsalis-Diomidis 2005). All his caretakers believed that these places had a salubrious effect. The numerous votive offerings (see Figure 1.1) in the temples of Asclepius throughout the Graeco-Roman world indicate that the experience of Aristides was representative. Similarly, the treatise of Vitruvius (first century BCE) on architecture, *On Architecture*, and that of Vegetius (fourth century CE) on military matters, *Epitome of Military Science,* suggest that the notion of inter-relation between environment and health was widespread.[2] Some of these understandings were based on experience, others were founded in theory; both marked the environment pertinent to healthcare.

The aim of this chapter is to enquire into the relevance of the environment on health and healthcare in classical antiquity. Questions to be raised include: (i) how did ancient physicians perceive the impact of the environment on the human constitution? (ii) How widespread were these notions? Were they restricted to medical practitioners and medical discourse or did they trickle down to other forms of discourse and to audiences other than physicians? (iii) Were they expressed by works of art and architecture? Writing a cultural history requires going further than medical sources alone, as they offer only limited information as to how pertinent the ideas they manifested shaped habits, forms of life and governmental actions. Hence, the sources hereby used include an ethnographical work, a forensic speech, legal sources, a textbook on warfare, and various others, alongside medical works. They all addressed different

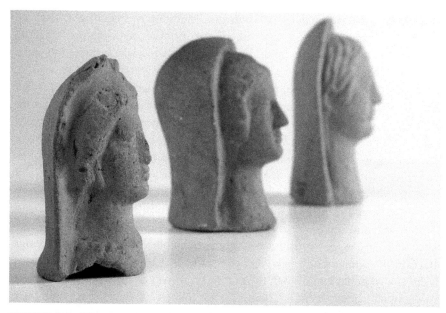

FIGURE 1.1: Three terracotta votive offerings representing heads, Roman, date uncertain. There are numerous examples of such votives in the Wellcome collection. Courtesy of Wellcome Images.

audiences and pursued altering goals. However, they all disclose vital information both on the impact of the environment on health, and on how Graeco-Roman society reciprocated to this impact.

THE MEDICAL BACKGROUND

Graeco-Roman medicine acknowledged the profound relevance of the environment on healthcare since at least the fifth century BCE and the publication of the Hippocratic treatise *On Airs, Waters and Places*.[3] In this work, the Hippocratic author showed professional doctors who were forced to pursue their profession as itinerant physicians how best to secure the trust of potential clients in the cities in which they arrived.[4] Such a skill was imperative as there was no official form of medical credentials throughout classical antiquity.[5] This treatise equipped doctors who arrived in a city where they were unknown with means to distinguish themselves from other healthcare providers. More specifically, it taught itinerant physicians how to make an accurate *prognosis* on the basis of the city's topography and climate. An accurate prognosis was the most trusted means in the Graeco-Roman medical marketplace for a heath care provider to demonstrate his skills.[6] The Hippocratic author assumed that the influence of the environment on the human constitution was significant. It caused certain ailments and discouraged others. An intimate acquaintance with the effects of the environment would, therefore, be able to yield accurate *prognosis* and, in consequence, secure the prestige of the doctor who provided it.

The Hippocratic author of *On Airs, Waters and Places* informed his readers that whoever wishes to pursue properly the science of medicine must consider the effects that each season of the year can produce (*On Airs, Waters and Places* 1). The next point is the hot and cold winds, both the winds which are universal as well as those which are particular to each region. It is equally crucial to learn the property of the local water 'for as these differ in taste and in weight, so the property of each is far different from that of any other' (*On Airs, Waters and Places* 1). The relevance of local water to the human constitution, and therefore to the work of the physician, goes further. Marsh water and hard water which comes from rocky places are also of particular effect on the human body. Taken together, the data collected from an analysis of the environment could teach the doctor on arrival at a town with which he is unfamiliar about its local diseases or the nature of those that commonly prevail (*On Airs, Waters and Places* 2). Moreover, as time passes, the doctor who is attentive to the environment could tell what epidemic diseases – which in the Hippocratic context mean plagues that are indigenous to certain places and that are caused by the environment – will attack the city either in summer or winter, 'for knowing the changes of the seasons, and the risings and the settings of the stars, with the circumstances of each of these phenomena, he (i.e. the itinerant physician) will know beforehand the nature of the year that is coming' (*On Airs, Waters and Places* 2). This treatise offers the first systematic analysis of the impact of the environment of the human body, alongside practical guidelines for doctors who were asked to treat ailments caused by it.

The Hippocratic view became commonplace throughout classical antiquity and beyond. Physicians, scholars and laypeople accepted the Hippocratic understanding of the impact of the environment on the human body and acted accordingly. Like other Hippocratic texts, the treatise *On Airs, Waters and Places* was habitually read by Greek, Hellenistic and Roman physicians and it guided their practice. Scholars, such as the philosopher Aristotle (384–322 BCE), the Greek philosopher, historian and scholar Posidonius (135–51 BCE) and the Roman author and scholar Marcus Terentius Varro (116–27 BCE) read it and acknowledged its validity (see Jacoby 1911; Pohlenz 1938; Heinimann 1945: 13–41). Tellingly, these ideas also guided professional practitioners in fields other than medicine, such as architects and military experts, who used the environmental works of Hippocrates both in their theoretical works and in their practice. During the High Roman Empire, and following the Hellenistic legacy, it was well known that the inhabited world encompassed various microclimates (see Horden and Purcell 2000), which shaped different cultural institutions.[7] Authors who wished to shed light on remote areas as explanation to their unique culture habitually discussed the environment.

Such, for example, is the habit of Tacitus in his *Germania*, who found the German environment pertinent to his exposition of the local culture and institutions. Tacitus' *Germania* is the only known Graeco-Roman work dedicated solely to a description of another people (see Gruen 2011: 159).[8] Moreover, the Germans epitomized the notion of 'barbarians' in Roman eyes (see Gruen 2011: 161). The connection between the character of the Germans and the landscape of their dwelling place, although not explicitly discussed, can be inferred from Tacitus' elaborate claim that the Germans were autochthonous as an explanation for their attributes and habits. Autochthony played a central role in Graeco-Roman historiography and anthropology (even if this title was yet to be coined). Herodotus (8.73.1; 4.171.1; 4.172.1; 4.109.1) and Thucydides (6.2.1) used it in their geopolitical surveys, often with a positive connotation.[9] Athenian autochthony in particular was seen as grounds for its democratic culture and political ideology (Plato, *Menexenus* 245d; see Lape 2010: 100–5).[10] The Germans must have been autochthonous, according to Tacitus both because they resemble no one else, and also because it seemed incomprehensible to Tacitus (*Germania* 2.1; 4.1) that anyone would choose to migrate to this landscape from Asia or Europe.[11] Hence it is the environment that shapes appearance and dictates habits. It was the cause of particular ailments and offers certain *materia medica* through vegetation, minerals and other substances. Such state of mind is also present in Tacitus' description of Britain in his treatise on his father-in-law, Agricola. After a short description of Britain's topography, Tacitus discussed its inhabitants. He is uncertain whether the Britons are autochthonous or whether they migrated from Spain or Gaul, as it is impossible to conclude, so Tacitus (*Agricola* 12) thought, if they resemble the people of Gaul because they share common ancestors or whether it is the similar climate that shapes similar people.[12] A generation earlier, Seneca (*On Providence* 4.14) had made a more explicit connection between German traits and the environment.[13] More generally, the widespread premise that the environment affects the human body, shapes human character and instigates certain political institutions was seen as relevant not only to physicians and other types of healthcare providers, but also to architects, military commanders and political commentators.

THE INFILTRATION OF MEDICAL NOTIONS CONCERNING THE EFFECT OF THE ENVIRONMENT OF THE HUMAN CONSTITUTION OUTSIDE MEDICINE

An understanding of the influence of the environment on the human body was not reserved exclusively to scholarly enterprises and to the works of physicians, ethnographers and philosophers. The notion of a connection between environment and the human body seems to have been commonplace amongst the general public and it guided artisans and policy makers, shaping recruitment policy to the Roman army and its influences could and still can be seen in architecture and landscape design. According to Vitruvius, Greek theories concerning the effect of the environment on health were widely acknowledged by professional architects in their practice. Vitruvius himself paid much attention to health-related considerations in his guidelines for city planning. He emphasized, for example, how important it was to choose a particularly airy location for the city's *forum*. The positioning of the *forum* was crucial because a large crowd of people habitually convened there, which therefore had the potential to turn public events into health hazards. Vitruvius (*On Architecture* 5.3.1) explained that the spectators, with their wives and children, who participated in these events, sat outside for the whole of the games, and the pores of their bodies, being opened by the pleasure they enjoyed, were easily affected by the air, which, if it blew from marshy or other noisome places, infused its bad qualities into the system. These evils were avoided by the careful choice of a situation for the theatre.

The work of Vitruvius, alongside archaeological evidence and other corroborative testimonies, which will be discussed below, attests to two ways in which the environment seemed to be relevant to health, according to architects, city planners and the general public. The first is the contribution of urbanism in general, and of civic architecture in particular, to healthcare during the High Roman Empire. Thus, the noticeable attention of Roman architects, military commanders and legislators to the relevance of the environment to health makes it meaningful to talk about 'environmental history' in the context of the history of medicine.[14] The second focused on climate, vegetation and terrain and their influence on the human constitution. However, much like in the case of Germanicus' soldiers mentioned above, this distinction is purely methodological and has no bearings on the actual phenomena concerned. It is impossible to discern architects' notions of the connection between the environment and health and the impact of their incorporating of these notions in their work and its influence on public health and public perceptions of environment and health. It is enough to note that the architect, according to Vitruvius, must be conscious of the environment when planning a city. Vitruvius' thoughts on health-related issues were far from being simply intuitive and he must have had at least a basic acquaintance with Greek medical theories. He was aware of the humoural system and of the effect of exercise upon the function of the various humours and on the balance between them (*On Architecture* 5.9.5). These notions, even if they reached Vitruvius in an abridged fashion through textbooks, were of Hippocratic origin and dictated that the city planner must be aware of the influence of the environment of public health.

Vitruvius further explained that in setting out the walls of a city the choice of a healthy situation was not to be disregarded: it should be on high ground, subject neither to fogs nor rains; its aspects should be neither violently hot nor intensely cold, but temperate in both respects. Proximity to a marshy place had to be avoided; for in such a site the morning air, uniting with the fogs that rise nearby, would reach the city with the rising sun; and these fogs and mists, charged with the exhalation of animals, would diffuse unwholesome effluvia over the bodies of the inhabitants and render the place pestilent. A city on the seaside, exposed to the south or west, would be insalubrious; for in summer mornings, a city thus placed would be hot, at noon it would be scorched. A city, also, with a western aspect, would be warm even at sunrise, hot at noon and of a burning temperature in the evening (Vitruvius, *On Architecture* 1.4.1). These guidelines reveal how such views were used as devisers for shaping Roman landscape. The effect of such places on the inhabitants' constitutions was explained to be devastating (Vitruvius, *On Architecture* 1.4.2). In addition, as in the Hippocratic treatise *On Airs, Waters and Places*, Vitruvius placed much emphasis not only on the climate but also on the changes between the seasons. He explained that, if one changed a cold for a hot climate, he rarely escaped sickness and was soon carried off; whereas, on the other hand, those who pass from a hot to a cold climate, far from being injured by the change, are thereby generally strengthened (*On Architecture* 1.4.3). Offering practical advice, Vitruvius therefore concluded that much care should be taken when setting out the walls of a city (*On Architecture* 1.4.4). Though there is little evidence as to the influence of Vitruvius on later Roman architects in general, and on later Roman city planners in particular, the work's popularity suggests that its influence was not unnoticed. Furthermore, the imperial recipient of the work suggests that its content was meant to echo imperial policy rather than to promote avant-garde architecture.

The connection between salubriousness and location, as explained by Vitruvius and derived from the Hippocrates *On Airs, Waters and Places*, also guided Roman generals in choosing encampment locations and in designing military camps (see Figure 1.2). Onasander (first century CE) warned Roman generals in his first century CE short treatise on the duties of military commanders (*Strategicos* 8.2) not to camp in marshy sites because the smell in such places caused illness and infection.[15] The foundation of a professional army by Augustus also meant that military units were stationed in permanent camps in potential conflict zones (on medicine in the Roman imperial army, see Israelowich 2016a). According to Onasander and other sources, choosing such a site was not guided solely by strategic considerations but also took into account environmental ones. The late antique military author Vegetius explained that camps should be built in a safe place, with a sufficient supply of firewood, fodder and water, and, if a long stay was planned, particular attention should be paid to choosing a pleasant site (*Epitome of Military Science* 1.22). The meaning of the site's salubriousness is later explained: the site should not be pestilential or near unhealthy marshes, nor in barren plains and hills. Tree cover is crucial, as the troops should not be unprotected from the elements (*Epitome of Military Science* 3.2). These comments call to mind the work of Celsus, a first-century CE author of an encyclopedic work on medicine, whom Vegetius used as a source. In the first book of his treatise *On Medicine* Celsus explained that a healthy dwelling place is that which is lit, airy in summer and sunny in winter.[16] It should be far enough from rivers and marshes. Areas that are known to be pestilential should be avoided at all cost (*On Medicine* 1.2.3). Vitruvius also discussed the choice of a salubrious site and specified that it should be high and free from clouds and where the climate is temperate. Marshy neighbourhoods should also be avoided because they cause pestilence (*On Architecture* 1.4). Vegetius followed the recommendation of Celsus and Onasander and suggested that soldiers should not camp in pestilential areas or in proximity to unhealthy marshes. In addition, Vegetius (*Epitome of Military Science* 3.2) noted that generals must take notice of the water supply, the seasons, medicine and exercise as being crucial for

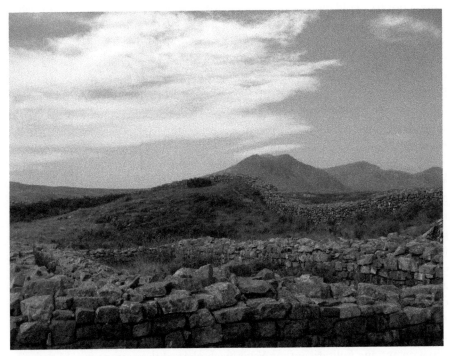

FIGURE 1.2: The Roman military fort at Hardknott Pass (Mediobogdum), Cumbria, United Kingdom, was built in a salubrious, but rather wet, location. ©Laurence Totelin.

controlling the health of the army. All of these considerations of the impact of the environment on health originated from the work of Hippocrates and other physicians. They were influential throughout classical antiquity in various disciplines, which had to take public health into their considerations.

ENVIRONMENTAL PSYCHOLOGY

Another Hippocratic legacy, which concerned the connection between the environment and health, revolved around the shaping of the human character. The Hippocratic author of *On Airs, Waters and Places* assumed that difference in climate between various regions causes a difference in the nature of all its inhabitants and even vegetation. The inhabitants of mild climatic regions will therefore be

> well nourished, of very fine physique and very tall, differing from one another but little either in physique or stature. This region (i.e. the mild regions of Asia), both in character and in mildness of its seasons, might fairly be said to bear a close resemblance to spring. However, courage, endurance, industry, and high spirit could not arise in such conditions either among natives or among immigrants, but pleasure must be supreme.
>
> —*On Airs, Waters and Places* 12

Throughout the second part of the work *On Airs, Waters and Places* (chapters 12–23), the Hippocratic author enumerates the ways in which the environment shapes human character. This view, which was often studied by modern scholars as a potential source of racism in classical antiquity, was nevertheless prevalent in the Graeco-Roman world (see Isaac 2004: 60–9). In fact, the second-century CE Latin author Apuleius had to rebuke an accusation in court that his behaviour was dictated by his place of origin. Apuleius was charged in the court of the Roman proconsul of Africa at 159 CE with the accusation of practicing *magia*. Apuleius said:

> About my homeland . . . After all, it's not a man's origins but his habits that ought to be inspected, not in what region but in what fashion he chooses to live his life. It's the habit of the vegetable-grower and the innkeeper to praise vegetables and wine on the basis of the excellence of their native soil – hence 'Thasian' wine and the 'Phliasian' vegetables.
>
> —Apuleius, *Apology* 24[17]

This comment of Apuleius is made in the unusual context of him being accused on the charge of *magia*. The Latin rhetor who arrived in the North African city of Oea, where he allegedly used *magia* in order to compel an older wealthy widow to marry him in order to get hold of her possessions, was an odd voice in classical antiquity concerning his attitude to the intrinsic connection between place of birth and character traits. Benjamin Isaac's work on the invention of racism in classical antiquity (2004) has demonstrated that proto-racism, prejudice against ethnic groups and xenophobia were widespread throughout the Graeco-Roman world and were actively advertised by most key Greek and Latin authors. The peculiar Greek notion of 'barbarian' demonstrates how effectively Greek culture was able to mark its 'other' and describe it as morally and culturally different to itself. Originally a Greek term, the word 'barbarian' initially referred to those who do not speak Greek.[18] Furthermore, Isaac was able to demonstrate that the view of Greek and Roman authors towards ethnic groups such as Phoenicians, Carthaginians, Syrians, Egyptians, Parthians, Roman views of Greeks, Mountaineers and Plainsmen, Gauls, Germans and Jews bore clear traces of the Hippocratic ideas which were first expressed in *On Airs, Waters and Places*.

In fact, Apuleius' *Apology* cleverly plays on this theme of proto-racism. By telling the influence of the environment on humans and other living beings apart Apuleius uses terminology and a form of argumentation derived from Hippocrates and his successors:

> The flavour of this fruit of the earth is much improved by the fertility of the region, the rainy sky, the gentle wind, the warm sun and moist soil. And yet, since the mind moves into the home of the body from without, how can one of these earthly aspects enhance or diminish malice or virtue? Don't you find differing dispositions among all peoples, though some may have a reputation for dullness or cleverness?
>
> —Apuleius, *Apology* 24

This alleged innocent refutation of an accusation made must have aimed to revoke the Hippocratic tradition of *On Airs, Waters and Places*. Apuleius played throughout his *Apology* with Hippocratic themes, demonstrating his abilities as a rhetor.[19] If anything, it can be used as evidence for the tenaciousness of these ideas amongst the educated elite, whom Apuleius was currently addressing. Likewise, the following catalogue of renowned figures who did not represent the ethnic group from which they originated demonstrates the wide spread of ideas connecting the influence of place of origin on the shaping of the human character and physique:

> Wise Anacharsis was born among the idiot Scythians, the shrewd Athenians produced the block-head Meletides. And I don't say this out of shame for my country. For even though we were once a city belonging to the king Scyfax,

when he was overthrown we were given as a gift of the Roman people to the king Masinissa, and now, with the recent arrival of resettled veteran soldiers, we have become a magnificent colony. In this colony my father was duumvir, the equivalent of a princeps, who held every office of honour. Now I uphold his rank in that republic with an honour and a respect, I hope, in no way inferior, and have done so since I began to take part in public affairs. Why did I offer this information? So that from now on, Aemelianus, you may be less offended by me, and so that you may extend your good will and forgiveness, if by some negligence I didn't select your Attic Zarat as my birthplace.

—Apuleius, *Apology* 23

Apuleius argued in his *Apology* that airs, waters and places were relevant in the growing of vegetables or the making of wine (Apuleius, *Apology* 24). However, he contended that the effect of the environment on human character is unfounded: 'And yet, since the mind moves into the home of the body from without, how can one of these earthly aspects enhance or diminish malice or virtue?' (*Apology* 24). As proof, he claimed that throughout time and in every place, there were people of different qualities who were raised in similar conditions. As a rhetor and a sophist, it seems probable that Apuleius' use and abuse of the Hippocratic theme of environmental determinism should not necessarily be taken as a testament of his own beliefs, but rather as a tour de force of a scholar who has perfect command of the Greek *paideia*. Such demonstration of skill was expected from a sophist of his stature and of a rhetor who expected to take disciples. Be Apuleius' belief as it may, his speech was a refutation of allegations raised against him. This was the argument of the prosecutor whom Apuleius had to meet in the court of a Roman proconsul. Intrinsic connection between environment and character was a serious enough claim to be used in a murder trial during the second century CE.

Moreover, Apuleius must have been an odd voice. Vegetius seemed less critical of this form of ethnography. When discussing recruitment policy, he referred to the regions from which they should be levied; the advantages and disadvantages of recruits from the country or city; and how better ones could be recognized at selection by their face and physical posture as most important during recruitment. Vegetius (*Epitome of Military Science* 1.3–7) explained all these issues in medical terms and his conclusions were attributed to past authorities.[20] Following Hippocrates, Vegetius concluded that all people who dwelled near the sun, being parched by great heat, were more intelligent but had less blood. They were therefore less capable of fighting at close quarters because they were conscious that for them every wound could be mortal. The people from the north, who were far remote from the sun, were less intelligent but had more blood. It is therefore Vegetius' recommendation that recruits should be levied from the more temperate regions. The plenteousness of their blood allowed 'contempt for wounds and death' but they would not be lacking in intelligence, as unintelligence 'prevents discipline in camp and is of no little assistance with counsel in battle' (*Epitome of Military Science* 1.2, translation: Milner). It is noteworthy that Vegetius was not a general himself, and that his work was based on secondary sources of late Republic and early Principate period. The appearance of this type of ethnography, which depicts a causal connection between a place of birth and one's character, must have been derived from Vegetius' earlier sources. In addition, by presenting his work to an (unnamed) emperor Vegetius confirmed that the content of his treatise reflected current ideology.

SALUBRIOUS PLACES AND MEDICAL TOURISM

Another aspect of the environment, which is relevant to a cultural history of medicine in classical antiquity, concerned the reputation of various places as particularly salubrious, while other places were perceived as detrimental to health. The various temples of the healing deity Asclepius resided in locations which were seen as beneficial to health. Here too, it is worth repeating the dual nature of this enquiry – perceived and real effects of the environment – and to emphasize that it is only a methodological duality. Modern archaeologists have recorded more than thirty temples of Asclepius in Asia Minor alone, all of which were situated in places that share similar qualities (see Croon 1967: 239). They attracted worshippers from throughout the Graeco-Roman world. In fact, the major temples were often visited by people who travelled great distances to convalesce in them. Strabo (*Geography* 8.6.15) and Pausanias (2.27.3; 7.27.11) depicted Epidaurus, Cos and Tricca as vibrant places, visited by worshippers from far and wide.[21] For Aelius Aristides, encountering visitors from Alexandria and Rome in the Asclepeion in Pergamum seemed natural.[22] Inscriptions from Pergamum and other Asclepeia confirm that worshippers seeking cures spared no effort in travelling great distances to find remedy. This form of medical tourism was conscious of the connection between health and the environment. Plutarch, a contemporary observer without any known special bond with Asclepius, reported that the worshippers of Asclepius were keen to build temples in airy, clean and high places (*Roman Questions* 286D).[23] All known temples of Asclepius were built in proximity to a water source believed to have held curative qualities (see Croon 1967; Ginouvès 1994; Lambrinoudakis 1994; Jones 1991). While this might be in tune with a more general trend of early Greek religion of the archaic period, the source of curative water was a dominant part of the cult of Asclepius, and was perceived even during the Roman Principate as a reason for locating temples in their particular settings. The central role of cleansing in Asclepius' cult turned water into an important feature of the temple. This was the case in Athens, where the Asclepeion resided next to two water sources with curative properties on the south slopes of the Acropolis and dated back to 420 BCE (Martin and Metzger 1976: 347). The temple of Asclepius in Corinth was located close by to the springs of Lerna (Martin and Metzger 1967: 79). The Asclepeion in Troezen resided near the springs of Heracles, which produced water rich in minerals (Ginouvès 1962: 361). The temple of Asclepius in Messene was built around the spring of Arsinoë (Mee and Spawforth 2001: 248). Proximity to a well-known therapeutic spring was also the case in the Asclepeia in Delos and Lebena (Israelowich 2015: 117). The temple of Asclepius in Acragas was placed about 5 kilometres inland from the southwest coast of Sicily next to a crossing of two rivers, the Hypsas and the Acragas, where a spring existed, whose water enjoyed a reputation of being curative since the archaic era (Israelowich 2015: 117). Perhaps the most famous spring attached to an Asclepeion is that of Epidaurus (see Figure 1.3), which, according to archaeologists, was known to have therapeutic qualities since the third millennium BCE, and all temples of Asclepius recorded by modern scholars were associated with a spring of curative water (Ginouvès 1962: 370; Lambrinoudakis 1994: 225). The environment, it appears, played a vital role in temple medicine. The worshippers of Asclepius, who frequented his many temples since the classical era and well into late antiquity, did so also because of the salubrious location in which it was set. Modern scholars who studied the inter-relations between temple medicine and the one practised by laypeople noticed that 'the god seemed to have learned medicine' (Horstmanshoff 2004). In other words, the type of healthcare practised in the Asclepeia and the one practised by physicians who claimed to have understood the *modus operandi* of the human body were similar in terms of methodology, curative measures and professional language. The environment had an important role to play in the cult of Asclepius, in the form of hydrotherapy. As the experiences of Aelius Aristides portray, physicians operating within the temple wholeheartedly approved the commands of the god regarding journeys to healthy locations (*Orationes* 48.19–20 Keil).

All contemporary commentators were conscious of the importance of fresh water to health. In fact, the rise of Hippocratic medicine occurred simultaneously to the rise of hydrotherapy and medical tourism to certain springs whose water were reputed to be curative. Ralph Jackson (1999: 107) noted that:

In the Roman world numerous forms of medical treatment were available, administered by a wide range of healers. Many of the treatments were unpleasant; some were dangerous; few were predictably and consistently beneficial. Given this uncertainty and discomfort, it is not difficult to understand why hydrotherapy held such an appeal.

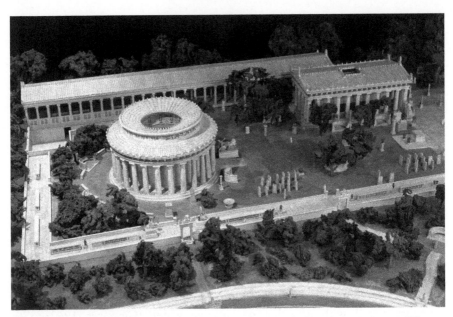

FIGURE 1.3: Plaster and wood model of the Asclepeion of Epidaurus, Greece. The sanctuary's spring had therapeutic qualities. This model was made in 1936 after the reconstruction of the French architect Alphonse Defrasse. Scale 1:66. The Science Museum, London, object number A632959. Courtesy of Wellcome Images.

As bathing (see Figure 1.4) was both a daily activity in the Roman world and as physicians advocated for hygiene, bathing and hydrotherapy for health, journeys to salubrious water sources or attempts to bring healthy water into the city became commonplace in the Roman world (see Israelowich 2015: 118–24). Hygiene was an important facet of Greek and Roman medicine. Already in the fourth century BCE Diocles (fragments 176–7, 188, 191, 195, 200, 222–3, 225, 228–9, 233 van der Eijk) composed an elaborate treatise bearing this title, in which he predominantly discussed diets. Later works on the subject, by authors such as Soranus and Galen, presented hygiene in a more holistic manner. When addressing its relevance to medicine they emphasized, in addition to personal cleanliness, the importance of diet and a healthy lifestyle (see Nutton 2013: 298). Medical tourism as an attempt to change one environment for a healthier one, or attempts to alter an unhealthy civic environment into a healthier one by importing fresh water into it both allude to an understanding of an intrinsic connection between environment and health. As mentioned before, the Hippocratic tradition of *On Airs, Waters and Places* assigned certain qualities to waters. Indeed, physicians and lay scholars discussed the waters of places such as Baiae and Cumae; the *Thermae Neronianae*; sulphur baths on the bay of Campania; the Simbruine springs in

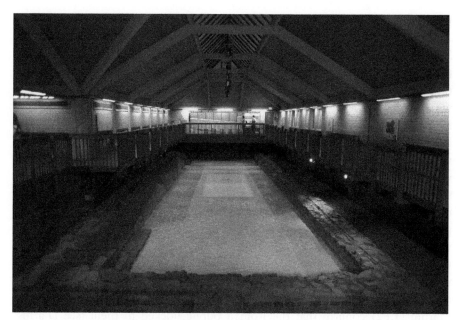

FIGURE 1.4: The natatio (swimming pool) at the Roman baths of Caerleon (Isca Augusta), Wales, United Kingdom. The baths at Caerleon also included a frigidarium (cold bath), tepidarium (lukewarm bath) and caldarium (hot bath). Bathing was an important aspect of the life of the Roman legion stationed at Isca Augusta. ©Cadw.

the district of Simbuvium near Tivoli (see Tacitus, *Annals* 11.13; 14.22; Strabo, *Geography* 5.4.7); and those at Cutilia which Pliny (*Natural History* 31.6) described as exceptionally cold and biting due to the presence of carbonic acid gas which lay between the Via Nomentana and the Via Salaria.[24] Some locations enjoyed the reputation of their salubrious waters, as did *Aquae Cutiliae*, near Rome (Celsus, *On Medicine* 4.12.7; Pliny, *Natural History* 31.6), and *Aquae Albulae*, which lay between Rome and Tivoli (Vitruvius, *On Architecture* 8.3.2; Strabo, *Geography* 5.3.11; Martial 1.12; Suetonius, *Augustus* 82.2).[25] Travelling to convalesce near one of these springs was unanimously celebrated a therapeutic.

An understanding of the role of the environment in general, and of certain water sources in particular for healthcare was ubiquitous. According to Pliny,

> Everywhere in many lands gush forth beneficent waters, here cold, there hot, there both, as among the Tarbelli, an Aquitanian tribe, and in the Pyrenees, with only a short distance separating the two, in some places tepid and lukewarm, promising relief to the sick and bursting forth to help only men of all the animals.

> —Pliny, *Natural History* 31.1–2

Pliny was not an odd voice. More than one hundred therapeutic springs called *aquae* are known to have been active during Roman times, and they enjoyed a huge popularity (see Jackson 1990a: 1). Vitruvius (8.4–5; 8.17) and Pliny (*Natural History* 31.3–8; 31.32–3) distinguished between various types of thermal and medical springs: sulphur springs, whose waters 'refresh muscular weakness and sinews' by heating and burning poisonous humours from the body; alum springs, immersion in which was used as a treatment for paralysis, because their warmth opened the pores and restored health; bitumen springs which provided draughts to purge and to heal 'interior defects'; alkaline springs, whose waters were taken to purge and lessen 'scrofulous tumours'; and acid springs, draughts of which were drunk to dissolve bladder stones. Vitruvius explained that this effect occurred 'by nature, because a sharp acid juice is present in the soil, and when water currents pass out of it, they are tinctured with acridity'. The works and comments of these two Latin authors show how widespread the environmental notion of health springs was in the Roman world. The remains of Baiae and other spas, alongside comments of Celsus (*On Medicine* 2.17.1), Strabo (*Geography* 5.4.5), Pliny (*Natural History* 31.2) and Martial (1.62) confirm that the Roman public flocked to them (see D'arms 1970: 139–42).

Seawater also seemed relevant to healthcare. As part of the environment, they were perceived to have a strong effect on health and healthcare (see Celsus, *On Medicine* 3.27; 4.2; Pliny, *Natural History* 31.14; 31.33). Pliny (*Natural History* 31.8–9) explained that the waters of Campania were known to cure barrenness in women and insanity in men. Other conditions also required a change of environment. According to Celsus (*On Medicine* 3.21.6), some ailments were best treated by sweating in a bath or a spa, such as the one found in the myrtle groves above Baiae. For a wasting disease (*tabes*), especially if the condition was acute, such as true *phthisis*, Celsus (*On Medicine* 3.22.8) advised a long sea voyage, for patients who could endure it. In tune with the Hippocratic tradition of *On Airs, Waters and Places*, Celsus thought that the sufferers of wasting diseases might benefit from a change of air into a denser climate. He advised a voyage from Italy to Alexandria. Celsus (*On Medicine* 3.2.9) recommended *phtisis* patients should take a sea voyage, because the rocking would be beneficial. Literary and archaeological sources confirm that environmental treatments soon gained popularity. Medical tourism, motivated by an understanding of the importance of a healthy environment for recuperation was responsible for the growth of hotels, restaurants and other hospitable establishments on the roads towards these destinations and within them (see Yegül 2010: 50). Places such as Baiae in the bay of Naples (see Celsus, *On Medicine* 2.17.1; Strabo, *Geography* 5.4.5; Pliny, *Natural History* 31.2; Martial 1.62) and Allianoi near Pergamum (see Yegül 2010: 50–1) were associated with environmental benefits for the sick, and also known as fashionable vacation destinations. Furthermore, the successful application of cold-water therapy by Antonius Musa to Augustus soon marked the springs of a physician by the name of Charmis, in the city of Massilia as a destination for medical tourists (see Pliny, *Natural History* 29.5.10; Dio Cassius, *Roman History* 53.30.3).[26] The prestige of Antonius Musa and the belief that some locations offered waters of unique curative qualities is thought to have caused the brushing aside of the *laconicum* and the conversion of the Stabian Baths (see Wallace-Hadrill 2008: 183). Likewise, Horace (*Epistles* 1.15.2–11) noticed a growing preference for Clusium, Gabii and the cold sprigs over the myrtle and sulphur springs of Baiae.[27]

The Roman governing institutions also acknowledged the connection between the environment and public health. The Roman legislator assigned the responsibility of civic hygiene to the civic *praetor*. According to the *Digest* (43.23.1.2) it was his responsibility to clean and repair the drains because this task pertained to the health of the citizens and to their safety.[28] For drains filled with filth threaten pestilence of the atmosphere and ruin if they are not repaired. Guaranteeing a healthy civic environment was the motive behind other Roman institutions: the aqueducts and the *curator aquarum*. Both institutions originated from the Graeco-Roman practice of benefactions and both were in tune with prevailing medical ideas concerning the health hazards of the civic environment. Providing aqueducts to cities was an act of benefaction affordable only for the wealthiest of citizens. In Rome, this benefaction was so important that Augustus and future *principes* felt obliged to preserve it for themselves in the interest of civil order. This was the ground for the establishment of the office of the waters (*curator aquarum*). This responsibility was initially entrusted to Agrippa in 33 BCE, but it was turned into a permanent *cura* in 11 BCE (see Rodgers 2004: 15). The choice of Augustus to appoint a well-respected person for this position, Messala Corvinus, indicates the importance the Roman imperial government assigned to it. Future emperors followed Augustus' path. In 52 CE Claudius could celebrate the completion of two further aqueducts, which added more than one hundred miles of water channels and doubled the water supply to the city. Like Agrippa before him, Claudius created an administrative system for the maintenance of the Roman water system. These monuments indicated that the emperors were concerned about public health and that they were aware of environmental hazards.

We are fortunate to have a treatise on the construction of aqueducts by one Iulius Frontinus, who had a distinguished career under Domitian, Nerva and Trajan before being appointed as *curator aquarum*. Frontinus (*On the Aqueducts of Rome*, preface 1) described the scope of this position as pertaining to 'not merely the convenience but also the health and even the safety of the city and which has always been administered by the most eminent men of our state'.[29] He explained that the Romans have for long assumed that water, particularly spring water, was therapeutic. He referred to the water of the springs of

Camenae, of Apollo and of Juturna as having healing powers, thus confirming that originally Greek ideas about the connection between the environment and health guided Roman imperial policy (on sanitation and health see: Scobie 1986; Shaw 1996). As a *curator aquarum* it was Frontinus' responsibility to secure the water supply into the city and ensure a healthy environment within it (*On the Aqueducts of Rome* 1.17). Frontinus (*On the Aqueducts of Rome* 88) explained that the safeguarding and maintenance of the water supply system was immediately responsible for improving the health of the inhabitants by amending the impurities caused by a civic environment. Following the Hippocratic notions regarding the provenance of water, Frontinus reported that water brought from springs is far superior to the water that could be produced from wells within the city. Similarly, the civic environment held certain dangers, which the *curator aquarum* had to diffuse. It fell within his responsibilities to maintain the city's sewage. The *curator aquarum* was similarly responsible for ensuring that 'the city is cleaner, the air is purer, and the causes of the unwholesome atmosphere, which gave the air of the city so bad a name with the ancients, are now removed' (*On the Aqueducts of Rome* 88).

Roman legislation reflected current medical thought regarding the effect of the environment and particular health hazards of city life. Galen (*On the Preservation of Health* 1.11), perhaps the most distinguished of all physicians working during the High Empire, used the example of water becoming polluted once a sewer from a city or a large military camp has been poured into it as a safety warning for those responsible for water systems and sewers.[30] A later medical author by the name of Oribasius, who worked during the fourth century CE, included in his treatise, *Medical Collections*, some otherwise unrecorded authors of the first and second century CE who held very similar views about environmental medicine to Vitruvius in his first book *On Architecture* (see Nutton 2000: 69). Athenaeus of Attaleia, Oribasius' earliest source, emphasized how in cities the movement of air was blocked by buildings. The result was that the air was thick, enclosed and, when combined with the exhalations of the city's dwellers, unhealthy (Oribasius, *Medical Collections* 9.5; 12).[31] A later medical author, Antyllus, followed a similar line of argument concerning environmental hazards within cities to those raised by Galen in his commentary on Hippocrates' *On Airs, Waters and Places* (Antyllus, cited in Oribasius, *Medical Collections* 9.9; 11; Galen, *Causes of Pulses* 1.5, K9.10).[32] Similarly, Oribasius (*Medical Collections* 9.15–20) cited the writings of Sabinus, Galen's contemporary and self-confessed follower of Hippocrates, who claimed that he himself paid considerable attention to the architectural attributes of a healthy city. His ideal city had straight roads, oriented north–south and east–west, without obstructions, and with clear straight roads leading into them from the suburbs. Thus, medical authors during the High Empire were well aware of the environmental effects of cities and they encouraged architects and the government to take due measures to ensure that cities were appropriately planned and, once set, were consciously managed.

The civic environment was not necessarily detrimental. If properly built and adequately maintained it could offer a healthier environment than its surroundings. This understanding drove Severus Alexander to lead his soldiers from their camp near the Euphrates frontier in Northern Syria to the city of Antioch. It is reported by Herodian (6.6.2) that Severus' army had all fallen ill in the stifling air during the year 232 CE.[33] Herodian explained that Severus' army also included soldiers who were recently transferred from Illyrium who were unaccustomed to the local climate. The emperor therefore decided to move his army into the civic environment of Antioch. The city offered cool air and good water. According to Herodian, the soldiers in the camp fell ill because of their nutrition and climate. Herodian's narrative is therefore consistent with the explanation of contemporary physicians as to the effect of the environment on the human body, emphasizing the active role of a man-made civic surroundings, and demonstrates that these medical ideas guided Roman policy makers (see Nutton 2000: 65).

This chapter set out to examine whether beliefs about the environment influenced attitudes towards health and medicine in the Greek and Roman world. It appeared that a Hippocratic conceptual grid habitually guided health-related activities. It taught the benefits of climate and natural resources, such as water, vegetation and minerals; it clarified all health-related distinctions between town and country, and it even explained how these environmental attributes shaped the human character. The Hippocratic tradition encouraged doctors to learn to analyse the environment as part of their professional practice. Independently, temple medicine too advocated the benefits of a healthy environment and the use of natural resources in the therapeutic procedure. These notions percolated into other disciplines, such as architecture and military affairs, thus shaping the man-made environment into a pattern believed to hold curative or at least preventative attributes. In Roman times, the belief that the environment had direct influence on public health drove the Roman government to take active measures for keeping environmental hazards to a minimum, and exploiting environmental resources, such as water, wind and topography for the benefit of public health.

NOTES

1. *Stomacace* is a disease of the gums. *Scelotyrbe* is lameness in the ankles or the knees. This and all citations hereafter of books 24 to 27 of Pliny's *Natural History* are from the Loeb Classical Library edition by Jones (1956).
2. This and all citations hereafter of Vitruvius' *On Architecture* are from the Loeb Classical Library edition by Granger (1931). This and all citations hereafter of

Vegetius' *Epitome of Military Science* are from the Oxford Classical Texts edition by Reeve (2004).

3. This and all citations hereafter are from the Collection des Universités de France edition by Jouanna (1996). An English translation by Jones (1923a) is also available in the Loeb Classical Library.

4. The Hippocratic physician should be seen as an artisan rather than a scientist or a scholar. As such, physicians paid much attention to their professional conduct, to the technical skill they possess, and to the theoretical foundation of their discipline (see Nutton 2013: 87; Edelstein 1967: 87–110; Horstsmanshoff 1976; Temkin 1977: 137–53; Jouanna 1988: 168–90; Pleket 1995).

5. The only exception to the unofficial nature of the medical profession was that of the 'public physician', whose tasks are still baffling. However, the 'public physician' was elected by a formal procedure, and therefore, enjoyed the acknowledgement of his skills the city expressed. On public physicians see Plato, *Gorgias* 455b and 456b (citation from the Loeb Classical Library edition by Lamb 1925); Xenophon, *Memorabilia* 4.2.5 (citation from the Loeb Classical Library edition by Marchant, Todd and Henderson 2013); Pohl (1905); Cohn-Haft (1956); Nutton (1977).

6. On the importance of prognosis for securing patients' trust see, in addition to the Hippocratic treatise *On Prognosis*, Edelstein (1967): 65–85.

7. For the habitual attempts to explain human character as being shaped by ethnicity and place of origin see Isaac (2004).

8. This and all citations hereafter are from the Loeb Classical Library edition by Hutton et al (1914).

9. This and all citations hereafter of Herodotus are from the Loeb Classical Library edition by Godley (1920–1925). This and all citations hereafter of Thucydides are from the Loeb Classical Library edition by Smith (1919–1923).

10. This citation is from the Loeb Classical Library edition by Bury (1929).

11. Gruen (2011: 162) rightfully draws a comparison with Thucydides (1.2) and the Athenians.

12. This and all citations hereafter are from the Loeb Classical Library edition by Hutton et al (1914).

13. This citation is from the Loeb Classical Library edition by Basore (1928).

14. The term 'environmental history' was coined by Nash (1972). It refers to the 'interaction between human cultures and the environment in the past' (Worster 1988).

15. This and all citations hereafter of Onasander's *Strategicos* are from the Loeb Classical Library edition by the Illinois Greek Club (1928).

16. This and all citations hereafter are from the Loeb Classical Library edition by Spencer (1935–1938).

17. This and all citations hereafter are from the edition, translation and commentary by Hunink (1997).

18. See Homer's description (*Iliad* 2.867) of the Carians as those who speak barbarian. Herodotus (2.57) compared the sound of barbaric languages (i.e. not Greek) to those of animals. He later juxtaposed barbarian lawlessness and ferocity with Greek nature (4.3 ff; 8.837).

19. Apuleius was a teacher of rhetoric.
20. For an English translation of Vegetius, as well as short commentary, see Milner (1993). For the Latin text see Reeve (2004).
21. This and all citations hereafter of Strabo are from the Loeb Classical Library edition by H. L. Jones (1917–1932). This and all citations hereafter of Pausanias are from the Loeb Classical Library edition by W. H. S. Jones (1918–1935).
22. For an English translation of Aristides' *Sacred Tales* see Behr (1981–1986).
23. This citation is from the Loeb Classical Library edition by Babbitt (1936).
24. This and all citations hereafter of books 28 to 32 of Pliny's *Natural History* are from the Loeb Classical Library edition by Jones (1956).
25. This and all citations hereafter of Book 1 of Martial's *Epigrams* are from the Loeb Classical Library edition by Shackleton Bailey (1993). This citation to Suetonius' *Augustus* is from the Loeb Classical Library edition by Rolfe and Bradley (1914).
26. This citation of Dio Cassius is from the Loeb Classical Library edition by Cary and Foster (1917).
27. This citation is from the Loeb Classical Library edition by Rushton Fairclough (1926).
28. For an English translation of the *Digest* see Watson (1998).
29. This and all citations hereafter are from the Cambridge Classical Texts and Commentaries edition by Rodgers (2004).
30. This citation is from the Loeb Classical Library edition by Johnston (2018).
31. This and all citations hereafter are from the Corpus Medicorum Graecorum edition by Raeder (1928–1933).
32. This citation of Galen's *Causes of Pulses* is from the tenth volume of Kühn's edition, abbreviated as 'K10'.
33. This citation is from the Loeb Classical Library edition by Whittaker (1970).

CHAPTER TWO

Food

JOHN WILKINS

INTRODUCTION

Food and nutrition in antiquity are a vast and complex area of study, with much more attention focused on food supply and transport than nutrition. 'Antiquity' of course can span millennia from the Neolithic age (Mee and Renard 2007; Valamoti 2009) to Byzantium (Dalby 2011). The period under review here is from Homer, notionally the eighth century BCE, to the late antiquity of Oribasius (fourth century CE) and Aetius (sixth century CE) (see Wilkins 2012 and 2015 for this periodization). Further stimulus has come from the emerging discipline of Food Studies, which draws on approaches based in history and the social sciences (see Clafin and Scolliers 2012, and especially Wilkins 2012).

The Mediterranean region is vast and varied, with many microclimates, particularly in Greece and the Aegean (Hordern and Purcell 2000; see also Luce 2000; Chandezon and Hamdoume 2004). The impact of place and climate on health is brought out vividly by medical authors from the Hippocratic authors to Galen of Pergamum (see Figure 2.1). The first observe in *On Airs, Waters and Places* 3, 'a district which is sheltered from northerly winds but exposed to the warm ones ... will ... have ... inhabitants ... [with a constitution that will] usually be flabby and they tolerate neither food nor drink well'.[1] Galen, 600 years later, rehearses in detail the variation in cereals (see Figure 2.2) grown in Asia Minor and Thrace, according to soil and climate: primitive wheats such as einkorn and emmer are best in Mysia, rye in Thrace (*On the Properties of Foodstuffs* 1.13, see Bertier 1972: 48–56).[2] Bread wheat may have been the most nutritious cereal (in the view of Galen and many

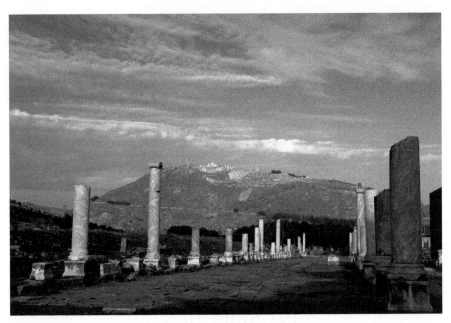

FIGURE 2.1: Galen's home city of Pergamum, view from the Asclepeion. ©Cenk Durmuskahya.

others), but there was no point planting it if the conditions were not right. Garnsey (1988: 10–14) notes that on average, wheat failed one year in four, barley only one year in seven. The solution, for small farmers at least, was to diversify, and to grow legumes as well as cereals, so that there was a better spread of risk (Foxhall and Forbes 1982; Gallant 1991; Sallares 1991). Galen knew that peasants had to send the best grain to the cities (see below); but cities too had problems with supply. Studies of the grain supply have followed wheats (Jasny 1944; Kokoszko et al 2014), processing mills (Moritz 1958), grain stores (Rickman 1971) and historical and demographic approaches (Garnsey 1988). There have been studies, too, some with farming experience (White 1970; Fitch 2013), of the agricultural authors from Columella (first century CE) to Palladius (fourth–fifth century CE) and, in the Byzantine period, the *Geoponica*; studies too of fish supplies and fermented fish, not least the fermented fish sauce, *garos/-um* in Greek and Latin (Curtis 1991; Mylona 2008), again with much archaeological corroboration.[3] All of these important approaches, linked with archaeological science have brought an understanding of ancient nutrition which Garnsey summarizes in his valuable 1999 overview of food and society. He finds that Galen's view is broadly in line with the modern assessment, and this has recently been confirmed by archaeology: the plants as we understand them are broadly the same as those declared significant

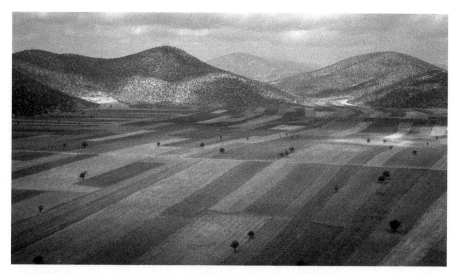

FIGURE 2.2: The cereal plains of Turkey. ©Cenk Durmuskahya.

by Galen (Rowan 2014). There are methodological disputes along the way, as I discuss below.

The complement to these studies of production, distribution and processing, and consumption are studies within Ancient Medicine, of which Ludwig Edelstein and Georg Wöhrle are the most important for the study of nutrition. The first is particularly significant in methodological terms since he wrote first in 1931 (reprinted in Edelstein 1967: 303–16) and is driven by a belief in scientific progress as the means to combat hunger in Europe and other continents. With this went a low estimation of preventive medicine if it meant excessive attention to one's own wellbeing, as Plato suggested (*Republic* 405c–408e).[4] Nearly a century later, when industrial processing and distribution through supermarkets has not only cured food shortage but expanded the incidence of such diseases as diabetes and heart disease, a different perspective is possible: wellbeing, lifestyle and control of purchase and cooking has its importance once more. This will affect how we now read the Hippocratic Corpus and Galen.

Nutrition from the Hippocratic doctors through to Galen and his successors has a major part to play in ancient medicine that is almost entirely lost to modern biomedicine. Nutrition constituted a third of therapy according to Celsus (*On Medicine,* proemium 8) and Galen (*On the Properties of Foodstuffs* 1.1): nutrition, along with pharmacology and surgery, were the chief resources available to the doctor.[5] Nutrition and pharmacology were closely related as disciplines, especially in Galen's system, and based on a largely similar *materia medica*, with plants predominating over animal products, and some minerals in drug categories only. When Galen considers *preventive* medicine, which includes, among other things (see below), food and drink along with exercise, sleep and good breathing, prevention constitutes half of the medical art, to complement a therapeutic half. As I understand it, nutrition barely appears in the curriculum of modern medical students: nutrition is important, but diverted to a subsection of medical practice and not strictly part of the doctor's skills. While leaving space for major areas such as viral and bacterial infection, surgery and chemotherapy, this division has left medicine in difficulty when presented by cultural practice in calorie intake and low rates of exercise. This is a major challenge to biomedicine, which perhaps fails to take nutrition seriously enough. Whether classed within 'public health' or 'medicine', health professionals are well aware that they need to restore control of health to patients in order to reduce the incidence of diabetes, heart disease, depression and other illnesses partly induced by 'life-style'. Better living could reduce health costs and the level of avoidable disease. This idea lies behind Galenic and Hippocratic medicine, which offered a theorized version of the effects of diet on the body, viewed over centuries, each with their own case studies added. The Hippocratic Corpus and Galen will be our main sources, but Diocles, Mnesitheus, Phylotimus and Asclepiades of Bithynia will be in there too.

A further influential approach, both ancient and modern, is the linking of food with luxury, desire and appetite. Authors from Plato (*Republic* and *Gorgias*) to Athenaeus (*Deipnosophists*) decry the dangers of pleasure, particularly to the wealthy and young who may be tempted away from traditional values at the sensual meeting place of the symposium (Murray 1990). James Davidson (1997) has emphasized the corrupting power of expensive wine, fish and sex on the mind of the young in this strand of ancient thought, tempting them from frugality and preserving ancestral wealth. I address the issue below through ideas of taste and pleasure, since, while the doctors shunned the tempting concoctions of specialist chefs, they knew that taste was a key influence on the 'humours' and balance of the body, and that what tasted unpleasant was unlikely to benefit physiological equilibrium.

Greek nutrition in the written record begins with the poems of Homer. Heroes wearied by fighting on the battlefield need rapid restoration. Heroes too long at sea are desperate for sustenance and sink down the food chain to eat wild animals and fish. Denied the high-status beef of the heroic code, they are reduced to fishing and hunting. Such nutrition is distinguished from the Egyptian drugs that Helen supplies in *Odyssey* (4.219–32) to calm the mental anguish of the heroes as they remember their dead comrades at Troy.[6] Energy replacement and pharmacological properties remained at the heart of the ancient understanding of nutrition for the next two millennia, and indeed until well into the Islamic and Early Modern periods.

THEORIES ANCIENT AND MODERN

Differences between ancient and modern nutrition and their respective understanding of human physiology have led to some serious misunderstandings, to the detriment of the ancient nutritionists. The key difficulty lies in the blithe modern assumption that modern science is right and ancient wrong. I give two examples, from two very good historians. David Wootton (2006: 33) comments on the Hippocratic author of *Epidemics* (1.18–19), who describes

> an outbreak of *causus* (perhaps enteric fever) in the autumn. Those affected suffered from fever fits, insomnia, thirst, nausea, delirium, cold sweats, constipation, and they passed urine 'which was black and fine'; death often occurred on the sixth day, or the eleventh or the twentieth.
>
> 'The disease was very widespread. Of those who contracted it death was the most common among youths, young men, men in the prime of life, those with smooth skins, those of a pallid complexion, those with straight hair, those with black hair, those with black eyes, those who had been given to violent and loose living, those with thin voices, those with rough voices, those with lisps and the choleric. Many women also succumbed to this malady.'
>
> Much of this seems irrelevant to us; and reading through this list it is hard for us to avoid the impression that anybody and everybody died of the disease.[7]

Wootton has been economical with the evidence. The full text mentions 'haemorrhage through the nostrils, copious discharges by the bladder of urine with much sediment of a proper character; disordered bowels with bilious evacuations at the right time; the appearance of dysenteric characteristics', as symptoms which led to recovery. The author also clearly states that all did not die, but that those with successive symptoms recovered 'in every case'. In the full text, *causus* is clearly not one thing, but plural, and these are linked with *phrenitis* which is characterized as a brain disorder with a high temperature. Wootton mocks detailed observation of skin, hair and complexion: if the Hippocratic doctor was not allowed to investigate the inside of the body, what was he to do? Wootton has obliterated much minute and acute observation, of which a modern doctor would be proud. The note-taking is exemplary, even if the theoretical underpinning is not our own.[8] If Wootton believes all Hippocratic medicine was 'bad', why the misrepresentation? A little later, Wootton continues (2006: 37),

> in the ancient world bloodletting had its opponents. The followers of Erasistratus . . . thought bloodletting was dangerous, and preferred to get rid of excessive blood by fasting. But the main disputes were over where to let the blood from . . .

Wootton's evidence comes from a series of treatises by Galen, who argues about the advantages and disadvantages of bloodletting. We shall see below a case where it was not advised, and Galen frequently offers alternatives that he or the patient might prefer. Again, the modern critic of ancient medicine has been misleading. Let us note for the moment that many of the symptoms identified by the Hippocratic author were linked with his understanding of nutrition (thirst, nausea, diagnosis by urine, bowel movements and dysenteric symptoms) and that many of the other symptoms, such as sleeplessness and despondency were linked with nutrition in ancient discussions that I mention below.

Censure of a different kind comes from Peter Garnsey, who writes (1999: 105–6), on ancient treatment of pregnant women,

> whether the 'science' is ultimately independent of the ideology is a moot point, but it does have a life of its own. The list of foods judged suitable for women reflects bizarre physiological theory rather than male prejudice and the social subordination of women. The two of course coexist and are intertwined.

Earlier, on nutrition specifically, Garnsey comments (1999: 45),

> We might expect informed comment on [malnutrition] from the medical writers of antiquity. But their preoccupation was with the health of the upper classes . . . Food was thought of as a medicine. Food maintained the health of their clients . . . slimming diets . . . There is little sign that Galen, Soranus etc saw chronic malnutrition as a medical or social problem, if they had conceptualised it at all.

Garnsey's words are strongly expressed and reveal, I suspect, frustration with a medical system that appears to have done harm to women's health, unnecessary harm in Garnsey's view. Galen, however, as we shall see, wrote repeatedly about the lower classes; he thought food was a food as well as a medicine – strictly a drug was a substance that introduced change to the body, and this he wrote about in *On the Powers of Simple Drugs*, while a food sustained the body's energy and he wrote about this aspect in *On the Properties of Foodstuffs*.[9] In Galen's mind, foods and drinks were related but not the same. Furthermore, what Garnsey calls 'slimming diets' are not diets to lose weight that a modern reader might be familiar with, but substances to thin thick 'humours'.

It is important to note that Garnsey's estimation of Galen as an observer and reporter of peasants' strategies to deal with annual food shortages is high. He notes Galen's evidence for the choice of grains and the range of grains that a farmer might plant (1988: 51–2), as also storage and preservation methods

(1988: 53–5). His acceptance of Galen's evidence is mirrored in Gallant, who notes (1991: 116–7) that Galen has the 'best discussion of the use of gathered "famine foods" in the ancient world'. Galen too has evidence for the variety of fruits and vegetables grown, that confirms comparative evidence gathered by anthropologists and historians (Gallant 1991: 68).

One response to Garnsey's impatience with ancient doctors is to ask what medical historians will say centuries hence about the inability of modern medicine to deal with diabetes, heart disease and depression, all diseases generated largely by a wealthy and sedentary lifestyle. To some extent this is Wootton's approach, who complements his frustration with pre-modern medicine with an acid overview of modern medicine in Appendix 1.

Let us turn to some details and examine a passage of Galen that Garnsey has discussed elsewhere (1988: 26; see also Wilkins 2015). Galen is addressing the effect of bad juices on the body, particularly among the peasants who had to send the best grains and pulses – the most nutritious food – to town:

> The food shortages that have frequently and for no few successive years befallen many of the subject peoples of the Romans have clearly shown to those who are not completely unthinking what power bad juice has in the generation of disease. For people living in towns, as it was their custom to prepare straightaway after the summer sufficient food for the whole year following, by taking from the countryside all the wheat along with the barley and the beans and lentils, left for the countrymen all the other grains, which they call pulses and legumes, after taking not a few of these too to the city.
>
> —Galen, *On Good and Bad Juices* 1[10]

This valuable demographic observation belies claims that Galen is concerned only with the rich. Galen continues with what the peasants were forced to eat, details which supplement observations elsewhere (I emphasize observation once again since this is a strength of ancient, indeed of modern medicine, which must be underlined in response to Wootton's and Garnsey's charges that the ancient doctors were not 'scientific'):

> So these foods that were left to them the country people use up during the winter, and are forced to use foods of <u>bad juices</u> for the whole of the spring. They eat twigs and shoots of trees and bushes, and bulbs and roots of plants with bad juices and consume the so-called wild greens, whichever happens to be in good supply, without sparing until they are satisfied, just as they boiled and ate whole green grasses which they had never tasted, even to try them. It was possible to see some of them in the last days of spring and almost all of them at the beginning of summer afflicted with numerous sores

taking shape on their skin, not all taking the same form. For some of them
were *erusipelatōdē*, others *phlegmonōdē*, others *herpēstika*, others *leichēnōdē*
and *psōrōdē* and *leprōdē*. The softer kind of them as they flowered on the
skin emptied the bad juice/humour out of the organs and the depths of the
body. In some cases, they became charcoal-like and *phagedainika* and killed
the patient with fevers over a long period, with only a few barely surviving.

—Galen, *On Good and Bad Juices* 1

Poor people were forced by hunger to head down the food chain and to eat
foods damaging to the human body, Galen tells us. One consequence was a host
of skin conditions, observed in detail, which Galen believed indicated juices/
humours collecting in the wrong place in the body as *perittōmata* or residues or
misplaced juices/humours.[11] Appropriate methods to relieve these problems
might be massage and red wine (see below). Galen continues:

Apart from the skin conditions, many fevers developed, bringing malodorous
and biting gastric emptying that ended up as *teinesmoi* and dysentery, and
urine that was bitter and malodorous and damaged the bladders of some . . .
Of very few did some of the doctors dare to cut the vein at the beginning of
the disease (for they feared, rightly, to use this remedy because of pre-
weakening of bodily strength), but they saw good blood was taken from
none of them.

—Galen, *On Good and Bad Juices* 1[12]

Note here, that, in contrast to Wootton's claims, Galen does *not* counsel
bloodletting for weakened bodies. More important, he moves to internal
conditions, namely fevers, and diagnostic methods for identifying these,
including taste and smell. Diagnosis by the senses is central to Galen's diagnostic
art, and is not confined to nutrition and matters linked with food and taste in
that sense. The taste of the food and the nature of the 'humour' in the body are
intimately linked, as I discuss below. Dismissal of such observation and reasoning
as pseudo-science is itself an unscientific method in my view. It is the science
which Greek and Roman cultures produced and we as historians need to
understand that if we are to understand those cultures.

   Ancient nutrition is not ours, but in the words of Vivian Nutton (2013: 283),
'most of Galen's recommendations would meet with the approval of a modern
dietician, with one major exception. He placed an almost total ban on fresh
fruit . . .' With the exception of the caveat about fruit, which is overstated, I
propose to follow Nutton's overall positive assessment of Galen's nutrition.[13]
We have seen that this is a big advance on Edelstein (1967), who expresses
some fears that ancient dietetics were all about hypochondriacs. This was not
the view of Galen or the many medical authors who wrote on the subject.

Unlike Plato's division of the soul from the body,[14] body and soul were intimately linked for the doctors. I discuss psychology and diet in the context of 'necessary activities' or 'non-naturals' below.

We can see something of the similarities and differences between Galen and the earlier tradition in the evolution of ancient nutrition. As early as Mnesitheus in the fourth century BCE, Aristotelian categories had worked their way into medicine. In the same century, Diocles had isolated certain properties from certain consequences: in a nuanced discussion Philip van der Eijk (2000: 331–3) evaluates how Diocles appears to have integrated (or not) plant properties with causation in physiology. Diocles' position seems to resemble the Hippocratic *On Regimen*, which also argues that flavours such as sweet and salty do not all have a fixed outcome:

> which power (*dunamis*) of each food and drink must be identified according to their nature and which by the medical art are as follows. The people who have undertaken to speak in general about sweet foods or fatty foods or salty foods or any power of such foods do not identify them correctly. For sweet things do not all have the same power as each other, nor do fatty foods or any other such foods. For many sweet foods are laxative, but some are constipating; some dry the body, others moisten it. And so it is with all the others.
>
> —Hippocratic Corpus, *On Regimen* 2.39[15]

At all events, Galen draws on Diocles to show the importance of experience and experimentation in evaluating the *dunameis* of foods; and on Mnesitheus (fragment 23 Bertier, preserved by Galen, *On the Properties of Foodstuffs* 1.1, Wilkins 2013: 5, lines 19–22) to show how the parts of plants vary in *dunameis* just as do parts of animals (ears, trotters and so on). This comes out well in Galen's discussion of beet (*gongulis*):

> The part of the plant that is proud of the earth is vegetable-like and the root contained in the earth is hard and inedible prior to boiling. When boiled in water, I would be surprised if it was less nourishing than related plants [e.g. the arum lily]. People prepare it in multiple ways, going so far as to preserve it in salt or vinegar. It imparts to the body a juice (*chumos*) that is thicker than balanced juice. Consequently, if a person eats too much of it, especially if that person digests it on a needy stomach, it will collect the so-called raw juice (*chumos*).
>
> —Galen, *On the Properties of Foodstuffs* 2.60

I discuss below whether Galen means the word *chumos* to indicate 'humour' or the 'juice' rendered here.

A further area in which Galen resembles Diocles is in his *comparative* evaluations of one plant against another, and in emphasis on preparation of the raw foodstuff as crucial (van der Eijk 2000: 332, and see below). Diocles (fragment 191 van der Eijk) declares, 'charcoal-bread is *softer* than wafer bread'; and in a further fragment, which Galen quotes, we are told: '*Dolichoi*[16] are *no less* nutritious than peases, and they are about as non-flatulent, but they are *less* tasty[17] and pass *less* easily' (fragment 193a van der Eijk; translation van der Eijk). Some of the fragments of Diocles and Mnesitheus survive only in Athenaeus, on whose importance see below. A Hellenistic doctor who wrote on nutrition and who survives only in Athenaeus, so far without a scholarly edition, is Diphilus of Siphnus (Gourevitch 2000). As physician to Lysimachus, one of the successors of Alexander, Diphilus is one of those distinguished medical writers promoted by Hellenistic monarchs, such as Andreas, Mantias and Crateuas, who were major contributors to medical botany and nutrition and pharmacology, and predecessors of Dioscorides of Anazarbus, a key source (often unacknowledged) for Galen in *On the Properties of Foodstuffs* and for *On the Powers of Simple Drugs*.[18] These authors anticipated Galen in addressing new foods arriving in the Mediterranean from the Far East after Alexander and Theophrastus, such as the citron. Galen's nutrition was largely based on native plants, but there was room in the imperial system for new arrivals, of which the good doctor is supremely aware.

Despite Galen's protestations, many seem to have been in agreement about nutrition. Among the Empiricist doctors, he mentions Heraclides of Tarentum with approval; and for all Galen's dismissal of Asclepiades of Bithynia, much of what Galen says agrees with Celsus who appears to draw heavily on that author. The view of Edelstein (1967), that there is much stability in ancient dietetics over the long period from Hippocrates to Oribasius and beyond appears to be right. Consistency in broad treatment, though not in theory or in detail. Nutrition remains always important, and not confined to treatment of the rich, as Galen makes very clear.

WHAT CONSTITUTES FOOD?

As I set out at the beginning, there is much agreement between historical and archaeological sources on food production and agriculture in antiquity. The archaeological sources now include what we might call 'not food', that is eaten material excreted by the body as unnecessary for nutrition. From an understudied area (Scobie 1986), research into sewers and drains has moved forward strongly. Erica Rowan (2014) presents findings from Herculaneum, and the broad coincidence between findings and ancient texts corroborates Garnsey and his fellow historians. Rowan has gone on to study food remains on Graeco-Roman sites in three continents (Herculaneum, near Naples, Aphrodisias in Western

Anatolia and Utica in North Africa), finding much continuity of diet, with some local differences. It is now possible to integrate the study of nutrition from the plant in the soil or animal eating fodder, through eating and digestion to blood making of some nutrients and excretion of food materials surplus to requirement. To this picture we should add the observations of Mitchell (2005) on olive oil, which was much more important for bathing and massage than for cooking in Asia Minor under Roman administration. Galen confirms this at length in discussions in *On the Preservation of Health* and in *On the Powers of Simple Drugs*. In the introductory books to the latter, in particular, olive oil contributes greatly to oiling the skin and freeing of the pores to release any residues causing problems in subcutaneous tissue. Galen's nutritional text, *On the Properties of Foodstuffs*, derives from *On the Powers of Simple Drugs*, and that division enables Galen to define nutrition more narrowly than a modern equivalent would do. Foods for Galen provide *both* energy to replace that lost in muscles, *and* pharmacological properties in small amounts to regulate other physiological needs. For Galen, cannabis is a food as well as a drug, as is juniper, cedar and (more surprisingly to the modern eye) onions.

Van der Eijk (2015, with valuable accompanying bibliography) has argued that mixtures (*kraseis*) are more important than 'humours' (*chumoi*) in Galen's dietetic and pharmacological works. Mixtures, based on the biological elements of hot, cold, wet and dry, prevail in Galen's analysis over the four humours of blood, phlegm, yellow bile and black bile, he claims.[19] I am less confident than van der Eijk in this matter. Both systems it seems to me operate powerfully in Galen's treatises on foods and drugs, and I am not yet clear on how he thought they interacted.[20] What Galen says is that a body should preferably be of good mixture (*eukratos*) and balanced in humours (*summetros*) and that foods ingested should be of good mixture (*eukratos*) and not of bad mixture (*duskratos*), and of good juices (*euchumia*) and not bad (*kakochumia*). A good food, such as lettuce is 'generative of blood'; a bad food will produce that worst of all things, 'raw humour/juice' (*chumos*) – that is food that the body has been unable to 'cook' or digest to transform it into blood preferably, or, failing that, into a blend of blood and other 'humours'. As far as I can see, *duskrasia* and *kakochumia* are equally undesirable and equally urgent for the doctor to disperse. For van der Eijk (2015), following Galen *On Mixtures*, touch is essential to diagnostic understanding; I agree, but touch is particularly important in diagnosing illness and in massaging residues from the pores. Foods and drugs, in contrast, have key tastes and textures, which are crucial in blood-making: emphasis on taste is also prominent in diagnosis, and that returns us to 'juices', 'humours' and '*chumoi*'.

When considering the properties of foods, Galen is concerned with *poiotētes* and *dunameis*. The former are based on the biological elements (heating, cooling, moistening and drying), while the latter is concerned also with flavour and texture, and these are closely related to the 'humours', as I discuss below. As mentioned above, a *chumos* might be a plant juice or a fluid in meat or fish, or a juice or 'humour' in the body of the human consumer. The treatise on good and bad juices quoted above focuses on these qualities of foods, and the dangers or benefits to the human body that absorbs them.

Let us consider some examples, comparing them with the passage below from *On the Powers of Simple Drugs* in which Galen sets out how different tastes in drugs produce or do not certain effects in terms of humours, *chumoi*.

> Lettuce is rather good in juices/humours (*euchumoteron*), . . . it generates blood . . . If it naturally generates the most blood, then it naturally produces none of the other humours.
>
> —*On the Properties of Foodstuffs* 2.40

> Beet distributes a thicker juice (*chumos*) to the body than is balanced. Therefore if a person eats it to excess, and especially if he digests it in a needy stomach, it will collect the so-called raw humour (*chumos*).
>
> —*On the Properties of Foodstuffs* 2.60

> Beef generates a thicker blood than is fitting and if a person is by nature more given to black bile in their *krasis*, he/she will fall victim to one of the black bile illnesses if they go too far, such as *karkinos* and many others.
>
> —*On the Properties of Foodstuffs* 3.1[21]

> Digestion (*pepsis*) in the stomach and blood-making in the liver and veins and assimilation into each of the parts to be nourished is easier with softer [foods], and more difficult with firmer. These processes occur when foods are transformed, and softer foods are more easily transformed, because they are also more readily acted upon. And transformation is the experience of foods being transformed. So it is right to say that firm-fleshed fish are difficult to digest and right to say that they are generative of thick humour, for firmer nourishment has a thicker substance, while softer has a finer. We must now look at whether firmer nourishment produces salty humours/juices.
>
> —*On the Properties of Foodstuffs* 3.30

> The gourd (see Figure 2.3) is raw and unpleasant and extremely bad for the mouth of the stomach and indigestible . . . but when well boiled it has no clear property of humours/juices, unless you can call a humour/flavour what is neither pungent nor salty nor astringent nor bitter, nor revealing any other taste clearly, like water.
>
> —*On the Properties of Foodstuffs* 2.3

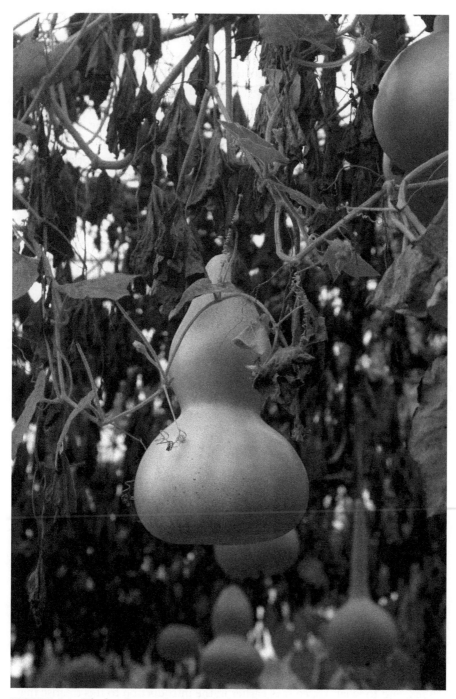

FIGURE 2.3: The bottle gourd. ©Cenk Durmuskahya.

This range of passages on nutrition from Galen's main treatise on the subject show three things: first, an assimilation of approaches through 'mixtures' and approaches through 'juices/ humours/flavours'; secondly, the juices/humours may be raw or cooked – well-concocted into blood or the reverse – and they also have tastes ('salty') and textures ('lighter in consistency'), as I am about to discuss. Thirdly, blood-making takes place in the liver and veins and is affected by elemental aspects (e.g. 'earth-like'), mixture aspects (e.g. heating, moistening) and 'humour/juice' aspects (e.g. thicker, thinner). An onion is thus a heating and a thinning food, illustrating that Galen's nutritional theory works through both 'mixtures' (*kraseis*) and tastes and humours (*chumoi*).

FOOD AND *DIAITA*

The properties of foods are many and varied, as Hippocratic authors and Galen have declared (above). Authors are frequently in disagreement on details, but Galen has (what he hopes are) authoritative guidelines on these apparent confusions. The difficulty lies, as the Hippocratic author of *On Regimen* book 2 (quoted above) and Diocles (quoted below) had observed, in matching general principles and detail:

> Generally speaking, one cannot properly test anything empirically without first accurately working out, by reasoning, the disposition to which he is applying what is being tested, be it food, drink or drug. For the knowledge of such dispositions is the stuff of remedies, not the remedies themselves; but since without knowing precisely the properties of the materials we use, it is impossible to help those who need them, it is necessary here to discuss the properties in the foodstuffs, as it was elsewhere to discuss those in drugs. Knowledge of them is achieved with difficulty by a defining test over a long time, and from the nature of the odours and flavours which the foods being tested appear to have; and as well from the consistency they have acquired in respect of viscidity, friability or loose texture; and solidity, lightness or heaviness.

> — Galen, *On the Properties of Foodstuffs* 1.1;
> translation Powell 2003: 38, adapted

As Powell notes (2003: 161–2) on this valuable passage, Galen's methodology falls squarely in the field of 'qualified experience' or experience mapped out by differentiating variables that is discussed by van der Eijk (1997: 50–1) in relation to both dietetics and pharmacology. Galen's methodology draws on Aristotle: much depends on both the nature of the foodstuff and the way it is applied, and to what. Galen says earlier in the introduction to this treatise that the same food can have quite the reverse effect on two different people if their 'disposition' or bodily state (*diathesis*) differs. Seasons, way of life, climate and gender can all have an impact.

PRACTICE AND FOOD PREPARATION

Nearly all foods require processing before they can be digested. Such practical cooking skills, common to the cultures of most human peoples (Lévi-Strauss 1970), are central to the anthropology of the Hippocratic *On Ancient Medicine*:

> I am of the opinion that our present way of living and our present diet would not have come about if it had proved adequate for a man to eat and drink the same things as an ox or a horse and all the other animals. The produce of the earth, fruits, vegetables and grass, is the food of animals on which they grow and flourish without needing other articles of diet. In the beginning, I believe that man lived on such food and the modern diet is the result of many years' discovery. Such devising was necessary because, in primitive times, men often suffered terribly from their *indigestible* and animal-like diet, eating *raw* and *uncooked* food, difficult to digest. They suffered as men would suffer now from such a diet, being liable to violent pain and sickness and a speedy death . . . For this reason I believe these primitive men sought food suitable to their constitutions and discovered that which we now use. Thus, they took wheat and wetted it, winnowed it, ground it, sifted it, and then mixed it and baked it into bread, and likewise made cakes from barley. They boiled and baked and mixed and diluted the strong raw foods with the weaker ones and subjected them to many other processes, always with a view to man's nature and his capabilities.
>
> —Hippocratic Corpus, *On Ancient Medicine* 3; translation Chadwick and
> Mann 1978

Later, in the fourth century BCE, Diocles writes on preparation:

> Since most foodstuffs require additional preparation of some sort, and some become better if things are added to them, and others when things are withdrawn from them, and others again when brought into a different state, it is perhaps appropriate to say a little about these [processes]. Not least important among such [processes], both for health and for pleasure, is the purging of things that are still raw; and the first thing, as much as anything, to pay serious attention to is this, to remove what is useless and to purge anything in this [the food] that has some kinds of unpleasantness. All things are purged by being either boiled or soaked or washed many times; it is appropriate to boil foodstuffs that have a bitter or astringent [flavour] in water, and those that have biting pungency[22] in a vinegar mixture, to soak those that are salty . . . .
>
> —Diocles, fragment 187 van der Eijk; translation van der Eijk 2000: 333

This processing is essential to prepare and adapt food for successful digestion. It is central to a doctor's concern and discussed normally literally, but sometimes as an analogy. In a number of Hippocratic texts, the nature of blood is compared with the coagulation of mare's milk among Scythian nomads of the Russian steppes (Braund forthcoming). The milk was stirred at length as part of the processing, and it is that emulsifying of complex liquids that the Hippocratic doctors are using to understand the complexity and *texture* of blood.

Galen memorably illustrates from personal experience the importance of correct preparation. Wheat porridge has a very different impact on the body from properly baked bread:

> If I had not once eaten wheat [boiled in water], I should not have expected food from it to be of use to anyone. Not even in famine[23] would anybody come to this sort of use, for if wheat is in good supply, one can make bread from it. At dinner people eat boiled and roasted chickpeas (see Figure 2.4) and other seeds for want of so-called desserts, preparing them in the same fashion, but nobody eats boiled wheat in this way . . .
>
> But once when walking in the country not far from the city, with two lads of my own age, I myself actually came upon some rustics who had had their meal and whose womenfolk were about to make bread (for they were short of it). One of them put the wheat into the pot all at once and boiled it. Then they seasoned it with a moderate amount of salt and asked us to eat it. Reasonably enough, since we had been walking and were famished, we set to with a will. We ate it with gusto, and felt a heaviness in the stomach, as though clay seemed to be pressing upon it. Throughout the day we had no appetite because of indigestion, so that we could eat nothing, were full of wind and suffered from headaches and blurred vision. For there was not even any bowel action, which is the only satisfactory remedy for indigestion. I therefore asked the rustics whether they themselves also ever ate boiled wheat, and how they were affected. They said that they had often eaten it under the same necessity that we had experienced, and that wheat prepared in this way was a heavy food, difficult to concoct.
>
> — Galen, *On the Properties of Foodstuffs* 1.7;
> translation: Powell 2003: 46

Such is the importance of food preparation that alongside the Hippocratic drug recipes studied by Laurence Totelin (2009) and greatly elaborated in Galen's pharmacological works, doctors included food recipes in their treatises. Galen has a detailed recipe for making pancakes, for example, in *On the Properties of Foodstuffs* 1.4, and promises to write a cookery book. If he did so, it has not survived.

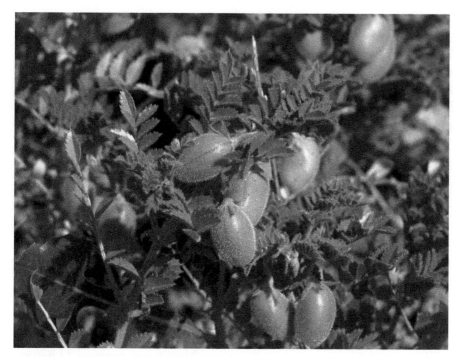

FIGURE 2.4: Chickpeas, an important addition to the cereal diet. ©Cenk Durmuskahya.

TASTE (AND PLEASURE)

Plato wrote influentially in *Gorgias* on the dangers of bodily pleasures, and limits acceptable food preparation to doctors who are beneficial, rejecting cooks as meretricious. Galen follows Plato, but has to concede a crucial modification:

> We physicians aim at benefits from foods, not pleasure. But since the unpleasantness of some foods contributes largely to poor concoction, in this regard it is better that they are moderately tasty.[24] But for cooks, tastiness for the most part makes use of harmful seasonings, so that poor rather than good concoction accompanies them.

— Galen, *On the Properties of Foodstuffs* 2.51;
translation: Powell 2003: 105

The importance of taste is a constant throughout the nutritional tradition reviewed by Edelstein (1967) and by Wöhrle (1990: see index s.v. säfte-medizin). Bertier (1972: 30–1) has observed that taste and daily regime are the only means doctors of this period had to determine the properties of foods and remedies. And the expression of categories of flavour is the only way to set out the results of this exercise. She remarks that there are many interconnections between nutritional texts such as the Hippocratic *On Regimen* 2 and Mnesitheus *On Foodstuffs,* and therapeutic texts such as the Hippocratic *On Affections* and *On Regimen in Acute Diseases*: taste and flavour were key indicators of *dunameis*. She notes (1972: 31 n. 6) that despite Galen's reservations about generalizations (echoing *On Regimen* 2.39), he declares,

> it must be remembered as a common feature (*koinon*) of all foods that pungent and bitter things give less nourishment to the body and that indeterminate and in particular sweet things give much, and still more so if they have a tight substance that results in their being neither moist nor spongy in structure.
>
> — Galen, *On the Properties of Foodstuffs* 2.62

Mnesitheus makes an earlier statement of a similar general kind,

> Salty flavours (*chumoi*) and all sweet flavours relax the cavity, while acidic and pungent ones release urination. Bitter ones are more diuretic, and some of them relax the cavity. Astringent ones . . . excretions.
>
> — Mnesitheus, fragment 22 Bertier

Galen had addressed the issue earlier in *On the Powers of Simple Drugs* where he devotes the fourth book to tastes and juices:

> So too[25] in testing pungent (*drimea*) drugs that are so on their own account, moving on to onion, garlic, pepper, *purethron*, ginger, *strouthion*, *helenion* and gypsum. For just as the person who mixes pepper with the juice of *struchnon* is not able to test either of them, nor can the person dealing with items that nature has mixed. In the same way, I think it right that you survey also the acidic property, along with the bitter and the sweet in their strong form and singly as far as is possible when taking them for testing and when seeking out their powers by experiment. And the notion of bringing to experiment everything that might be astringent or harsh or bitter, as if it will take on a test of astringency or harshness or bitterness in itself is terribly misplaced. For if it partakes of only one property, you will have the same test for the drug and for the property. But if it partakes of many, then the drug will clearly activate an activity composed of all of them, with the result that the activity of one of them singled out remains obscure. So if as was said before it is necessary to make a judgement, the assumption is not correct of those who believe that nothing at all can be revealed about the power of the flavours/humours, nor of those who make a judgement in the alternative way.
>
> — Galen, *On the Powers of Simple Drugs* 4.7, K11.642–3

Taste is essential in identifying the *poiotēs* or the *dunamis* of a drug, or a food. Here taste feeds into the understanding of *chumoi*, just as touch feeds into *mixtures* in the analysis of van der Eijk, as I set out above.[26] Tastes, and by implication juices/'humours' are key to how the food will act on the body, both in nutrition and in Galenic diagnosis more broadly, for which the senses – all of them – are the true guides in diagnostics. We can see this at work in Galen's discussion of myrtle berries (see Figure 2.5) and garlic in *On the Properties of Foodstuffs*:

> [the myrtle berry], like the juniper berry is devoid of nutriment, but it has the opposite property. For it is exceedingly astringent and as a result is constipating. Nevertheless it is not cold in property in proportion to its astringency, because not only has it astringency but some pungency has also been mixed with it. In common with all foods that have any strong *pharmacological* property, whenever it loses this by boiling, roasting or wetting, it contributes a small amount of nutriment to the body where formerly it gave none at all. The same thing also happens with onions and leeks.
>
> — Galen, *On the Properties of Foodstuffs* 2.18;
> translation: Powell 2003: 85

> People most often eat the roots of these plants [alliums], but very seldom the stem and leaves. In proportion to the root, the latter have a fairly pungent (*drimus*) property and are heating in the body and thin its thick humours, and cut the sticky (*glischros*) ones. Yet, when they have been boiled twice or even three times, they lose the pungency.[27] However, they are still thinning and give very little nutriment to the body. But up to the time they were boiled they gave none at all.
>
> —*On the Properties of Foodstuffs* 2.69; translation: Powell 2003: 114

Galen's understanding of taste is based on Aristotle's discussion in book 2 of *On the Soul*, where taste is classed as a subsection of touch (in contrast with vision and smell), wherein wetness is more important than flavour (*chumos*), and tastes are relative. Galen has greatly elaborated the Aristotelian basis. Galen's approach is not radically different from that of John McQuaid (2015), which is a summary of modern approaches to the science of taste. Here, taste is not genetic; it varies greatly between individuals; and in assessing the relative importance of tongue and brain in processing information on taste, the brain is important and uses the same part as other advanced functions. On bitterness, for example, McQuaid observes (50) that 'it tastes good . . . when combined with other flavors . . . Chocolatiers have spent the last 500 years since Cortes . . . brought cacao beans to Spain from Mexico tempering their natural bitterness with sugar and milk.' Of coffee he notes (51), that

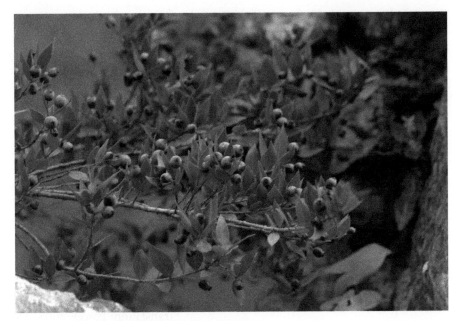

FIGURE 2.5: The myrtle. ©Cenk Durmuskahya.

'when raw, dried coffee beans are a pale green; they are seeds that have been removed from a reddish fruit, then soaked and cured. When chewed, they have a mealy consistency and a grassy taste that is not particularly bitter. Many substances contribute to coffee's bitter taste; the best known is caffeine. But roasting itself is responsible for most of it.'

SOCIABILITY AND RELIGION

Social and religious practices, such as sacrifice, are less prominent in medical texts than others but some have a strong presence, such as the symposium and temple medicine: in addition, Galen locates preventive medicine firmly in the daily life of the city. Even though the doctor is writing for an elite readership, the full animal body across the population is a key issue. Wealth was seen as helpful to health, but workers and scholars could stay healthy if necessary adjustments were made to lifestyle to balance abnormalities in the individual constitution. Indeed, on manual workers Galen writes that an athlete, a soldier, or anyone involved in agricultural or city work must have a good bodily mixture,

for these are the tasks of strong men and they would not be so without a mixture in proportion (*summetrōs kekrasthai*). And since they have mixtures in proportion they would have the greatest innate heat.

— Galen, *On the Preservation of Health* 5.12[28]

Manual workers *were* at greater risk, however:

> Emptying of the whole body necessarily follows those who work hard the
> whole day long at their normal activities (*oikeiai energeiai*). For the empty
> flesh snatches up from the stomach not only half digested fluids (*chumos*) but
> also completely undigested fluids, whenever they work after eating.
> Consequently, these people later suffer from very difficult diseases and die
> before old age. Not realising this, most people praise the strength of their
> bodies when they see them eating and digesting food which none of us could
> eat and digest. And since people who work hard sleep very deeply, and this
> contributes greatly to successful digestion, for this reason they are less
> harmed by bad foods. If you were to force them to stay awake for many
> nights in succession, they would instantly fall sick. These people thus have
> this one advantage for the digestion of bad food.
>
> — Galen, *On the Properties of Foodstuffs* 1.2

At the literary symposia of Athenaeus, Plutarch and others, doctors give a
particularly dietetic flavour to the discussion, as we have seen in citations of
Diphilus and Mnesitheus in Athenaeus, who also has Galen as a semi-fictional
symposiast in the *Deipnosophists*. It is, however, in the wine that was at the
heart of the symposium that we see how dietetics and sociability came together
most powerfully. Wine is both heating (if red) and diuretic (if white) and thus
complements massage as the main means to disperse residues (*perittōmata*, and
their Hippocratic equivalents). Three fragments of Mnesitheus of Athens, all of
them preserved by Athenaeus, bring this out well. In verse, and probably not in
the words of Mnesitheus himself, Dionysus the doctor, in Mnesitheus fragment
41 Bertier, integrates the medical and the sympotic: wine brings 'nourishment
to the drinkers and strength for body and soul'. It is possible that the quotation
comes from a comic version of Mnesitheus: comic verse and medicine shared
an interest in the festive and therapeutic potential of wine. Bertier (1972: 70–7)
brings out the shared interest in relative mixtures of wine and water as displayed
by Athenaeus in texts from Mnesitheus and the comic authors.

Wine was recognized as nutritious and restorative from Homer onwards
(Bertier 1972: 57–86, esp. 63–70). Galen identified wine as nutritious and a
drug, since it promotes urine and detoxification. Galen lists wine in his nutrition
text with the comment:

> Everyone agrees that wine is one of the things that give nourishment, and if,
> indeed, everything that nourishes is food, one would have to say that wine
> also would be one of the class of foods. But some physicians assert that one
> should not call it food . . . The properties of wine about which Hippocrates
> wrote in *On Regimen in Acute Diseases* are not properties *qua* food, but

rather properties *qua* medicament. Now I have explained these in the third of my commentaries on that book; in my treatise *On the Therapeutic Method*; and in my *On Hygiene*.

— Galen, *On the Properties of Foodstuffs* 3.39;
translation: Powell 2003: 149–50

Galen brings out the different categories of food and drink in medical discussion (mirroring the division of the Greek meal into *deipnon* and symposium); the nutritiousness of wine; the pharmacological properties predominating over the nutritional; and consequently the discussion of wine in his therapeutic works as well as in his works on lifestyle and food.

More surprisingly, Mnesitheus (fragment 45 Bertier) discusses the utility of heavy drinking in a special large sympotic cup (*kōthōn*). Unmixed wine damages body and soul, he observes, but heavy drinking over a few days purges the body and lifts the soul. Daily symposia give rise to 'pungent substances at the top of the stomach', which are cleansed by heavy drinking. The third fragment of Mnesitheus on wine declares: 'Black wine is the most nutritious, white the lightest and the most diuretic, and tawny wine is dry and assists more the digestion of foods' (fragment 46 Bertier). Ancient praise in medical authors for the diuretic qualities of wine and its ability to restore body heat is quite the reverse of the problematizing of alcohol in modern medicine (Mudd 2015).

I conclude this study of nutrition with Galen's discussions of the body's 'necessary activities'. These complement the 'natural activities' of growth, nutrition and reproduction: there are six of them, namely breathing air from the surrounding environment; eating and drinking; exercise and rest; sleep and waking; physiological balancing of the humours of the body ('filling and emptying' in Galen's terms); and good mental health. Galen devotes *On the Preservation of Health* to show how these activities must be kept in equilibrium and adjusted to the individual's constitution: this is achieved in the course of working, walking in the city, relaxing at the baths and masseur, and maintaining a calm mind. This done, a person can avoid trips to the doctor for much of life (*On the Preservation of Health* 6.14). These necessary activities are important to therapeutic as well as preventive medicine. In *On the Therapeutic Method* (8.2), in a discussion of fevers, Galen observes the blocking of the pores in bodies that give off not vaporous emanations that are of good juice/humour (*euchumoi*) but biting, bitter emanations like smoke or soot.[29] What is needed are 'baths of *eukratic* water, massage which rarifies, moderate exercise and food with sweet juices' and not 'cold baths that are astringent, remaining unwashed, vigorous exercise, either no massage at all or that which is hard, *kakochumous* foods, sleeplessness, anger, grief, anxiety, heatstroke and fatigue (*kopos*)'.

Galen confounds Erasistratean and Methodist rivals by combining bathing and massage and not using fasting therapy. Blocked pores, fatigue and excessive exercise are the problem, as they are in his treatise on preventive medicine. Galen (*On the Powers of Simple Drugs* 2.14, K11.494) could have used drugs for problems of *euchumia* and sweetness but did not.

On mental health, finally, Singer (2017) has shown that Galen's psychology was more physicalist than has been allowed. Hitherto in ancient medicine, psychology and mental health has (with important exceptions) been studied by philosophers, and anatomy and physiology by ancient medical scholars. This is the result of the stratification of the discipline of Classics, and is justified by Galen's following Plato's psychology of the *psuchē*. But as Singer now shows, Galen also maintained a causation of psychological states that went alongside diet, exercise and fever. Galen modified cause and explanation according to the matter in hand, and may never have felt called upon to integrate causation in mind and body fully. Perhaps he thought it wise not to do so.

NOTES

1. This and all citations hereafter are from the Collection des Universités de France edition by Jouanna (1996). An English translation by Jones (1923a) is also available in the Loeb Classical Library.
2. This and all citations hereafter are from the Collection des Universités de France edition by Wilkins (2013). An English translation by Powell (2003) is also available.
3. For Columella, see the Loeb Classical Library edition by Ash (1941–1955). For Palladius, see the English translation by Fitch (2013). For the *Geoponica*, see the English translation by Dalby (2011).
4. This and all citations hereafter are from the Loeb Classical Library edition by Emlyn-Jones and Preddy (2013).
5. This and all citations hereafter of Celsus are from the Loeb Classical Library edition by Spencer (1935–1938).
6. This citation to the *Odyssey* is from the Loeb Classical Library edition by Murray (1919).
7. Wootton quotes from the Penguin translation by Geoffrey Lloyd (1973).
8. On case studies and observation in Hippocrates and Galen see Lloyd 2009.
9. This and all citations hereafter of *On the Powers of Simple Drugs* are from the eleventh and twelfth volumes of Kühn's edition, thereafter abbreviated as 'K11' and 'K12' respectively.
10. This and all citations hereafter are from the Corpus Medicorum Graecorum edition by Helmreich in Koch et al (1923).
11. Van der Eijk on Diocles fr. 182.12, and index s.v. *Perittomata* are discussed in the *Anonymus Londinensis* but that part of the text probably postdates the fourth century BCE. See further below on 'mixtures', 'juices' and 'humours'.
12. Note that taking blood allows the doctor to understand the condition, as a modern doctor needs to do.
13. Fruits are reviewed in the second book of *On the Properties of Foodstuffs*, before vegetables. This implies that Galen thought them more nutritious than vegetables

since he has a descending nutritional value as he goes through cereals to weeds, fruits to onions and pork to fish in each of the three books. Fruit has little *trophē* (energy), but other important digestive powers, many of which need careful handling – which takes us back to Nutton's point.

14. On Plato's tripartite soul and Galen's engagement with it, see Gill 2010.

15. This and all citations hereafter are from the Collection des Universités de France edition by Joly (1967). An English translation by Jones (1931) is available in the Loeb Classical Library.

16. A type of bean, 'espèce inconnue', according to Amigues (see Wilkins 2013: 75 note 2).

17. ἡδονή: on the ambiguities of pleasure and taste in ancient nutrition see below.

18. On the Hellenistic medical botanists and physicians who tried to protect monarchs from poisoning see Scarborough and Nutton 1982; Hardy and Totelin 2016; Keyser and Irby-Massie 2008: 77–8, 491 and 525–6. Galen comments on their work at the beginning of *On the Powers of Simple Drugs* book 6.

19. 'Animal bodies are a mixture of hot, cold, wet and dry; and these qualities are not mixed equally in each case . . . When we say that bodies are a mixture of "hot, cold, dry and wet", we understand by this the extreme case of each of those qualities, in other words the actual elements: air, fire, water and earth. When we describe an animal or plant as hot, cold, dry or wet, on the other hand, we do not understand these qualities in that same sense. No animal is hot in the absolute sense, like fire . . .' (Galen, *On Mixtures* 1.1). This and all citations hereafter are from the Corpus Medicorum Graecorum edition by Helmreich (1904).

20. Cf. the Hippocratic, *On the Nature of Man* 2–4, the key text for Galen's development of humoural theory on what he believes to be a Hippocratic foundation. 'Humour' and 'mixture' appear to be combined in the explanation: 'physicians . . . say that a man is a unity, giving it the name that severally they wish to give it; this changes its form and its power, being constrained by the hot and the cold, and becomes sweet, bitter, white, black and so on . . . The body of man has in itself blood, phlegm, yellow bile and black bile; these make up the nature of his body, and through these he feels pain and enjoys health. Now he enjoys the most perfect health when these elements are duly proportioned to one another in respect of mixture, power and bulk, and when they are particularly mingled.' This translation is adapted from the Loeb Classical Library translation by Jones (1931).

21. This passage is noted by van der Eijk (2015: 676, n. 2), who recognizes the combination of the concepts of *krasis* and *chumos*.

22. 'Pungent acidity' in van der Eijk. I believe *drimutēs* is best translated as 'pungency', not least here where it is tempered with a mixture of acetic acid.

23. This is one of numerous references in *On the Properties of Foodstuffs* to famine foods that country people were forced to eat (especially in the spring), including acorns, bitter vetch and wayside plants.

24. 'Pleasure', 'unpleasantness' and 'tasty' are all in Greek based on the same root ἡδυν-/ἡδον-.

25. Galen is discussing heating drugs.

26. Van der Eijk quotes (2015: 682) *On Mixtures* 1, on the skin, where touch provides perfect diagnosis, and where massage and bathing can help with detoxification

through opening and closing pores in the skin. Foods need to bring taste into the picture.

27. Onions contain alicin, a pungent sulphurous compound that sweetens on cooking.

28. This and all citations hereafter are from the Loeb Classical Library edition by Johnston (2018).

29. This citation is from the Loeb Classical Library edition by Johnston and Horsley (2011).

CHAPTER THREE

Disease[1]

JULIE LASKARIS

OVERVIEW

Beginning with *Homo erectus* 1.9 million years ago, the greatest health threat to early humans was not plagues or predators, but parasites.[2] As ethnobotanist Timothy Johns ([1990] 1996: 252) puts it: 'Like most large mammals, instead of being consistently threatened by predators larger than ourselves, we are attacked by various parasitic micro-organisms and invertebrates that consume us from the inside out.' Traditional medical systems reflect this in typically employing emetics and laxatives to act as purgatives, some of which may in fact have reduced the parasite load. Their use may have been rationalized over time and extended to other conditions, such as to the infectious diseases that arose in the Neolithic (*c.* 10,000 BCE) in tandem with the domestication of plants and animals, the advent of irrigation, deforestation and other consequences of agriculture, and the rise of settled communities. Some deadly infectious diseases were in fact first transmitted to humans from domesticated animals,[3] though they and others may have appeared only sporadically until populations became dense enough to sustain them (Arnott 2005: 14). Urbanization increased exposure to parasites transmitted from human to human. These were often intestinal parasites, as the absence of proper sanitation would have led to urination and defecation in public places,[4] habits contributing to both parasite infection and contamination of water supplies (Arnott 2005: 15).[5] With some notable exceptions, parasites are not frequently fatal in themselves, but can cause or aggravate nutritional deficiency diseases that increase the risk of contracting other diseases and of dying from them. Pregnant women, with cell-mediated immunity suppressed to prevent spontaneous abortion (miscarriage), were already more vulnerable to disease; dietary deficiencies would have made maternal mortality figures climb (Demand 1994: 81). Certainly with maternal mortality today, childbirth is often the final straw for bodies already weakened by malnourishment and disease. Most Greek and Roman medical authors followed the pattern we see in traditional medical systems elsewhere in applying such purgatives as hellebore far beyond parasite control to the treatment of many conditions and to the maintenance of good health (see Hardy and Totelin 2016: 72–3 on hellebore). Some of the purgatives in the ancient pharmacopoeia in fact would have been reasonably effective at parasite control, though often with dangerous side effects.

A myriad other health problems existed in addition to parasites, of course; here, too, the conditions of the Neolithic – denser populations, unsanitary conditions and closer contact with animals – escalated their number and severity, though their precise identification is often problematic. Our ancient texts describe a variety of conditions, but since many diseases have similar symptoms, only when texts describe a unique or unusual symptom can a confident identification be made. We must adjust our concepts, as well; for example, in antiquity 'fever' (Greek: *kausos, pur, puretos*; Latin: *calor, febris*) is generally an illness in itself, not a symptom, and the formation of pus can be a positive sign in wound treatment, which is quite contrary to our way of thinking.[6] Finally, too, there is not necessarily a one-to-one correspondence between an ancient illness and a disease identified in modern medicine.[7] For example, the illness that is the subject of *On the Sacred Disease* is identified by some scholars as 'epilepsy' (see, e.g., Temkin [1945] 1971: 3–27; Grmek [1983] 1989: 40–1; Jouanna [1992] 1999: 182; Longrigg 2000), which is in part correct since the symptoms include seizures and the aura characteristic of epilepsy; the text, however, also lists kyphosis (hunchback) as a symptom, which is not a feature of epilepsy and can have numerous causes (*On the Sacred Disease* 6.1).[8] On the other hand, the text speaks of small children being left after an episode with classic symptoms of stroke – distortion of the mouth, eye, hand or neck – and stroke is a leading cause of death in children today (Jeong et al 2015) and may follow seizures (*On the Sacred Disease* 8.2). Clearly 'the sacred disease' denotes what for us are multiple conditions, only some of them the equivalent of diseases recognized by modern medicine. In short, we can base retrospective diagnoses on our texts alone only occasionally, and only if aware that ancient perceptions of illnesses are often completely different from our own.[9]

The art historical evidence must also be used with caution. Idealized figures were in vogue in classical Greece, for instance, and one would never know that anyone in that period suffered from a single malady if classical Greek sculpture were our only evidence. In periods that did favour greater realism, such as the Hellenistic, one may still not be able to arrive at a definitive conclusion. One

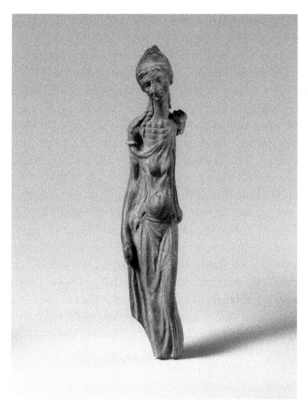

FIGURE 3.1: Terracotta statuette of an emaciated woman, Greek, from Smyrna, first
century BCE. The woman represented may look like an old woman, but is in fact a
young woman suffering from a severe disease. The Metropolitan Museum of Art, New
York, accession number 89.2.2141. Courtesy of the Metropolitan Museum of Art.

Hellenistic statuette depicts an emaciated woman (see Figure 3.1), but we cannot
know if the cause of her condition is famine, parasites, tuberculosis, cancer, or
some other disease, or is the result of the socio-economic ill of poverty.

Bioarchaeology can sometimes put us on surer footing, though with gaps in
our evidence remaining. For Greece and Italy, bioarchaeological evidence
consists of bone remains, with no opportunity for scientists to probe soft tissue
– a factor that limits findings. But limitations on our findings from bone remains
exist, too, arising from several issues: the practice of cremation – frequent in
Graeco-Roman antiquity – destroys evidence; the bodies of some may be treated
with less care than those of others, and the relative lack of their remains will
skew the results;[10] many skeletons are incomplete or damaged, in some cases
not preserved by archaeologists; viruses and certain other diseases do not leave
markers on bones, and a substantial period of illness is required for those that

do, with the result that evidence is unlikely when victims succumbed quickly (Fox 2005: 60; for a full discussion, see Roberts 2015). Bone remains can tell us about only three of the deficiency diseases: rickets and osteomalacia (Vitamin D deficiency) and scurvy (Vitamin C deficiency) (Grmek [1983] 1989: 75). Magnetic resonance imaging (MRI) and computed axial tomography (CAT) scans can now give us views inside the human body that were impossible in the past; advances in the study of ancient DNA (aDNA) have brought remarkable results and doubtless will continue to do so as techniques improve, but even here we may be left with a skewed picture, since the DNA of some pathogens deteriorates more rapidly than that of others.[11]

Bearing in mind these difficulties and limitations, and taking data from all sources into account, we can be reasonably certain that Greeks and Romans could suffer from the following major health problems: malaria; thalassemia, 'favism' (glucose–6-phosphate dehydrogenase), and possibly sickle-cell anaemia (genetic conditions associated with malaria); tuberculosis; brucellosis (a bacterial infection contracted from animals); pyogenic infections (e.g. staphylococcus and salmonella); dental disease; typhoid; pneumonia; pleurisy; leishmaniasis (a parasitic infection transmitted by sandflies); hepatitis; tetanus; diphtheria; pertussis; rheumatic fever; cancer; stroke; seizures; lead poisoning; poliomyelitis; dysentery; metastatic bone cancer; degenerative bone diseases (e.g. osteoarthritis, gout); osteoporosis; Paget's disease (abnormal bone growth); bladder stones; smallpox; cholera; leprosy (from the fourth century BCE); the deficiency diseases night blindness and xerophthalmia, osteomalacia, rickets, scurvy and iron-deficiency anaemia; with women additionally vulnerable to the dangers of childbirth, which were increased by the frequent custom of a young age at marriage.

With the growth of cities, mortality rates climbed from both consistently present (endemic) and suddenly appearing (epidemic) infectious diseases as well, since sanitation was lacking and populations became dense enough to sustain them. Periods that saw increases in trade, travel, immigration and conquest probably also saw mortality rates rise, since all three provided opportunities for the transmission of disease, including the advent of new ones.[12] As Mirko Grmek notes of Greece:

By virtue of its position at the crossroads of the continents, the Greek world forms a bridge between Asia, the northern coast of Africa, and central Europe, and the great routes of infectious disease went straight through it. Not only did the first great historical pestilences pass through Greece on their way north and west, but it also saw the slow, insidious penetration of endemic disease (like tuberculosis and malaria in the distant past and, more recently, leprosy). On the other hand, its temperate climate acted as a barrier against the diffusion into Europe of the so-called tropical diseases whose vectors or germs could survive only under specific physical or biological conditions. Sheltered from yellow fever, schistosomiasis, sleeping sickness, filariasis and perhaps acute cutaneous treponema infections as well, to cite only a few of the large number of diseases that ravaged lands with less merciful climates, the Greek world nonetheless suffered terribly from one African pestilential disease: malaria.

—Grmek [1983] 1989: 93

Warfare took an inestimable toll on ancient populations, with combat-related injuries and deaths minor factors relative to the impacts of famine and disease.[13] Famine frequently sailed into a population in the wake of war, weakening it and making it more vulnerable to disease, to which military personnel were then exposed. Soldiers and sailors then became both the victims and vectors of diseases that were far deadlier than any of the battles they endured. The Roman army, for instance, almost certainly transmitted the 'Antonine Plague', probably smallpox, west from the eastern Mediterranean (Duncan-Jones 1996: 166; Sallares 2002: 124; Nutton [2004] 2013: 24; Zelener 2012: 167–77). From 165–72 CE (with recurrences later) it spread rapidly throughout the Empire, killing perhaps ten to fifteen per cent of its population (discussed below).

Malnutrition and starvation occurred in peacetime, too, and disproportionately affected the poor and enslaved and – paradoxically – rural populations, who could not outbid wealthier city residents in competing for scarce food supplies. People weakened by malnutrition and perhaps burdened by parasite loads became more vulnerable to endemic and epidemic diseases. In addition, malnutrition or starvation would have harmed the health of girls especially, since they might not have grown large enough to bear children without increased risk of obstructed labour, which was also a factor whenever they were married off very young (discussed below). For pregnant and nursing women, malnutrition or starvation would have been a particularly severe problem.

Men's occupations could also bring injury, illness or death. Soldiers and sailors could suffer from wounds, but were even more likely to fall ill, living in close quarters as they did, sometimes without proper sanitation or diet, and exposed to unfamiliar microbes. Farming and fishing were common occupations and the risk of injury, with subsequent infection, was quite high. Shepherds and farmers were liable to contract parasites and tuberculosis from animals, as were butchers, tanners, hunters and anyone else who handled the raw remains of animals, domesticated or wild. Depending on where they lived, shepherds, farmers and fishermen were also more subject to malaria (see below). Mining and metallurgy were and still are dangerous occupations that expose workers and nearby people and animals to a host of toxic substances, including arsenic and other heavy metals. In fact, the earliest organic remains in Greece of a compound drug may have been concocted by Bronze Age metalworkers trying to combat the effects of arsenic poisoning (Arnott 2008). The areas surrounding mining and smelting were liable to heavy metal pollution, with humans exposed directly and through eating the plants and animals that also had absorbed the metals (Harrison et al 2010). Some ancient authors remark on this toxicity and the shortness of miners' lives (Lucretius, *On the Nature of Things* 6.808–17; Pliny, *Natural History* 33.98; Strabo, *Geography* 12.3.40).[14] Mining was so deadly that the workforce sometimes comprised criminals sold into slavery; their death rate could be so high that the cost of constantly replacing them could halt production (Strabo, *Geography* 12.3.40). Any repetitive job might cause degenerative joint disease, especially if heavy labour were required. As such, degenerative joint disease is found more frequently in male skeletal remains, though women were not exempt: osteoarthritis of the shoulder was found in the remains of a female weaver whose daily actions must have resembled those on a terracotta oil flask dating to the sixth century BCE (see Figure 3.2) (Grmek [1983] 1989: 79).

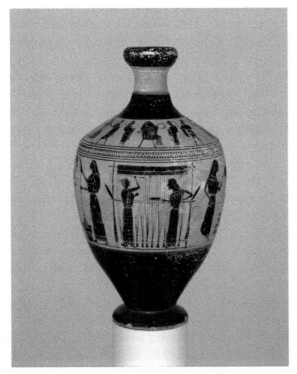

FIGURE 3.2: Women weaving represented on a black-figure lekythos (oil flask), attributed to the Amasis Painter, archaic Greek, 550–530 BCE. Working wool was one of the most important activities carried out by women in the Greek world. The Metropolitan Museum of Art, New York, accession number 31.11.10. Courtesy of the Metropolitan Museum of Art.

Wear and tear and other markers can reveal class differences, as well. These are shown starkly in two sets of male skeletal remains from Herculaneum, identified as Erc 27 and Erc 86. Both men were about forty-six years old when they died as the result of the eruption of Mt Vesuvius in Italy (79 CE) (Laurence 2005: 90). Erc 27 was ten centimetres shorter, and his bones were thin and flattened; seven of his thoracic vertebrae were fused and he had osteoarthritis. As Ray Laurence (2005: 90) notes, 'His body had been exposed to years of hard labour and had been worked beyond its strength.' He also had lost seven teeth and had four dental caries and four abscesses so painful that wear patterns on his teeth revealed that he chewed on only one side of his mouth. It is clear that he lived in daily agony. By contrast, Erc 86, though he did suffer from one abscess, had teeth that were generally in good condition, with solid bones and massive muscles not developed through day-long hard labour, but athletics (Laurence 2005: 88, 90). His height and condition show he was a well-fed member of the aristocracy with the energy and leisure for athletics.

Ancient healers were at their best in treating trauma, though challenged by haemorrhage and infection; anyone suffering serious trauma, especially to the head, chest or abdomen, was at risk (Majno 1975; Salazar 2000; Laskaris 2015).There is, however, early evidence for the expert setting of bones and for trepanation to alleviate pressure on the brain (Majno 1975; Arnott et al 2003; Petrone et al 2015). Healers did offer some beneficial treatments – and some that were believed to be so – but had little but palliative care to offer those suffering from occupational toxins, malaria, tuberculosis or any other major illness.

DEMOGRAPHY

Average lifespan figures for the ancient world are of little value since the very high rates of mortality for infants and young children skew the overall mean. Of greater value are life expectancy figures, which estimate how many more years a person who has survived to age x is likely yet to live. Demographers are hard-pressed to develop such figures because the sources for determining the age at death are few, unreliable and vary widely in accordance with region, social class and other factors (Frier 2000: 787–91; Scheidel 2012: 266–77; Scheidel 2013: 49–51; Hin 2013: 102–9). Nevertheless, scholars make tentative use of the available evidence, bolstering conclusions with comparative data from later and better documented periods, to arrive at a rough idea of life expectancy at any given age.[15]

Scholars have determined that mortality rates in Roman Italy (for which we have more abundant evidence than for Greece) fluctuated over the course of the year, which indicates a heavy toll exacted by seasonal infectious diseases and thus a low life expectancy; conversely, where there is high life expectancy, deaths occur fairly evenly throughout the year (Hin 2013: 103). There is general, though not universal, agreement that at birth a Roman baby had approximately twenty-five more years to live (Frier 2000: 788); if the baby made it through that risky first year, however, he or she might be expected to live thirty-five to forty-five more years.[16] In Rome itself, mortality remained high for those in their teens and twenties, and this is reflected in the life expectancy figures: According to one calculation, a fifteen-year old might expect to live to age forty-nine, but a thirty-five year old to fifty-eight (Hin 2013: 121–3). The period of greatest mortality in Rome was August to October, with death rates among adolescents and young adults just as high as in any other age group (Scheidel 2013: 47). Since malaria was doubtless the chief cause of mortality at that time of year, the death toll among what should have been the most resilient part of the population is puzzling: adolescents and young adults ought to have acquired a degree of immunity to malaria by that point in their lives and so should not have mortality rates equal to those of infants and young children (Scheidel 2013: 47). Walter Scheidel suggests that two factors may account for this phenomenon: strong exposure to particularly virulent forms of malaria coupled with immigration from non-malarial regions by adolescents and young adults who lacked immunity (Scheidel 2013: 47–8). Immigration may well have been a factor, but Scheidel also notes that malaria is synergistic with other seasonal diseases, to some of which adolescents and adults are more prone than are the very young; included in this group are typhoid and tuberculosis (Scheidel 2013: 48). These diseases would have increased one another's lethality to cause high mortality among Rome's youth in the late summer and early autumn. More tangible evidence of the risks children faced comes from the skeletal remains of nine inhabitants of the House of Julius Polybius (Pompeii), all of whom died in the eruption of Mt Vesuvius. Four were adults, aged approximately thirty-five to fifty, and five were children three to eleven years old (Scheidel 2013: 48). An analysis of the Harris stripes and enamel hypoplasia (both indicators of severe malnutrition or illness)[17] of these remains reveals that all but one had suffered at least one acute illness in childhood, and most had endured two or three episodes (Laurence 2005: 87). One child, by the time of his death at age eleven, had been so ill as to cease growing on four occasions between the ages of roughly four and seven, with two episodes only six months apart (Laurence 2005: 87). In sum, eighty-eight per cent of this small sample had suffered at least one childhood illness severe enough to cause growth to cease; this is comparable to the figure of eighty per cent for Pompeii as a whole, but well below that of fifty per cent for Herculaneum, where malaria may not have been as prevalent or at least not as virulent (Laurence 2005: 88).

Mortality rates throughout antiquity were sufficiently high that ancient urban populations could not grow without an influx of immigrants, including enslaved people, from outlying rural areas or elsewhere (for Italy, Scheidel

2007: 327). Robert Sallares (2002: 247–58) has even suggested that the failure of ancient populations to replace themselves was in large part owed to the death toll caused by malaria and its complications, which in his view spurred the growth of the institution of slavery in Rome, as the shortage in labour consequent upon endemic malaria combined with the desire of Roman citizens to avoid working in the well-watered and fertile fields located in malarial areas. Whether or not that is correct, there is no denying the heavy toll taken in antiquity by malaria, a disease that is today, though both preventable and curable, still a leading cause of disability and death (see Scheidel 2007 for a complex of factors that includes malaria).

ENDEMIC DISEASES

Endemic diseases exist in a population as part of the biological landscape of a region in the sense that they are a steady presence (with perhaps seasonal fluctuations). In some cases, an endemic disease may have entered a given population as a fast-moving epidemic but then, as its human hosts acquired immunity, 'settled in' to become part of the 'ecosystem' of diseases (see Grmek [1983] 1989 on this concept, which he termed 'pathocoenosis'). An indicator that this has happened is when children are the particular victims of an endemic disease, as they have not had the chance to acquire immunity. In other cases, an endemic disease may arrive slowly – perhaps because, like leprosy, it requires a great deal of exposure for transmission to occur – and take a long time, even hundreds of years, to become a major problem. Endemic diseases do not always attract the attention in primary or secondary sources that swiftly moving epidemics do, probably because they do not create the same degree of social, economic, and political upheaval, but they in fact cause the higher mortality, working steadily within a population year after year.

Malaria

While today malaria is associated with the tropics, in the past it was found in all climates. In Europe, malaria ranged from the Mediterranean to the Arctic Ocean (Faure 2014: 2), though the deadly falciparum form could not survive the cold climate of northern Europe (Sallares 2006: 21). Malaria wins the prize as the most lethal of all human diseases for at least the last 10,000 years and up to today, even though it is now preventable and curable. The five forms to which humans are subject are transmitted by the *Anopheles* mosquito, which draws blood from a person infected with a protozoan parasite of the genus *Plasmodium* and deposits it in the bloodstream of its next target. In ancient medical texts, three types of periodic fever are mentioned very frequently: tertian, quartan and semitertian; the first two occurred after two and after three days, respectively, while the third indicated a constant fever with spikes every other day. These categories correspond well with the forms of malaria most present in Greece and Italy: *P. malariae, P. vivax* and *P. falciparum* – with the last causing by far the greatest number of deaths. All forms of malaria, however, can cause lasting weakness and disability, including cognitive impairment in children (Fernando et al 2010). Malaria can also contribute indirectly to mortality rates by compromising the immune response of victims, making them more vulnerable to other serious diseases with which it sometimes acts synergistically.[18] While it is impossible to know the impact of malaria on ancient mortality rates precisely, there is evidence that it was highly significant, dramatically shortening the life expectancy of infants, children and youths, as already discussed, but impacting that of adults, as well (Sallares 2002: 151–67). Evidence for the indirect contribution of malaria to mortality rates can be seen in more recent times: Sallares (2002: 119–23) points to the example of the Italian village of Sermoneta where in 1925, only about twelve people had been diagnosed with acute malaria and in only eight per cent of deaths was malaria considered to be the direct cause, although all of the children had the enlargement of the spleen often found with chronic malaria. Once malaria was eradicated, however, the death rate was halved, a result that indicates how malaria contributes to mortality through such indirect means as co-infection and compromise of the immune response. Though there is hardly doubt that the eradication of malaria or its severe reduction lowered mortality rates dramatically, the eradication techniques themselves may have killed other parasites as well and so contributed to the reduction in mortality (Sallares 2005: 205).

Though malaria was endemic in Greece and Italy, one should note that not all areas of any given region will be malarial; on the contrary, mosquitoes do not travel far from their breeding grounds and do not tend to go uphill. In antiquity, people living in the mountains were not likely to be infected provided they did not descend to the lowlands. Many, however, spent at least part of the year tending to crops and herds in the lowlands where the better-watered and more fertile fields were often found. Moreover, sporadic exposure to malaria could result from rivers' flooding, since retreating floodwaters would leave behind pools of water ideal for mosquito breeding, as they contained no fish to eat the larvae (Sallares 2006: 23). This happened in Rome, whose low-lying districts along the Tiber often experienced outbreaks of malaria when the river flooded (Sallares 2002: 109–13). The alluviation of river deltas, deforestation and other changes in the landscape brought about by nature or human activity – most particularly the advent of agriculture – could also contribute to the creation of breeding sites for mosquitoes (Sallares: 2006: 24–5). While people in antiquity did not know that mosquitoes spread the disease – a causal connection that, as Elizabeth Craik (2017: 154–5) notes, would have been difficult to make since symptoms may not appear for many days or even months – they did associate it with the bodies of stagnant and often foul-smelling waters that are the insects' preferred breeding ground. There are numerous passages in Greek and Latin texts that reveal that living near marshes was recognized as undesirable; these include references to draining swamps and siting military camps and cities at a distance from marshes in order to avoid inhaling the foetid air or drinking the stagnant water that came from them; the illnesses to which one would reportedly be liable if exposed bear strong similarity to malaria (Craik 2017: 156–8). Despite such precautions, wells cisterns and reservoirs provided ample opportunity for mosquitoes to breed in close proximity to humans (Craik 2017: 158–9).

Continuous exposure to plasmodia parasites can produce partial immunity to both the parasite and the disease, though not protection that will last for even a year if exposure is not maintained continuously. The very high malaria mortality rate in infants and children under nine is in part owed to their not having developed immunity. Populations with endemic malaria generally have relatively high incidences of thalassemia and sickle cell anaemia, genetically passed diseases that confer at least partial immunity to those carrying the trait but not expressing it. That these anaemias are beneficial evolutionarily despite the terrible cost they exact is grim evidence of the severe toll malaria itself takes, since twenty-five per cent of children born to carriers of the gene have its full expression and, in antiquity, would have died horrible deaths before reaching puberty and reproducing.

Pregnant women, because of their higher metabolic rate, are particularly attractive to mosquitoes (Craik 2020: 92). Even those who acquired immunity before pregnancy are at increased risk for malarial infection, as pregnancy reduces their immune response; they thus endure both higher rates and greater severity of infection (Stivala 2015: 155). Mortality rates of infected mothers may be in the fifty to sixty per cent range (Stivala 2015: 155–6). Foetuses and newborns are also at high risk: spontaneous abortions are common today in regions with endemic malaria and the neonatal mortality rate high (Faure 2014: 2). In infected but asymptomatic women, the abortion rate can reach thirty per cent and in symptomatic women, fifty per cent (Stivala 2015: 155–6). There is no reason to believe that the figures for antiquity would have been significantly different. The dangers to pregnant women and children from 'intermittent fevers' are recognized in our medical texts and, as Craik (2020: 94–7) has so persuasively argued, by the cult activities surrounding the childbirth goddess Artemis, who frequently bears epithets connecting her with lakes and marshes. Archaeological evidence of the drastic toll taken by a falciparum malaria outbreak can be seen in the excavation of a late fifth-century mass burial of forty-seven newborns and aborted foetuses at a villa in Umbria, Italy, near the banks of the Tiber River. The burials were made in haste and accompanied by magical rituals, possibly intended to ward off evil; the lower layers of the excavation show the infants interred one or two at a time, but at the top they are buried in groups of up to seven (Soren 2003: 197).

Tuberculosis

Tuberculosis was endemic in Greece and Italy and pervasive (Grmek [1983] 1989: 177–97; Roberts 2015). Today, it kills more adults than any other infectious disease and is among the top ten causes of death (Gagneux 2012: 850). Tuberculosis occurs primarily among the poor, who are more likely to live in the crowded and unsanitary conditions that encourage transmission and to suffer from nutritional deficiencies that lower immune response. The eradication of poverty is an obvious step to control tuberculosis (Roberts 2015: S117), and all the more needed today as the evolution of antibiotic-resistant strains often makes the disease effectively untreatable medically. Pulmonary tuberculosis attacks the lungs and is the most frequent and infectious form of tuberculosis. Any organ, however, and the bones are vulnerable to tuberculosis; when it attacks the spine (Pott's disease), it will cause adjacent vertebrae to break down and form a distinctive angular hump (angular kyphosis), which is a sure indicator of the disease (see Figure 3.3). Among the symptoms of pulmonary tuberculosis are persistent cough, spitting blood and emaciation. That last symptom is reflected by the Greek word *phthisis*, which means 'withering or wasting away' and is found throughout our medical texts. When combined with other symptoms characteristic of tuberculosis, the existence of the word *phthisis* is a fairly sure indicator of the presence of tuberculosis in Greece and Italy (Grmek, [1983] 1989: 177–97). Nutton ([2004] 2013: 26) notes that Greek and Latin medical writers give *phthisis* as a prime example of a disease spread by close proximity to another person, and Phillips (1973: 99) points out that the author of the Hippocratic treatise *On Joints* (chapter 41) correctly associates tubercules in the lungs with kyphosis, though misunderstands the causal relationship.[19] *On Joints* also states that obese hunchbacks may live to a fair age, tacitly differentiating them, it seems, from the emaciated hunchbacks whose lives will be shortened by *phthisis*.

Apart from the distinctive angular kyphosis, tuberculosis is difficult to trace in the archaeological record since the evidence consists of lesions left in the skeletal remains, which developed only after a long period of illness.[20] When victims succumbed quickly – as children and the elderly so often did – the bone remains will not tell the story, nor will they if the person had an immune response sufficiently strong to survive; today, untreated tuberculosis can be observed on only three to five per cent of skeletal remains (Roberts 2015: S118–19).

Today, untreated tuberculosis kills fifty per cent or more of those infected (Gagneux 2012: 850), a figure that may give some indication of the mortality

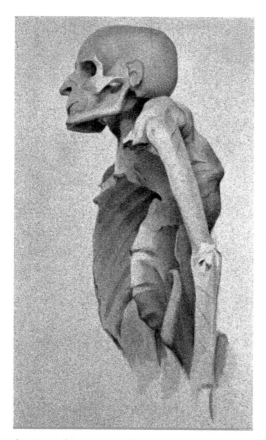

FIGURE 3.3: Line drawing of a mummy of a priest of Ammon of the Egyptian 21st Dynasty (around 1000 BCE) affected with Pott's disease. This priest shows angular kyphosis, one of the signs that the disease has attacked the spine. From: Grafton Elliot Smith and Marc Armand Ruffer (1910), Pott'sche Krankheit an einer ägyptischen Mumie aus der Zeit der 21 Dynastie (um 1000 v. chr.), Giessen: Verlag von Alfred Töpelmann. Courtesy of Wellcome Images.

rate in antiquity. In addition, an estimated 2 billion people have latent tuberculosis (Gagneux 2012: 850), which is not infectious; if it becomes active, however, it is infectious and thus debilitating or deadly. The chances that latent tuberculosis will become active are increased by malnutrition, cigarette smoking and other factors. In antiquity, we have already seen that malnutrition would have been a factor for many; the risk posed today by cigarettes may find its match in the ubiquitous exposure to smoke for those living in poorly ventilated buildings and heating and cooking with fires.

Tuberculosis is caused by a group of closely related bacteria known as the *Mycobacterium tuberculosis* complex. Two members of the complex – M.

tuberculosis and *M. africanum* (found in parts of West Africa) – are the primary cause of tuberculosis in humans. Genomic analyses have shown that *M. tuberculosis* and *M. africanum* arose in Africa at least 70,000 years ago and that the various waves of human migrations from Africa that began 67,000 years ago were each accompanied by their own strain of tuberculosis (Galagan 2014: 310–11).

M. *bovis* and the other strains of tuberculosis that infect cattle and other animals evolved from a clone of *M. tuberculosis* long before animal domestication (Galagan 2014: 311). Since humans can contract *M. bovis* through handling the raw meat, hide and bones of infected animals, it may also have existed in humans from hunter-gatherer days (Roberts and Buikstra 2003: 116). After animal domestication, humans – especially children – were additionally exposed to *M. bovis* through ingesting the raw milk of infected animals and the soft cheeses made from it. The rate of *M. tuberculosis* and *M. bovis* infection in both humans and animals very likely rose in the Neolithic, perhaps even dramatically, as both came to live in more densely populated and less sanitary conditions (Roberts and Buikstra 2003: 116–17).

EPIDEMIC DISEASES

Epidemic diseases are frequently found in tandem with famine, either because starvation makes a population highly vulnerable to disease, or because a highly infectious and lethal disease causes people to be incapable of providing food for themselves and may disrupt trade in food. The years immediately following an epidemic, however, may see some positive results. For instance, there is often a decrease in mortality because only those in excellent health survived the epidemic; reservoirs of other infectious diseases may be diminished, since those suffering from them very likely died in the epidemic; food resources may become more abundant, since there are fewer to feed; and wages may increase as the result of a shortage of labour. These benefits, though, hardly outweigh the devastation caused by epidemics, which was felt not only on the physical level, but emotionally, socially, politically and economically. Plague narratives often tell of a general breakdown of personal morals and the social order, and of the scapegoating of socially vulnerable groups, such as the Jews in medieval Europe during the first wave of the Black Death. Certainly, Thucydides' description of the Plague of Athens (2.47–55, discussed below) is an early example of such an account.[21] According to Samuel Cohn (2012), however, collapse and chaos are by no means a universal response to epidemics, which could sometimes serve to unify a populace.

We do not have full records from antiquity of when epidemics struck any given region. In no case do we have enough details of symptoms from our textual sources that scholars can be completely confident of an epidemic's identity, though sometimes the description in combination with other evidence can lead to a fair degree of certainty. We have more textual evidence for Rome than for other ancient western cities, and Livy is our main source for its early years. Richard P. Duncan-Jones (1996: 110–11; see also Wazer 2016) calculates that in the extant books of Livy, one epidemic is mentioned for every eight years from 490 to 292 BCE, and one for every four years from 212 to 165 BCE.[22] For the late Roman and early Byzantine Empires (304–750 CE), Dionysios Stathakopoulos (2004: 27–31) calculates from textual sources that Rome suffered thirty-six instances of epidemic disease or food shortage (sometimes famine), which averages to one devastating episode every 12.5 years, a marked improvement over the earlier years, especially considering that Stathakopoulos is counting periods of food shortage as well as epidemics. Rome is not typical, however: it was one of the larger and more densely populated cities of the ancient world and was more exposed than most to influxes of new pathogens via trade, travel and immigration; Stathakopoulos' data (2004: 27–31) reflect this, with only Constantinople (modern Istanbul), the centre of the Byzantine Empire, approaching the same figures. Stathakopoulos (2004: 31) remarks, however, that concentrating on the mean average (as above) does not reflect the reality of long disease-free periods followed by a series of closely spaced epidemics. The former allowed the city to develop in ways that it could not have done had it in fact been struck by a severe epidemic every dozen years, while the latter were surely horrifically devastating, coming as they did at such close intervals. For the Empire as a whole in this period, Stathakopoulos (2004: 177–386) catalogues 222 instances of epidemic disease and/or food shortage or famine: roughly one major catastrophe every other year somewhere in the Empire.

The Plague of Athens

In 430 BCE, while it was besieged by the Spartans, Athens was struck by an epidemic disease that lasted for four years, abating from time to time, but never disappearing entirely. Most of the population was infected and approximately twenty-five per cent died (75,000–100,000), including high percentages of certain military units and Athens' leader, Pericles. An account of the plague's symptoms and of its impact on the Athenian population was offered by the war's chronicler, Thucydides (2.47–55), who himself had fallen victim to it but survived. Though Thucydides intended that his description would permit identification of the plague if it struck again, that has decidedly not been the result: scholars' retrospective diagnoses have included measles, ebola, bubonic plague, typhus, typhoid, malaria and smallpox.[23]

At the time of the plague, the population of Athens had at least doubled and possibly quadrupled to 200,000–400,000, as refugees fled the countryside for the protection of the city. This influx provided the conditions for the plague, as sanitation was poor, and the population became sufficiently dense to maintain an extended epidemic. Thucydides (2.47–8) says that the plague struck Ethiopia first and then advanced through North Africa and the Near East before coming to Athens. The plague's swift spread and the high mortality that Thucydides describes have led scholars to believe that this was a 'virgin soil' epidemic: the population affected had never experienced the disease before and had no immunity to it.

The Antonine Plague

In 165 CE, a fierce epidemic broke out in the Roman world, almost certainly carried to the West by Roman soldiers returning from Lucius Verus' eastern campaign, and it reached Rome in 166 (Duncan-Jones 1996: 118–20). While ironclad certainty is not possible, most scholars agree that it was smallpox and that it was a virgin soil epidemic. If this is accurate it may have killed as much as a third of the population of Rome (Scheidel 2013: 52) and up to twenty per cent of the Empire as a whole (Duncan-Jones 1996: 117, 136). Dio Cassius' report of an epidemic causing 2,000 deaths a day in Rome in 189 CE may indicate a resurgence of this disease, and a mass burial just outside of Rome may have resulted from this or a later episode; as Scheidel says

> a series of rooms filled with large numbers of tightly stacked corpses that had been deposited at the same time and clad in garments decorated with gold threads and amber points to a sudden event that required the unceremonious disposal of numerous deceased individuals of not inconsiderable standing, quite possibly an epidemic in the late second or early third century AD that might even have been a resurgence of the 'Antonine Plague'.
>
> —Scheidel 2013: 52–3

While these facts are generally agreed upon, dissension exists concerning the epidemic's impact, with some seeing it as very great and as the beginning of Rome's decline, and others as calamitous, but not quite to that degree.[24] Recently, some scholars have investigated the broader context in which the Antonine Plague occurred, and point to drought, volcanic activity, food shortages, military threats, civil unrest and other epidemics as additional factors having a lasting and negative impact on the Roman world (see, for example, Rossignol 2012 and Elliott 2016).

PREGNANCY AND CHILDBIRTH

The Greeks and Romans tended to marry off their girls as soon as they reached menarche, which textual sources indicate was at twelve to fourteen years, though this may be accurate only for elite girls who, because of better diet, may have reached menarche earlier than others (Amundsen and Diers 1969: 125–32; Hin 2013: 151). Pregnancy-related mortality rates go up significantly when the mother is under eighteen years of age; if the mother is as young as twelve or thirteen, the risk of serious disease, injury or death increases dramatically; the risks can be sensed in a votive offering to a healing deity for a good outcome for mother and child (see Figure 3.4). As mentioned above, obstructed labour was very likely a major cause of disability and death for young mothers in particular. Obstructed labour occurs when delivery is blocked physically. Most cases arise when, because the mother is so young, or her growth has been so stunted by disease or malnutrition, the pelvis has not grown large enough for the baby to pass through; other causes include the baby's being very large or in an abnormal position, the latter mentioned as a problem in ancient medical texts (e.g. *On the Nature of the Child* 30; *On Diseases of Women* 33; Soranus,

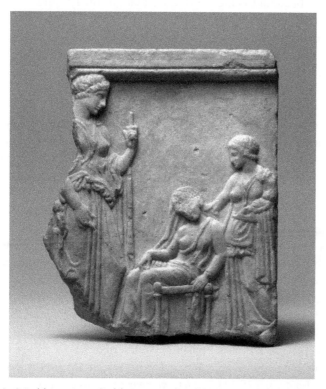

FIGURE 3.4: Marble votive relief fragment of goddesses, mother, nurse and infant, Greek, late fifth century BCE. This votive might have been offered to a healing deity in thanks for the survival of mother and infant at a time of high perinatal mortality. The Metropolitan Museum of Art, New York, accession number 24.97.92. Courtesy of the Metropolitan Museum of Art.

Gynaecology 4.1–6).[25] Without competent medical intervention, obstructed labour can last for several days, or even a week, and the baby will usually die. The mother may die, as well, very possibly from infection or obstetric haemorrhage, or she may be left with such severe chronic conditions as anaemia or obstetric fistulas (discussed below). One of the victims of the eruption of Mt Vesuvius was a pregnant sixteen-year-old (Erc 110). She had not finished growing and her pelvis was too narrow for the baby to pass through; she and the baby would almost certainly have died after days of suffering had they not died quickly that day from the pyroclastic surge (Laurence 2005: 89).

Post-partum (puerperal) infections are a possible consequence of obstructed labour, though they can have a variety of causes. They are bacterial infections of the reproductive organs to which women are especially prone if they are anemic; have undergone repeated pelvic examinations (especially if hygiene is lacking); or have suffered pre-eclampsia, protracted labour, traumatic delivery, retention of the placenta or obstetric haemorrhage. Any tear in the woman's tissue permits bacteria to enter the bloodstream or the lymph system and cause potentially fatal septicaemia, cellulitis or peritonitis. The conditions in which women gave birth in antiquity would have made them, and especially the young mothers, at high risk for puerperal infection (Demand 1994: 78–80).

Pregnant women were at risk, too, for pre-eclampsia and eclampsia, the root causes of which are unknown. In the former, the blood pressure spikes, and there may be swelling of the extremities, protein in the urine and other indications of organ dysfunction. With the advent of coma or convulsions, the condition is termed 'eclampsia', and can be fatal even today. In antiquity, of course, the death toll would have been higher, and especially among teenaged mothers who are even today at higher risk for these conditions (Demand 1994: 80–1).[26]

Obstetric haemorrhage is a leading cause today of maternal mortality, especially in developing countries, where it is responsible for twenty to thirty-six per cent of maternal deaths (Say et al 2014: 327). The most frequent type is post-partum haemorrhage, a major contributor to maternal mortality rates also in developed countries, with survivors sometimes left with severe anaemia. The Hippocratic Corpus contains references to obstetric haemorrhage (*Epidemics* 5.11 and 13 and possibly *Epidemics* 7.25), and Soranus (*Gynaecology* 3.40–2) describes in detail how doctors might seek to staunch 'the sudden and measureless flow of blood'.[27] *On Diseases* I (chapter 3) describes haemorrhage in a woman as 'necessarily long' and of uncertain outcome, which does imply that she might live;[28] in the *Epidemics* (5.11), in fact, we hear of a patient surviving a forty-day long siege of haemorrhage and fever. Greek and Roman mothers shared some of the major risk factors for post-partum haemorrhage with mothers in present-day developing nations, such as giving birth before age eighteen and past thirty-five, and having multiple births, but with no hope of benefiting from blood transfusions, caesarian sections and other life-saving medical treatments that women in developing countries today do sometimes receive. A conservative estimate for antiquity is that roughly ten to fifteen per cent of live births were complicated by moderate to severe post-partum haemorrhage.

Mothers who survived childbirth could suffer lasting health problems, such as anaemia (from haemorrhaging) or obstetric fistulas. Fistulas are holes that develop between two organs, forming a connection between them.[29] Obstetric fistulas generally arise from obstructed labour and so are yet another serious health complication for young or underdeveloped mothers (Lewis and de Bernis 2006: 3). During obstructed labour, the baby's head presses tightly against the vaginal walls, reducing the blood supply to the tissue, which may cause necrosis and one or more fistulas (Lewis and de Bernis 2006: 4). An additional cause is the practice traditional in some regions of female genital cutting, where sections of vaginal and vulval tissue are removed; this results in the formation of thick scar tissue, which can lead to obstructed labour (Lewis and de Bernis 2006: 7). The most common types of obstetric fistula connect the vagina with the bladder or with the rectum and leave the victim with uncontrolled urinary or fecal incontinence through the vagina (Lewis and de Bernis 2006: 3). Traumatic fistulas are the same in effect as obstetric fistulas, but are usually caused by unsafe abortions or sexual violence (Lewis and de Bernis 2006: 4). They are seen most frequently in war-torn regions where rape is used as a weapon of war, but also in the context of marital rape especially (though not solely) in the same countries that favour a very young age at marriage (Lewis and de Bernis 2006: 8). Fistulas also bring about great emotional suffering for the women who, having just lost a baby, are shamed and stigmatized because of their incontinence and are often rejected by their husbands and even their birth families (Lewis and de Bernis 2006: 4). Most do not receive corrective medical care and frequently develop complications that can be debilitating or fatal; some die by suicide (Lewis and de Bernis 2006: 4). The World Health Organization conservatively estimates that today two million women live with fistulas (Lewis and de Bernis 2006: 4).

The conditions that favour obstetric and traumatic fistulas are precisely those that obtained for many girls and women in Graeco-Roman antiquity, including marriage before growth is completed and vulnerability to sexual violence.[30] In addition to the passages referring to obstructed labour mentioned above, one Hippocratic treatise (*On Airs, Waters and Places* 4.3) describes a region of Greece where childbirth is so violent that women often wasted away as the result of 'ruptures' from it, and another (*On Barrenness* 1 and 35) mentions post-partum incontinence.[31] Soranus (*Gynaecology* 4.3), in his extensive discussion of difficult and obstructed labour, refers to possible injury to the mother's uterus if the body of a dead foetus has decomposed and the bones are exposed, or if the flesh is torn off of a foetus' body while it is being inexpertly extracted. This is clearly a situation in which fistulas could be caused either by necrosis of the mother's tissue, or by direct injury from the foetus' bones. Several passages describe extraction of a dead foetus by the gruesome operation of embryotomy: the dismemberment of the body while it is still within the birth canal.[32] The knives, hooks (see Figure 3.5), cranioclasts, spikes, forceps and claws used for this operation and the bones of the dead baby itself could have created fistulas (Bliquez 2014: 41–4 and 255–9). Manipulating a living but abnormally positioned baby may also have caused fistulas, as may have surgical instruments used on women for other conditions, such as bladder or kidney stones (e.g. see Bliquez 2014: 34, 82–3 and 104–5 for knives to treat anal fistula; 135 for knives to treat bladder stone; 220–4 for use of metal catheters with different designs for men and women). While female genital cutting is unknown in the Greek classical period, post-Hippocratic gynaecological works

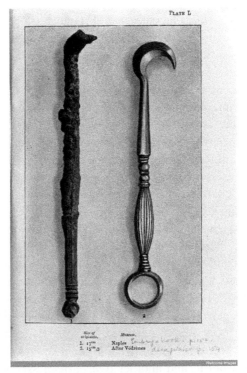

FIGURE 3.5: Illustration of Greek or Roman embryo hook and decapitator. This instrument was used to perform embryotomies, the cutting up of foetuses in the womb in order to extract it them more easily. The practice may have caused gynaecological fistulas. From: John Stewart Milne (1907), Surgical Instruments in Greek and Roman Times, Oxford: Clarendon Press. Courtesy of Wellcome Images.

describe surgical remedies for imperforate hymens (Celsus, *On Medicine* 7.28; Bliquez 2014: 105 with n. 145, commenting on Paul of Aegina 6.72.1 and Muscio 2.92) and for what were judged to be excessively large clitorises (Hanson 1990: 333–4);[33] either procedure could have produced the sort of scar tissue that leads to obstructed labour, and the former had the potential to damage internal structures. That incontinence is seldom mentioned in our texts should not lead us to believe that obstetric and traumatic fistulas were a rare occurrence. Since the conditions to which women were subject with respect to childbirth and sexual violence in Graeco-Roman antiquity were precisely those that lead to fistula, we can be confident that many suffered from this horrific condition.

CONCLUSION

Our understanding of the disease landscape of Greek and Roman antiquity and its impact on human lives is necessarily limited by the gaps in ancient evidence. Growing sophistication in demographic analysis, however, will no doubt continue to yield useful results, as will advances in aDNA analysis and genomics, scanning and other technology. In addition, work on the human microbiome (the communities of microbes that exist in or on the human body) will almost certainly bear fruit in the future for our understanding of health and disease in antiquity. Our current state of knowledge will let us conclude, however, that our earliest ancestors suffered significantly from parasites but, with the possible exception of tuberculosis, probably relatively little or only sporadically from infectious diseases. With the domestication of plants and animals, humans became additionally subject to endemic and epidemic diseases that took a great toll on their vitality and caused high mortality, particularly among children and pregnant women. The Greeks and Romans were particularly affected by endemic malaria and tuberculosis and their ramifications, which included higher maternal and neonatal mortality. Famine and epidemics, though they claimed many lives, were likely not responsible for as many deaths as the endemic diseases; they more than made up for this by causing greater social, economic and political upheaval.

NOTES

1. I am grateful to Elizabeth Craik for sharing with me her some of her work, at the time forthcoming or just-published, and to Laurence Totelin, whose *maia*-like editorial skills brought a much stronger chapter into the light. Naturally, she is not responsible for its remaining flaws.
2. I am restricting the use of 'parasite' to the protozoa, helminths (e.g. flatworms), and ectoparasites (e.g. lice) that use humans or other animals as hosts and am not including the fungi, viruses and bacteria that may also be classified as parasites.

3. E.g. pertussis and some forms of influenza from pigs, and measles as a development from rinderpest, found in cows.
4. Public toilets existed in some places, but the communal use of toilet sponges would have contributed to the spread of parasites and disease (Fox 2005: 59–60).
5. Scheidel (2013: 54) notes that even Rome's aqueduct system did not necessarily ensure clean water, since stored water could become contaminated by bacteria before consumption.
6. For the concept of 'good pus', see e.g. the Hippocratic texts *Aphorisms* 7.44–5 (this citation is from the Loeb Classical Library edition by Jones 1931); *Prognostic* 7 (this citation is from the Loeb Classical Library edition by Jones 1923b).
7. For the use of 'illness' for conditions as they are experienced within a particular cultural context and of 'disease' for those identified in modern biochemical research, see Demand (1994: 74–5).
8. This and all citations hereafter are from the Collection des Universités de France edition by Jouanna (2003). An English translation by Jones (1923b) is also available in the Loeb Classical Library.
9. Helen King (e.g. 1998: 205–46) is among the scholars who question the usefulness of retrospective diagnosis. Her objections arise with respect to the proclivity among some scholars to establish a one-to-one correspondence between conditions described in ancient texts and diseases recognized in medicine today. While those objections are clearly valid, I argue that there are occasions when scholars may legitimately use textual, bioarchaeological and other evidence, usually in combination, to make a reasonably secure case for the presence of a given disease in the ancient world, though without necessarily finding that there is an exact (or indeed any) correspondence between it and a condition as described in our texts. In the present example, for instance, we can say that epilepsy and stroke were present in ancient Greece on the basis of the passage discussed from *On the Sacred Disease*, though 'the sacred disease' does not match any modern disease entity.
10. Foetuses, infants and young children may not, for instance, have received full burial rites. See Liston and Rostoff (2013) for a dramatic example from Hellenistic Greece.
11. Bianucci et al (2015: 179) note that the aDNA of the plasmodium parasite responsible for malaria deteriorates relatively rapidly and that current analytical techniques are imprecise; it is expected that technical advances will give greater insight in the future into the impact of malaria in antiquity.
12. Duncan-Jones (1996: 136) points to the communication made possible by the creation of the Roman Empire as permitting universal epidemic.
13. Salazar (2000) is the only full-scale study of the treatment of war wounds in antiquity.
14. This citation of Lucretius is from the Loeb Classical Library edition by Rouse (1924). This citation of Pliny's book 33 of the *Natural History* is from the Loeb Classical Library edition by Rackham (1952). This citation of Strabo's *Geography* is from the Loeb Classical Library edition by Jones (1917–32).
15. 'Optimistic' and 'pessimistic' camps exist regarding assessment of life expectancy; see Kron (2012) and Scheidel (2012) for an example of the debate, with much of the relevant bibliography.

16. Males may have had a slightly higher life expectancy than females, which meant that the probable imbalance in the sexes at birth, with 105 males presumed born for every 100 females, continued through adulthood (Frier 2000: 795–6). See Demand (1994: 6–8) on the likelihood that baby girls were more often the victims of exposure or infanticide than boys, which would have created a greater imbalance yet. For textual sources on infant exposure, see Germain (1969).

17. Harris stripes form in the bone when growth is checked by periods of malnutrition or acute disease, which can also cause enamel hypoplasia of the teeth – lines of thinner enamel. According to Laurence (2005: 86), malnutrition was not a factor for the inhabitants of the House of Julius Polybius, so these markers indicate bouts of severe disease.

18. 'Synergy' here refers to co-infection where the diseases benefit each other. See also Sallares 2002: 123–40, Sallares 2005, and Faure 2014 for malaria's interactions with other diseases.

19. This citation is from the Loeb Classical Library edition by Withington (1928).

20. Skeletal evidence for the 'Old World' is collected in Roberts and Buikstra 2003: 129–86.

21. This and all citations hereafter are from the Loeb Classical Library edition by Smith (1919–23).

22. Of Livy's original 142 books, only thirty-five remain.

23. Hundreds of books and articles are devoted to identifying the Athenian plague. Sallares (1991: 221–94) and Littman (2009: 458–9) provide two of the more recent surveys.

24. Examples of the high-impact group are Duncan-Jones 1996 and Scheidel 2012, of the low-impact, Bruun 2012.

25. This citation of the Hippocratic treatise *On the Nature of the Child* is from the Loeb Classical Library edition by Potter (2012). This and all citations hereafter of the Hippocratic treatise *On Diseases of Women* are from the Loeb Classical Library edition by Potter (2018). This and all citations hereafter of Soranus' *Gynaecology* are from the Corpus Medicorum Graecorum collection by Ilberg (1927); an English translation by Temkin (1956) is also available.

26. Malinas and Gourevitch (1982: 753–5) think that eclampsia is behind Hippocratic descriptions of hysterical suffocation during pregnancy.

27. Laskaris (2015: 283–6) discusses the applicability to combat care of experience in treating obstetric haemorrhage. The Hippocratics also mention retained placenta, which can cause haemorrhage (e.g. *On Diseases of Women* 46). This and all citations hereafter of books 5 and 7 of the Hippocratic *Epidemics* is to the Collection des Universités de France edition by Grmek and Jouanna (2000).

28. This citation is from the Loeb Classical Library edition by Potter (1988a).

29. The Hippocratic treatise *On Fistulas* (this citation is from the Loeb Classical Library edition by Potter 1995) describes treatment of anal fistula, which is a hole between the perianal area and the rectum. Ancient doctors may have used similar techniques to treat obstetric fistula, though we have no direct evidence for this.

30. See King (1998: 76–7) for the violence inherent in the Greeks' notions of female maturation. For women as victims of gender violence in warfare, see Deacy and McHardy 2015.

31. This citation of the Hippocratic *On Airs, Waters and Places* is from the Collection des Universités de France edition by Jouanna (1996). An English translation by Jones (1923a) is also available in the Loeb Classical Library. This citation of the Hippocratic *On Barrenness* is to the Loeb Classical Library edition by Potter (2012).
32. Bliquez (2014: 42–4, 255–9) provides a full explanation with references to the primary sources, including the Hippocratic *Excision of the Foetus*; Soranus, *Gynaecology* 4.9–11; and Celsus *On Medicine* 7.29 (this and all citations hereafter are from the Loeb Classical Library edition by Spencer 1935–38).
33. This citation of Paul of Aegina's is to the Corpus Medicorum Graecorum edition by Heiberd (1921–4). This citation of Muscio is to the Teubner edition by Rose (1882).

CHAPTER FOUR

Animals[1]

CHIARA THUMIGER

INTRODUCTION

Medicine is one of the human arts *par excellence*, granted as gift to mankind by a divine concession, and taught as a *technē*, to be practised and learnt (see the Aeschylean or pseudo-Aeschylean narrative at *Prometheus Bound*, 436–506, and in particular 477, for the use of the word *technē*).[2] As such, it is firmly located past the threshold below which the distinction between human and animal can be blurred in ancient cultures, as mythological or religious discourses show. In short, medical knowledge and practice are among the defining markers of human civilization. And yet, in the construction of medicine as activity and science, in the authorization of medical figures of power, and in the perceptions of patienthood as human experience, the use of animal bodies and the component of animality are everywhere to be seen, more overtly in popular and non-technical representations, but also in professional contexts, in various forms.[3]

Animals in ancient cultures have attracted much attention in the last two decades. Readers of ancient texts have looked at animal–human interactions (see Fögen and Edmunds 2017); at animals as image for the human or as imagery, as literary device (see for instance Clarke 1995; Heath 2005); as philosophical conundrum (see e.g. Osborne 2007; Campbell 2008); as concrete presence in human life, provider of food or labour, as well as company or status (Wilkins 1995; Dalby 1996: 26–32; Wilkins and Hill 2006); as object of scientific knowledge and biological inquiry (Debru 1994, 1995; Grmek 1996; von Staden 2012, 2013); finally, as reverse, or trespassing of what 'man' is supposed to be, as the unthinkable other, in various post-human perspectives (see e.g. Payne

2010). This chapter will limit itself to a selection of topics under the umbrella 'animals and medicine', in an attempt to account precisely for the variety of uses and implications that the 'animal' brings to the realm of medicine. Focusing on Graeco-Roman medical cultures, I shall confine my efforts to the following specific spheres, broadly proceeding from the most concrete to the most abstract: the concrete presence of animal bodies in Greek medical practice, beginning from the most concrete – animals as dietetic item and pharmacological ingredient – to then consider the observation of animal bodies and their states of health in a medical perspective. I shall focus on medicine, following a (somehow artificial) separation between medical and ancient biological sciences; nonetheless, I will also succinctly survey the development of a veterinary art in antiquity, with its points of contact and mutual exchanges with medicine. Finally, I will analyze the topic of bodily pain and suffering as irreducible point of exchange between human and non-human animals as important presence in ancient cultures.

THE MATERIAL USE OF ANIMAL BODIES IN ANCIENT MEDICINE

This includes dietetics and everyday nutrition (see Wöhrle 1990; Wilkins 2015), on the one hand, and pharmacology on the other; the boundaries between these two are however far from easy to establish, especially when it comes to individual substances such as milk or honey, both sources of nutrition and active ingredients.

Animals and health: animals as dietetic items

Dairy products, meat and to a lesser extent fish were key sources of protein in the ancient diet, with the first being by far the heaviest presence. In particular, meat must have played a more limited role in the diet of the Greeks than literary emphasis suggests: for the majority of the population its consumption must have been limited to special occasions such as religious or civic festivals. The slaughter of animals was primarily conceived as offering to the gods, occasions in which the meat of the sacrificed victim was shared by the participants and the fat and bones offered to the flames. These meals were framed as ritual occasions, and usually reserved to the male members of the community.[4] From the available sources we can gather that meat was mostly provided by domestic animals – especially adult sheep, pigs and goats. Kids and lamb were expensive delicacies, while donkey and horse were consumed only rarely. Wild animals were only an occasional feature of the diet, and game remained a rare treat for most: hare (also treated as gift for special occasions, see Dalby 1996: 62), wild boar, wild goat, deer and even bears and lions are mentioned (for instance, in connection with the cult of Artemis, whose domain includes the hunting and killing of wild beasts, see Wilkins and Hill 2006: 108). Birds, represented in great variety, and poultry were the most common sources of meat for the poorest; and snails and cicadas an even less valued complement. Fish, finally, constituted somehow a class apart, considered a delicacy as well as a luxury and an extravagance (see Davidson 1995, 1997; Chandezon 2015 for a survey; Mylona 2015). Fish was not normally sacrificed (with few exceptions, see Wilkins and Hill 2006: 106–7, 142; Sparkes 1995: 154–9), arguably due to its small size that made it unsuitable for the shared meal. Its lesser presence in the regular diet can also be explained through its ambiguous cultural significance, perceived as both a precious luxury and an unworthy, debasing food to consume (Wilkins 1995; Purcell 1995; Sparkes 1995; Davidson 1995, 1997; Dalby 1996: 66–7; Wilkins and Hill 2006: 154–60).

In the medical texts the consumption of animal food is an important topic in dietetic discussions, and considered an element to be monitored in clinical cases. *On Regimen*, the most extensive ancient dietetic treatise to survive, lists a variety of animal meats as part of the diet, commenting on their qualities and hazards (for a summary, see Bartoš 2015: 71). Thus, at *On Regimen* 2.46 we read that

As to animals who are eatable, you must know that beef is strong and binding, and hard of digestion, because this animal abounds with a gross thick blood. The meat is heavy to the body, the flesh itself, the meat and the blood. Those animals who have a thin milk, and the blood the same, have flesh too of the like nature. Goats' flesh is lighter than these, and passes better by stool. Swine's flesh affords more strength to the body than these and passes well by stool . . .[5]

The author continues along similar lines commenting on beef, pork, lamb, goat, ass, horse, dog, wild boar, deer, hare, fox and hedgehog. Birds, a drier kind of meat for the author, are discussed in chapter 2.47; fish and other water animals, the driest meat of all, at 2.48. There follows an interesting account of 'Tame and wild animals' (2.49); in the former case, meat dryness or moisture varies depending on the labour the animals perform and on the environment in which they are reared; on the fodder, age, as well as body part. Eggs (2.50) and cheese (2.51) are considered; honey (2.53); and meat preparation, with various instructions and theoretical considerations (2.56). It emerges clearly that for this author animal products form a category neatly separated from vegetable-based meals, and especially capable of impacting on human health through the variation of dryness and moisture, a fundamental one in the treatise's vision of human physiology. Comments are also found on less common meat choices, such as boiled puppy or birds.

Dietetic considerations about meat are also present in case histories. For instance, the patient Apollodorus (in the Hippocratic *Epidemics* 3.17, case 13), prior to falling ill, followed an 'unhealthy regime', with 'excessive meat consumption'.[6] Avoidance or prescription of animal products are more often part of therapeutic and dietary prescriptions than vegetarian recommendations, precisely because of the greater strength and power of the animal ingredients. Fish is considered too: octopus and freshwater crab are used for gynaecological recipes in the Hippocratic texts (see Bourbon 2008), and in his *On the Properties of Foodstuffs* Galen analysed the impact of fish intake on the human body (see Wilkins 2017).[7]

Dairy produce – essentially cheese – accounted for a much greater part of the ancient diet than meat. From what we know about the reality of ancient human diet, milk and butter were not a central element in Greek and Roman everyday nutrition, possibly for reasons related to preservation and climatic factors; they are found as ingredients endowed with pharmacological properties, rather than emphasized as part of a regular diet (see Figure 4.1). When recommended,

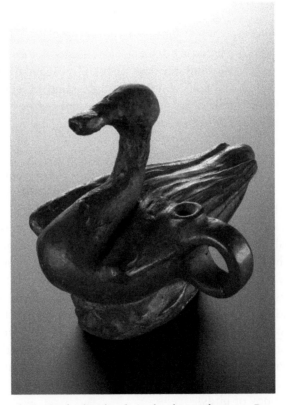

FIGURE 4.1: Earthenware feeding bottle in the shape of a swan, Roman, date uncertain. This bottle may have been used to feed young children milk or water. The Science Museum, London, object number A660399. Courtesy of Wellcome Images.

ovine rather than bovine milk is the first choice – and possibly the most readily available produce. On the whole, the main source of dairy intake was rather represented by cheese which in fact features prominently as an object of dietary recommendations.

Animals and illness: animal ingredients and pharmacology

A more remarkable role is played by animals as suppliers of specific ingredients for the preparation of medicaments. Animal ingredients are central in matters of pharmacopoeia and toxicology, and more than herbal ingredients they appear to be located in the grey area between scientific procedures (in the sense of recipes devised within the conventional boundaries of professional medicine), magic and the so-called 'Dreckapotheke', the use of ingredients openly perceived as disgusting, but regarded at the same time as powerfully active. These practices are located at the crossroad between professional medicine and popular practices, often dismissed as superstitious spells or despicable habits by professionals, but nonetheless sometimes included among the accepted therapeutics. Let us start by surveying the more conventional uses, namely those animal substances which are shared with the more ordinary dietetics in ancient Mediterranean cultures.

Honey, milk, butter Honey, and to a lesser extent milk are the two animal ingredients that feature both in everyday diet, as sweetener or condiment, and in medicine: honey is applied to the treatment of respiratory ailments and cough, as is evident in the short recipe preserved by Theophrastus in his *Enquiry into Plants* (9.20.3) and already, for instance, in the Hippocratic *On Regimen in Acute Diseases (Appendix* 34, L2.466.1) where it is prescribed 'for the *peripleumoniē*'.[8] More generally, in the Hippocratic texts the frequent mention of honey reflects its popularity in Greek culture overall: it features in particular in the pharmacology of the gynaecological treatises, as excipient as well as curative substance (see Byl 1999: 120–2). In addition, honey is a corrective of taste, and is used as a laxative and as an ingredient in recipes to cure ailments in children's mouths in papyrological sources (see Gazza 1956: 106).

In particular, two preparations based on honey are central from classical medicine onwards: hydromel or melicrat (a solution of water and honey) and oxymel (vinegar and honey), with a variety of applications. As in all active substances, the powers of honey are not always beneficial, and could trigger illnesses (See Byl 1999: 123). Certain types of honey even appear as powerfully psychotropic, such as the toxic or maddening honey from parts of Pontus.[9]

Although a substance featuring in usual diet, milk, an easily perishable product, has a more limited application than honey in the preparation of pharmaceutical products (see Laskaris 2005). Its use and valorization can be interpreted, at least in part, in the light of milk's symbolic significance as

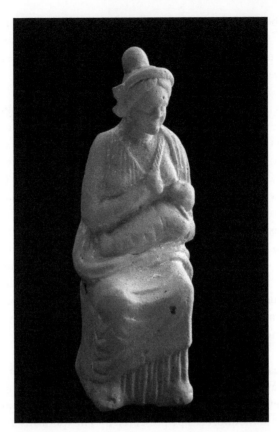

FIGURE 4.2: Terracotta votive offering representing a seated woman breastfeeding a child, Roman, 300–100 BCE. The Science Museum, London, object number A634990. Courtesy of Wellcome Images.

spiritual nutriment, as Mercedes López Salvá explores (1992: 251; see also Leven 2005: 615–18), which may explain its disparate therapeutic applications in the Hippocratic sources. In *On Regimen* (2.41) different types of milk are distinguished and prescribed (bovine, ovine, equine – of horse and donkey – and even produced by dogs and human mothers, see Figure 4.2). Other treatises confirm similar specifications (see Totelin 2009: 37–9) and a preponderance of gynaecological uses (if not gender-specificity) of milk for patients: for instance, donkey milk is recognized as laxative; horse milk serves for pulmonary ailments; that of dog is a remedy against menstrual disturbances and has the power to provoke the expulsion of the foetus (*On the Nature of Woman* 8).[10] In general, donkey, cow and goat milk are the most frequently used, and for all these the prescription is obviously nutritional as much as, or perhaps more than, therapeutic; at the same time, it carries strong magical and symbolic associations as first nutriment for the infant and 'miraculous' substance produced by the mother. Butter is also mentioned by papyrological sources, for instance as emollient for lesions; Galen (*On the Powers of Simple Drugs* 10.19, K12.292) describes the properties of butter, which 'some call *schiston* (curled milk)' for dysentery and ulcers;[11] and Paul of Aegina (7.3, see Gazza 1956: 106) also praises the virtues of *bouturon* for its ability to promote digestion and perspiration; as unguent against swollen nodules;[12] for children's aching gums and to heat the chest. In Pliny (*Natural History* 28.34–6) butter is mentioned as astringent, emollient, repletive and purgative; cheese is also praised for its therapeutic properties, both consumed as cure for the stomach among other things, and applied externally to remove spots from the skin; likewise, *oxugala* (sour milk).[13]

Other animal pharmacological ingredients   More notable is the use of animal substances considered active, and specifically pharmacological, outside any common nutritional use: specific bodily parts, fluids and secretions (such as bile), fat, dung from rare or exotic creatures or from more common animals. We can discuss this material as follows: first, the use of animal parts and secretions as pharmacological ingredients; secondly, the so-called iology, the art of protecting from venomous bites or curing their effect; thirdly, and cutting across both categories, recipes that qualify specifically as Dreckapotheke, the use of animal ingredients specifically notable for their disgusting character such as excrement or urine. The line between this last category and other, more 'regular', pharmacology is thin, often blurred and possibly reflecting the historian's perceptions more than an ancient categorization. Although it makes sense to address the use of dung and other repulsive ingredients for its cultural specifics, we should remember that these remedies are partly accepted (if with some unease) by official medicine and pharmacology.

As to the first, a summary of the tradition, reporting material lifted from Rufus, Galen and Oribasius among others, is provided by Aetius of Amida, the sixth-century CE medical compiler who discusses at length, in the second book of his *Books on Medicine* (2.84–195), the 'benefit from animal' that medicine and pharmacology can extract.[14] Before Galen and the information he offers in his *On the Powers of Simple Drugs* we know of a Sostratus (first century BCE), author of a treatise devoted specifically to animal drugs; more importantly Dioscorides (first century CE), an authority to the physician from Pergamum in pharmaceutical matters, gathered in the second book of his *Materia Medica* a repertoire of animal ingredients sampled during his military travels, some of which are exotic and rare (panther and lion fat, for instance), from a variety of species (including insects, eggs, caterpillars, elephants, as well as the most typical European varieties), bodily parts (liver, wool) and substances (blood, saliva, dung, bile, fat).

The richest source is however non-technical: Pliny's *Natural History* (books 28–32), which preserves a multifarious and wondrous repertoire of animal ingredients, from the ordinary to the most surprising (on Pliny's reliability as source on actual medical practice, in fact, it is legitimate to have doubts).[15] We find animal fat (suet and lard of various creatures, some of which exotic); marrow; gall; blood; and several other animal ingredients, some of which do not otherwise feature frequently in pharmacological and medical texts (wool, wool-grease, eggs and insects) (*Natural History* 28.29–41). This discussion is intertwined with notices on the magical and exotic formulas that can be associated with the recipes (on this tradition, see Davidson 1995). Matching information on these comes to us also from the medical papyri; here we find, for instance, otter kidneys, insects such as the cantharis and viper fat. Among the most common animal ingredients found both in medical recipes and popular sources are bile and other secretions of various animals, notably the *castoreum* (Gazza 1956: 76; 106–10), an unguent allegedly extracted from the testicles of beavers (Barbara 2008; Totelin 2009: 161–2), known to be therapeutic in cases of wounds in the belly, and especially in gynaecological contexts.[16] In some cases, a sexual symbolism might explain the perceived effectiveness of certain animal (and vegetable) ingredients, as evident in comedy but also in the Hippocratic gynaecological pharmacopoeia reflecting in both, if to different extents, widespread popular beliefs, as Totelin (2009: 199–208) analyses: a woman's chorion with worms' heads is used to promote conception, for instance (*On Diseases of Women* 1.75.9); animal genitals (a stag's penis and beaver testes) work against sterility (*On Barrenness* 12); and so on.[17]

These associations are mostly based on suggestions by analogy, and several instances in comic or iambic poetry confirm the thinking at work behind these pharmacological worlds. In some cases, however, another, 'rational' mode of animal-to-human channelling through pharmacological or dietetic means is recognized: the possibility of absorption of venomous substances through the flesh of animals which had fed on them, or the curative properties of the milk drawn from animals which had grazed on specific curative plants (see Amigues 2008). The example of the honey from Pontus we offered above also falls under this 'food chain' pattern; similarly, Galen (*Commentary to Hippocrates' Epidemics VI* 35, K17B.306) remarks that many inhabitants of Thessaly suffer from muscular cramps since they eat quails, 'because these feed on hellebore'.[18]

Iology, the science concerned with the effects of snake poisons, was also widespread; Christine Salazar suggests that interest and fascination with poisons and antidotes emerged with particular strength in the Hellenistic period and continued through to late antiquity, surviving into the middle ages.[19] Ancient iology comprised a rich repertoire of magical and folkloristic remedies, as documented in its earlier phases by the two surviving poems by Nicander, the second century BCE *Theriaka* and *Alexipharmaka*, describing over twelve types of snakes, as well as spiders and scorpions, and the remedies to their venoms (see Amigues 2008; Jacques 2008; Overduin 2015). As reptiles are monstrous and powerful creatures, the antidotes needed against them have a wondrous character. For example, a special power is suggestively attributed to beeswax or stag horns, whose smoke repels snakes (*Theriaka* 36); as Nicander explains later (*Theriaka* 141–4) the perennial enmity between deer and snakes is in point here (Spatafora 2007a: 116).[20] The *castoreum*, already mentioned, was also considered protective against snake bites (see Barbara 2008). Another association is of a homeopathic kind: a preparation of scorpions' flesh could be used to cure the bite of the animal, as explained by Dioscorides (*Materia Medica* 2.11), according to the principle that the similar cures the similar (*similia similibis curantur*), just as in the former case of the deer and the snake the principle was that *similia similibus evocantur* – i.e. an animal substance might symbolically evoke qualities antagonistic to the source of malaise – a tropic procedure that has much in common with the magical thinking that is behind the preparation of filters and potions.[21] Such symbolic mechanisms also appear to be at work in several pharmacological recipes (Totelin 2009: 208–9; Rumor 2016: 69–70). On the other hand, the discussion of animal poisons becomes integrated into works of professional medicine, such as in Paul of Aegina's medical treatise (5.1–26, on which see Salazar forthcoming).

Behind many, if not most of these cases of animal ingredients whose apparent value is not explicitly nutritional, the rationale must remain enigmatic. The deeper question – how could a pharmacological tradition establish itself so firmly, in which a large part of the ingredients were inert or even harmful – is culturally-historically naïve and impossible to answer. The more superficial issue, however – how the semiotics of the animal element works to establish a taxonomy of substances and assign pharmacological powers to them – is worth pursuing and in part possible to answer. In some cases, a well-known mechanism of 'coding' might explain some of the most extraordinary animal ingredients: the use of animal labels as symbolic, a disguise for herbal or other less extreme ingredients. Maddalena Rumor (2015: 217), for example, explains several features of the Greek use of Dreckapotheke as the later misunderstanding of earlier Near-Eastern sources and their nomenclature; this is obviously the case for several of her examples (see also Desch 2017). Such coding could also be explained by an intentional attempt to disguise powerful and dangerous plants from laypeople, or from those who might want to put them to evil use: the 'code name', she notices, is always of animal, human or divine origin.[22] In addition, there is the general belief that animal ingredients would be more powerful than plants, so that their inclusion would be reassuring for patients and a boost for the medicine's perceived efficacy (see Laskaris 2005: 176). It is impossible to give firm answers and choose between these possibilities, each plausible in individual cases. As Totelin (2016a: 145) rightly notes, however, it would be a step too far to use the coding hypothesis to discount altogether the material that falls under Dreckapotheke, and to avoid the problem posed by the most absurd and striking pharmacological ingredients such as excrement, whose meaning is to be inquired in deep-seated cultural attitudes. We now turn precisely to this most extraordinary part of our material.

Dreckapotheke, the 'disgusting pharmacology' that is transversally present in ancient medical science but features most extensively in non-technical and popular sources (such as Pliny's account, or the magical papyri) comprises medical therapeutics employing a range of excremental substances, secretions and discharges of animal origins (see Desch 2017: 44–5 for a discussion of the concept). These are notable for their repulsive nature, appearance, taste and smell or their association to life-cycle events considered impure (evacuation, menstruation, birth) and it is interesting to notice, alongside the emotional and cultural quality of these remedies, that they are all have animal origins.[23]

This kind of medicine had been widespread in the Mediterranean since its early records, and would enjoy a longstanding presence in Western medicine (see von Staden 1991, 1992b; Rumor 2015: 4–7; Harris 2020). In particular, it played a role as ingredient in female cosmetics, where animal dung is a notable ingredient (Totelin 2016a: esp. 143–6), and in gynaecology (von Staden 1992b). The use of ingredients largely inactive and (we may suppose) with recognized disgusting qualities (excrements are generally avoided as contaminated in human cultures) defies a unitary persuasive explanation.[24] Heinrich von Staden (1991; 1992b: esp. 9–15) famously explored the cultural significance of these ingredients perceived as polluted, degrading and defiling and their gender specificity. In gynaecological texts of the classical period we find in fact remedies such as 'fumigation of the uterus with the smoke of cow dung', and insertion of a suppository with blister beetle (*On Diseases of Women* 1.59), one of many similar passages that show cow dung as active against sterility; mouse excrement for the expulsion of the foetus (*On Diseases of Women* 1.78.41); bird excrement and eggs feature among the ingredients for a suppository against air in the uterus (*On Diseases of Women* 2.68 = chapter 177 in the Littré edition); and even mule excrement mixed with wine is found, to be drunk against offensive vaginal discharges (*On Diseases of Women* 2.83.18 = chapter 192 in the Littré edition); or fumigations with bull's urine, again against sterility (*On the Nature of Woman* 109). Von Staden (1992b: 15) interprets these Hippocratic practices in terms of a contact between a phase of ancient science and elements of ritualistic, non-scientific healing; in parallel, we see at play a male drive to control the female reproductive parts and functions perceived as 'impure' with impure ingredients, through a homeopathic move. In this way, the animal element catalyzes the alterity and impurity inherent in gynaecological matters and uses it in a therapeutic function. A comparable association is found behind the use of animal dirt in cosmetics, again a specifically female sphere and a characteristically stigmatized one. Totelin (2016a) recently explored the employment of dung in this respect, emphasizing female embellishment as dubious activity, marred by fraud and deceit from early on in Greek culture (see Hesiod's *Works and Days* 65–80; Semonides 7, esp. 56–69; Lucretius, *On the Nature of Things* 4.1175–82; Pseudo-Lucian, *Affairs of the Heart* 39).[25]

The gender polarization in the history of Dreckapotheke as far as the use of animal products is concerned (as pharmaceuticals or cosmetics) appears to weaken under the Roman Empire (see Laskaris 2005: 183–6).[26] Still, it would be wrong to think of these remedies in an evolutionistic frame as merely residual of ritual and magic practices, in clear-cut opposition to scientific medicine. It is thus no surprise to find Galen discussing several such ingredients in his monumental *On the Powers of Simple Drugs* (chapter 10.10, K12.292–3), from the blood of various animals to urine and dung, including human excrement, to the so-called *konisalon*, the mixture of sweat and sand to be collected from wrestlers' gyms after training; Galen claims to be able himself to testify to the miraculous properties of canine dung in the case of malign ulcers. On the other hand, in the same treatise (*On the Powers of Simple Drugs* 10.10, K12.248–50 and 284–6) he insists that medical uses of bodily discharges (urine, faeces and sperm) are ghastly and despicable practices; the drinking of urine is especially dreadful. We notice a tension, and even a contradiction concerning these practices: while obviously repulsive, such animal ingredients were, after all, at least in part traditional in official medicine from the Hippocratics onwards. Thus, Scribonius Largus (first century CE), the court physician of the emperor Claudius, also mentions the use of excrements as remedies or protection on two occasions (*Composite Remedies* 127 and 163); in the second passage in particular he describes the procedure as effective and expresses no reservation. Most significantly, he states (*Composite Remedies* 17) clearly that certain extreme remedies (the drinking of one's own blood, or the consuming of human bones or organs) remain 'outside the territory of medicine, even though they are apparently effective'.[27]

Plain disgust or a sense of professional elitism were not the only drives behind the ambivalence of official medicine towards certain animal ingredients and the exploitation of their powers to the service of human health: an ideologically grounded condemnation can be found in the words of the Christian author Tatian (second century CE), who turns in particular against animal ingredients in his criticism of *pharmakeia* (magic) and the knowledge about animals' self-healing properties as expression of humanity's misplaced faith in matter:

why would the person who believes in the healing power of the matter not trust in god . . . instead of healing like the dog does through grass, the deer with snake, the pig with crabs, and the lion with the monkey? *Why do you turn the things found in the cosmos into something divine?*

— Tatian, *Address to the Greeks* 18.4, my translation[28]

In summary, this material, however controversial, was to an extent integrated into professional pharmacopoeia. A stable category 'Dreckapotheke' thus becomes more the construct of the historian's perception than a concept of objectivity: if dung and urine can be safely taken as universally impure, when it comes to sweat, hair or burnt horns the line remains more blurred.

Anthropotherapia   We mentioned above a recipe from *On Diseases of Women* (1.75.9), where a woman's chorion was included among the ingredients for a cataplasm of gynaecological use. An interesting sub-group among animal substances is constituted of human ingredients – placenta, menstrual blood, urine, sweat, kourotrophic milk; these are also perceived as ambivalent and possibly to be interpreted, at least in their original conception, in the same homeopathic and apotropaic function as other animal ingredients of the Dreckapotheke. The most extreme elements of 'anthropotherapia', perhaps originally associated with a ritualistic and magic component (or to an external, perhaps Egyptian, influence, see Laskaris 2005: 177) also have a special application to female health in classical Greek medicine. Human milk, while being the natural nutrient for human babies, has in fact a repulsive quality in Greek culture, being variously associated with uterine blood as its putrefied or converted form (Laskaris 2005: 182–3).[29] Woman's milk is mentioned several times in the Hippocratic texts. It may be given to drink as a test for a woman's fertility (e.g. *On Barrenness* 2), or used for cleansing and softening vaginal pessaries (e.g. *On the Nature of Woman* 30 and 109). Kourotrophic milk (the milk of a mother who has borne a male child) is a special case within this group; it follows however the same pattern of purposes and practices (see López Salvá 1992: 259–61; Laskaris 2005: 180–1).

The most elaborate source on human ingredients is offered again by Pliny's *Natural History*. In book twenty-eight, Pliny discusses specifically the 'medicinal uses of the human body's own products'. He explicitly declares the necessity to extend his sources to the world of barbarians to discuss this topic, and his list of remedies reflects on the whole an othering ethnographic posture (28.5–6). A selection: drinking the blood freshly spilt from gladiators as cure for epilepsy; eating a friend's or an enemy's skull against various ailments; human gall against cataract; pills made from the skull of a man who had been hanged against the bite of a mad dog.[30] Human breastmilk is then mentioned as a true remedy, an abomination for Pliny; as well as spittle or contact with the human body (28.2). Turning to foreign populations and their powers, Pliny mentions the virtues of the spit and sweat of the Ophiogenes, a population from Cyprus, and their ability to keep off snakes. The idea is that an exotic population accustomed to the danger of poisonous bites and immunized through habituation is somehow capable of transmitting this immunity: by contact, through their voice, or through the water in which they have washed their hands.[31] It is difficult to assess the spread and popularity of these remedies, however, and the lengthy treatment given by Pliny is no proof of these being common or even used.[32] The employment of human excrements and urine is especially problematic and medical writers distanced themselves from its use: Aetius of Amida (2.110; see also 2.84) follows Galen in condemning these as hateful practices, revealing a particular unease with the human ingredient *qua* human.

All in all, our knowledge of the actual diffusion of Dreckapotheke and anthropotherapy as practices is sparse and limited. It is safe, however, to locate these in large part across the division between professional pharmacology and folk medicine; if we can assume that anthropotherapy remained more ambivalent, especially in the imperial era, woman's milk retained its place in professional pharmacopoeias, since Dioscorides (*Materia Medica* 2.70) includes it in his list of animal ingredients.

ANIMALS AS INSTRUMENTS OF STUDY AND RECIPIENTS OF CARE

We move now to the more abstract use of animals as instrument: the scientific observation of animals for the purpose of understanding human physiology and anatomy, based on the comparison between human and non-human animal. Although all sorts of animals were dissected by physicians, our topic here applies largely to mammals, and among mammals more often to specific categories that were privileged for observation and dissection for medical (i.e. not broadly naturalistic-biological) purposes; these are beyond the scope of this chapter.

Studying animal bodies

Observation and dissection of animals is documented from early on in Greek science, if in *On the Sacred Disease* reference to observing the brain of beasts of the flock is made to illustrate the humidity in the brain of those affected by epilepsy:

> This you may ascertain in particular, from beasts of the flock which are seized with this disease, and more especially goats, for they are most frequently attacked with it. If you will cut open the head, you will find the brain humid, full of sweat, and having a bad smell . . .
>
> — Hippocratic Corpus, *On the Sacred Disease* 11.2[33]

This kind of observation, however, leads to a confirmation of the already known or assumed, rather than engendering an inductive procedure, the backbone of the experimental method; a similar case is the comparative monitoring of the development of 'twenty or more' fertilized chicken eggs as model for human embryonic development described in *The Nature of the Child* 18.[34] Similar anecdotes are reported about Presocratic figures such as Anaxagoras (Plutarch, *Pericles* 6) and Democritus (Hippocratic *Letter* 17; see Rütten 1996), although by later sources.[35] The observation of the effects of certain drugs and herbs on animals mentioned by Theophrastus (*Enquiry into Plants* 9.10.2), instead, is truly incremental in nature: for him the powers of hellebore were discovered by humans by looking at sheep eating it and being purged as a consequence, and, likewise, by noticing how other animals are aware of the need to avoid dangerous plants (Laskaris 2016: 149; see also Holmes 2017: 238–40).

The first physician for whom activities of purposeful dissection and observations of animals are documented is Diocles of Carystus (fragment 17 van der Eijk), a physician from the fourth century held in high regard in antiquity, who is reported by Galen to have written a treatise on animal anatomy.[36] Diocles (fragment 24b and c van der Eijk) is reported to have compared the uterus of mules to that of women as sharing the same cause of sterility, and a similar extension from animal to human is reported with reference to Praxagoras (fragment 13 Steckerl).

Our earliest direct evidence comes from Aristotle, where the study of animal bodies and physiology finds its first systematic and developed expression: in *History of Animals, On the Parts of Animals* as well as variously in the *Parva Naturalia* the philosopher focuses in great detail on animal bodies, including their shapes and functions (see Kollesch 1997; von Staden 2013: 113–19). Moreover, Aristotle refers to a book on *Dissections* (now lost) he had written, which appears to have contained drawings of dissected animals (see Nutton 2013 [2004]: 120). If we look for the development of experiments in particular, the philosopher mentions mutilating animals in order to conduct investigations on their physiology (see von Staden 1989: 147, note 19), and in the Hellenistic *On the Heart* (chapter 2) we can read about an experiment conducted on a pig (see Figure 4.3), consisting in cutting the animal's throat open while it drinks, to observe the route followed by the fluid inside the body.[37] In the context of medicine, where it served to explain and cure the human body, the impact of animal observation is thus later to come, and the reference above from *On the Sacred Disease* is a well-known isolated case in Hippocratic and fifth-century sources. Greek science did not, in its earlier stages, have a sense of empirical observation and experiment, as argued by Mirko Grmek in his classic analysis (1996: 17–23). The first sustained activity in a medical sense is that conducted by Hellenistic physicians, famously Herophilus and Erasistratus, who not only

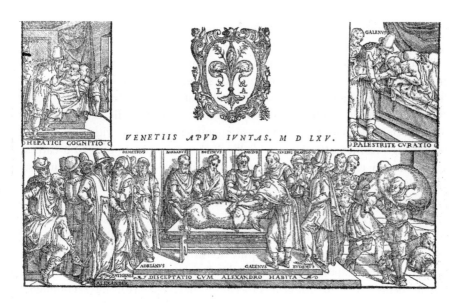

FIGURE 4.3: Frontispiece showing Galen dissecting a pig. This frontispiece adorned the fourth edition of Galen's collected works translated into Latin, which was produced in Venice in 1565. Courtesy of Wellcome Images.

dissected animals but also, uniquely in the history of Western science, vivisected human beings allowing enormous advances to the history of anatomy and medicine (see von Staden 1989: 140–53; 1992a).

Galen, as the physician who possibly practised dissection most extensively is the best source for us to gather an impression of the variety of animals used for dissection and vivisection (for bibliography, see Leven and Troehler 2005; see also Maehle and Troehler 1987). In his anatomical texts he reports using oxen, apes, sheep, pigs and goats, in particular for the study of the brain (see Rocca 2003; 69; von Staden 2013: 135–8). Although his *On Vivisection* is not extant we can gather an idea of his repertoire of activities from other works (see Rocca 2003: 67–76, especially note 107; see also Debru 1994, 1995; Grmek 1996: 101–22; Leven 2005; Leven und Tröhler 2005). Galen dissected different types of apes, the most prominent among the six classes of animals for him 'not far removed from the nature of man' (*On Anatomical Procedures* 4.2, K2.423): apes and ape-like animals; bears; pigs; saw-toothed animals; horned, two-hoofed ruminants; hornless, smooth-hoofed animals.[38] The choice of animal varied with the purpose of the individual research. The size of the animal is a key variable, as well as costs and availability (Grmeck 1996: 144). Apes, for instance, were apparently sometimes in short supply (see McDermott 1938: 93–100; Greenlaw 2011: 74–5). Galen dissected a huge number of animals in addition to these: from elephant to insects, to birds to various aquatic species.

We cannot expect to find in Galen any ethical question along the lines of current debates on dissection and animal suffering. Galen, as most ancients, shared the view of animals' lack of rationality and, to an extent, of their lesser ability to suffer by comparison with human beings.[39] His comments, for instance, on the convenience of vivisecting animals endowed with a loud voice, such as pigs, as they offer clearer feedback about the functioning of breathing and phonation, cannot but shock a modern reader for their ruthless pragmatism and lack of empathy (*On Prognosis* 5.8).[40] The question of empathy does arise, however, if in a utilitarian frame: the sight of the excruciating pain of animals during dissection may be a potential source of distress and distraction for the scientist. Thus, Galen (*On the Usefulness of Parts of the Body* 2, K4.126) expresses a kind of 'anthropomorphic sensitivity' (Rocca 2003: 70) in the particular case of apes, whom he labels elsewhere a 'laughable parody of a human being' (*On Anatomical Procedures* 4.2, K2.416): he recommends avoiding them in vivisections of the brain in order not to have to see the 'unpleasing expression' they make. Even with a lack of explicit evidence, moreover, this tension must have been greater than our texts allow us to see, as Marco Vespa (2017) analyses with specific reference to Galen's *epideixeis* (the public vivisections in which the famous physician put on show his exploration of animal physiology for audiences of the rich and notable in Rome). The overelaborate rhetoric and the extent to which Galen wrote about these *epideixeis* suggest that they had a greater purpose than scientific or didactic communication: they worked at least as much as enhancement of the socio-professional status both of the performer and of the spectators, celebrating their shared intellectual and material privilege through the vivisection of a living animal – and through its corresponding decipherment – for the purpose of appropriating, scientifically and concretely, control over (here, non-human) forms of life.[41]

Veterinary medicine

The development of veterinary medicine as an independent discipline can be seen as a by-product of the advance of medical science, while the practice of veterinary care itself must have been as ancient as the existence of husbandry and the exploitation of animal labour. Moreover, the veterinary art was apparently held in low regard in ancient times by comparison with medicine: the two were not thought of as parallel disciplines.[42] The actual concept of diseases common to animal and man remained underdeveloped in ancient cultures and almost absent, for the obvious ideological reasons that place man on a separate ontological level from non-human animals. Veterinary science and medicine remained thus fundamentally separate, although in pharmacology, as we have seen, a traffic between the two worlds was present in the empirical extension of the effects certain plants have on animals to man, and of popular forms of 'testing' of ingredients on animals (see Zucker 2008). Also the observation of animals' ability to heal themselves belongs to partial mirroring between human *technē* and innate wisdom in the animal realm (see Bouffartigue 2008; Holmes 2017).

Late antique sources mention the centaur Chiron as initiator of the veterinary art (Isidore, *Etymologies* 4.9.12; see Touwaide 2002: 146).[43] Chiron features in Greek mythology as the teacher of many cultural heroes, such as Asclepius and Achilles, and is famous for his knowledge of medicine. A hybrid identity thus characterizes the birth of the veterinary discipline, located as it is between the activity of tending and healing domestic animals and beasts of flock, and curing man through empirically gained pharmaceutical knowledge and remedies of associative efficacy. Such a body of knowledge was surely long available to the laypeople in charge of looking after the health of livestock, although it is concretized in treatise form only later than classical medicine (Goebel and Peters 2010: 589; see also Bodson 2005). The first official mention of a veterinarian with professional status is that of *hippiatros* (a horse doctor) on a 130 BCE tombstone (see Goebel and Peters 2010: 591), but for the first treatises on agriculture and hippiatric topics we have to wait until the Roman empire. Veterinary texts in the Roman tradition are based on the works of the Carthaginian Mago (fourth century BCE, only surviving in fragments); Marcus Porcius Cato's *On Agriculture* episodically discusses veterinary topics (third–second century BCE), and Marcus Terentius Varro (second–first century BCE) devotes a section of his own *On Agriculture* to the medical care of animals.[44] Although they are mostly concerned with the health of the herd, and discussions remain rather superficial, in some cases these agricultural treatises offer more detailed knowledge, as in the case of Columella's *On Agriculture*, which stands out for its discussions of the diseases and therapy of domestic animals, including small surgical procedures (see Fögen 2016: especially 331–4).[45]

A second phase in the history of ancient veterinary medicine is represented by late-antique writings, both Greek and Latin, such as the fourteenth book of *On Agriculture* by Rutilius Taurus Aemilianus Palladius (fourth–fifth century CE) or the *Geoponica* (tenth century CE), dealing with various animal species; there are also several works on horse diseases, which constitute the largest group within veterinary sources, in part surviving through excerpts.[46] In this context, a key source is the *Corpus Hippiatricorum Graecorum* (CHG), a compilation dating to the fifth to tenth century CE, and partly organized from head to toe, following the same pattern as human nosology, and complete with therapy and prescriptions.[47]

On the whole, the animals considered of interest by the discipline are mainly those of value in an agricultural economy: cattle, sheep, goats and horses (the latter also for their military importance); dogs, mentioned especially in discussions of the fatal disease named *lussa* or *hudrophobia* by ancient authors (it resembles the viral disease known as 'rabies', still incurable nowadays; see Metzger 2015), of which they were seen as the main carriers; poultry and bees. Healthcare included not only therapeutics, but also maintenance activities such as castration and birth assistance. Veterinary doctrine largely followed the principles of human medicine: mostly humoural and including practices such as dietetics, bloodletting, pharmacology and surgery (see Goebel and Peters 2010: 589).

MEDICINE, SUFFERING AND THE CONTINUITY OF ANIMAL EXISTENCE

So far, we have had the chance to observe the multifarious appropriations of the non-human by the human animal: whether as source of nourishment and active substances, or as living model for the physiology of the human animal, the move is one of annexing the animal to the human based on an analogy or a contiguity between the two realms.[48]

We move now to the reversal of this act of association, and away from material culture and bodies of technical knowledge, to consider the domain of imagery and symbolical suggestions which, from a different angle, also shed light on the role played by animals in medical cultures and medical psychology. In particular, in several popular, non-professional contexts an animalization of the human is used to construct the actions – and passions – of healing figures as well as victimized patients. These experiences of interference with the normal state of health of the human body, whether from the point of view of the healer or of the patient, are perceived as miraculous and unnatural and significantly entrusted to a hybridization of the human into the animal. This hybridization evokes the belonging to a common, ineluctable natural order in the latter case, the endangered patient, or a closer connection to that supernatural core from which therapy is originally dispensed, in the case of the practitioner of the medical art.

For example, animal identities are associated with healing figures: consider the mythological Chiron, the centaur proverbial for his medical doctrine and knowledge of herbs and drugs, whom we have mentioned as initiator of veterinary science. An (albeit different) hybrid status quality is associated to the titan Prometheus, who first taught the medical *technē* to humanity and fell pray in turn to an 'animalized' disease, the excruciating mauling of his liver by an eagle, as told in the well-known myth. The god Asclepius himself, who would become the chief divinity associated with medicine in the ancient world, is celebrated in association with two symbolic animals (see Figure 4.4). First, the snake, a reptile which sheds its skin and is thus capable of self-renewal;

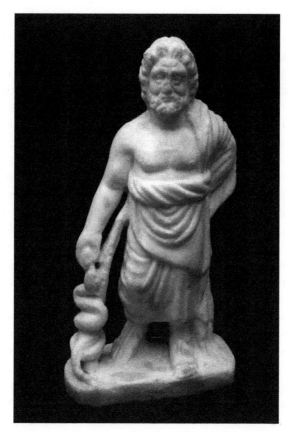

FIGURE 4.4: Marble statue of Asclepius, Greek, 400–200 BCE. The god is represented
with his staff around which a snake is coiled. The Science Museum, London, object
number A105412. Courtesy of Wellcome Images.

moreover, through its poison the snake is a repository of pharmacological
powers. Secondly, Asclepius is associated with the dog, whose licking is
considered capable of healing the wounds of the sick (*Inscriptiones Graecaea*
IV2, 1 121, lines 125–6; IG IV2, 1 122, lines 35–8; for Babylonian parallels for
this iconography, see Rumor 2015: 44–7). Another animal with important
connections to medicine is the horse, with its chthonian links to the underworld
and the restoration of strength to the dead. The centaur Chiron, as well as
several other Indo-European figures of horse-men healers exemplify this
association, most famously the Dioskuroi; the name Hippocrates (literally,
'master of horses'), as Valérie Gitton-Ripoll (2006: 232) suggests could be seen
as suggestive in this sense too.

Most prominent, however, is the surfacing of animality and animalization
when it comes to patienthood and to that subjectivity of medical suffering that

the narrative of medicine appears programmatically to eschew, especially in its classical, Hippocratic phase, in two senses: materializing the illness as a feral entity attacking its victim; and casting the suffering patient as a helpless animal, a mirror of degradation, weakness and impotence. Tragedy, a genre committed to the exploration of human suffering and human vulnerability, offers many examples (see Thumiger 2014): Medea's attacks of derangement make her 'turned into a bull . . .with respect to her eyes' (Euripides, *Medea* 92). Disease can also assume bestial characteristics, as in the case of Heracles, who has worn the tunic poisoned by the Centaur's blood and is now in agony as his flesh is corroded by the flames. His screams and agitation evoke bestial behaviour (Sophocles, *Women of Trachis* 1024–111), as he appears to be attacked by a monstrous entity: the 'fierce disease' (*agria nosos*) leaps at him (1026–30), his is a 'devouring plague', a *diaboros nosos* (1084), and indirectly his suffering is compared to the monsters he fought in his labours (1058–63, 1089–100).[49] The idea of a disease that is 'feral' and devouring (see also Philoctetes' 'foot infested by beasts' at Sophocles, *Philoctetes* 468), is present in a technical sense in the Hippocratic texts too, as Jacques Jouanna ([1990] 2012) explores, corresponding to ulcerous wounds and gangrene; the association is however obviously wider and traditional.[50] The most aggressive and sudden of illnesses are beastly in nature and characterization, as is the case of the panic attack with the screams and spasms it causes (see Charpentier and Pàmias 2016), or the disease *lussa*, a form of madness (personified as a winged, monstrous divinity in the case of the Heraclean attack in Euripides' *Heracles*) that takes canine form (Metzger 2015), and that later nosology will make synonymous to *hudrophobia*, the partly mental disease brought about by dog bites.[51]

A tragic character we just mentioned is, however, our best example of this animal characterization of patienthood and bodily suffering: Philoctetes, and in particular his Sophoclean representation. Philoctetes' character is challenged and debased on all levels of humanity from the point of view of a Greek, as I explore elsewhere (Thumiger 2019), but especially with respect to his differentiation from animals as a human. This is realized through the avenues of disgust, fear and hope(lessness) which are familiar aspects of the experience of illness throughout history. Philoctetes is famous as the unique fully rounded patient of ancient mythology: while other mythological patients are known – Heracles, Prometheus – their partly superhuman status, and the acuteness of their ordeal make them different from the painfully chronic and human experience of Philoctetes, his proper 'clinical case'. Philoctetes suffers from a wound in his foot, caused by the bite of a snake. The wound is putrid and gangrenous, and the smell it gives off, together with the hero's horrible cries of pain, induces his companions to abandon him on the deserted island of Lemnos, where he is left to carve out his own living with his bow and arrow, hunting animals, having animals as his only interlocutors, and turning, in many ways, into an animal himself. He is isolated from the rest of humanity: 'far from all others, with beasts dappled or hairy, and pitiable in his pain and hunger' (184–5), and addresses his surroundings, 'oh society of mountains beasts, oh jagged rocks . . . I know no other to speak to . . .' (936–40). He becomes part of a basic food chain, in a very direct way, when, deprived of his weapons, in his sickness and weakness he has no means to defend himself: 'come, you timorous creatures in the sky that once feared me, through the piercing breeze!' (1092–4); 'oh my winged prey and tribes of bright-eyed beasts . . . no longer need you fear me – now it is easy to sate your mouths in revenge upon my quivering flesh' (1145–53). Most explicit is the reversal announced at the end, his complete, material animalization: 'I myself shall die and provide food for those off whom I used to live, and those I used to hunt will now hunt me!' (955–62). Human language, that marks man against animals, also abandons him: the screams and grunts of the suffering hero are famous in ancient theatre, and his exceptional crying and screaming is often commented on by other characters; his suffering is substantiated into an element of savagery (see Worman 2000; Allen-Hornblower 2013, 2016; Männlein-Robert 2014).

CONCLUSION

Human appropriation of the animal domain, evident in Graeco-Roman medicine as much as in other realms of ancient cultures, takes place in our case study along three routes: first, the well-known exploitation of animals, on various levels – as source of nourishment and pharmacological ingredients, motivated on utilitarian grounds; next, within a wider relationship, where through symbolic associations animals are endowed with magical healing powers, to be seen in popular practices as much as in 'professional' pharmacopoeia; finally, in the scrutiny, more or less aggressive and invasive, of animal bodies as speculum of human physiology, from the early naturalists' and Aristotle's observations and dissections to the detailed work of the great anatomists, from the physicians of Hellenistic Alexandria to Galen.

Through all these moves and activities, ancient man arrogated the animal to himself in his search for medical understanding and therapeutic solutions. In a complementary way, the ancients also thought of their own medicalized suffering as a form of reduction to the animal, a move that belongs to the symbolic realm, and is most evident in non-technical literatures.[52] When the author of the gynaecological treatise On Diseases of Women (1.6) compares the copious bleeding that is healthy in a maiden to the blood of the slaughtered victim at the altar he is precisely resorting to the same equation between human (perhaps not by chance, female) and animal when it come to the fundamentals of physiology, such as the menstrual flow on which much of female health is based. It is in this sense that we can understand the animal symbols peculiar to the medical realm. Thus, through material exploitation as much as via the complex tropes through which Graeco-Roman cultures defined themselves largely against animals, our medical tradition was shaped in the exclusively anthropocentric form with which we are all familiar.[53]

NOTES

1. I would like to thank the Alexander von Humboldt Foundation and the Wellcome Trust for financing my research during the work on this chapter; the editor, Laurence Totelin, for her precious feedback; Christine Salazar for her help on various related topics; and Philip van der Eijk for his support.
2. This and all citations hereafter are to the Loeb Classical Library edition by Sommerstein (2009).
3. A simplistic opposition between 'popular' and 'high' medicine should be avoided; what I mean here is the distinction between a professional and self-styled scientific medicine and less systematic and organized beliefs and practices widespread among the population. On the definition of 'popular' medicine see Harris (2016).
4. See, however, Naiden (2012) on Spartan meat for a reassessment of this generalizing view; Wilkins (1995: 103–4) on gender and the control over meat production as a 'control of the symbolic' too.
5. This and all citations hereafter are from the Collection des Universités de France edition by Joly (1967). An English translation by Jones (1931) is available in the Loeb Classical Library.
6. This citation is from the Loeb Classical Library edition by Jones (1923a).
7. This and all citations hereafter are from the Collection des Universités de France edition by Wilkins (2013). An English translation by Powell (2003) is also available.
8. This and all citations hereafter of Theophrastus' *Enquiry into Plants* are from the Collection des Universités de France edition by Amigues (2006). This citation of the Hippocratic treatise *On Regimen in Acute Diseases* is from the second volume of the Littré edition, abbreviated as 'L2'.
9. I follow here the discussion in Forbes (1966: 90–2), who mentions pseudo-Aristotle, *On Marvellous Things Heard* 18 (831b24–5, citation from the Loeb Classical Library edition by Hett 1936; cf. Xenophon, *Anabasis,* 4.8.18, citation from the Loeb Classical Library edition by Brownson 1998), where it is said that 'all soldiers who ate this honey became mad, vomited and had diarrhoea, and could not stand upright', and Strabo (*Geography* 12.3.18, citation from the Loeb Classical Library edition by Jones 1917–1932) on the 'crazing honey' of the Heptacomitae. See also Pliny (*Natural History* 21.76, citation from the Loeb Classical Library edition by Jones 1951), where the quality of this honey is associated with the rhododendron flowers harvested by the bees.
10. This and all citations hereafter are from the Loeb Classical Library edition by Potter (2012).
11. This and all citations hereafter are from the eleventh and twelfth volumes of the Kühn's edition, abbreviated as 'K11' and 'K12' respectively.

12. This and all citations hereafter are from the Corpus Medicorum Graecorum edition by Heiberg (1921–1924).
13. This and all citations hereafter of books 28–32 of Pliny's *Natural History* are from the Loeb Classical Library edition by Jones (1963).
14. This and all citations hereafter are from the Corpus Medicorum Graecorum edition by Olivieri (1935–1950).
15. For a survey of animal ingredients in pharmacology, with anecdotal and paradoxographical elements see Pliny (*Natural History* 28.25–9), discussing elephant, lions, camels, hyaena, crocodile, chameleon, hippopotamus, lynx.
16. E.g. *On Diseases of Women*. 2.91 (= chapter 200 in the Littré edition), against womb suffocation; see Totelin (2009: 83–4) on otter-based ingredients. This and all citations hereafter of the Hippocratic treatise *On Diseases of Women* are from the Loeb Classical Library edition by Potter (2018).
17. This citation is to the Loeb Classical Library edition by Potter (2012).
18. This citation is from the seventeenth volume of Kühn's edition, abbreviated as 'K17'.
19. See Salazar (forthcoming), explaining the genre of treatises *Peri iobolōn* (literally 'about [animals] that throw/project venom') or *Thēriaka* ('[remedies] against wild beasts', quoting Galen's definition in his commentary on *Epidemics VI* (K17B.337): *Thēriaka* are 'what heals the bites of wild animals', while *alexipharmaka* counteract ingested poisons.
20. These citations of Nicander's *Theriaka* are from the Collection des Universités de France edition by Jacques (2002). See Pliny (*Natural History* 8.118; 28.149–50) on remedies against snakes made with burnt deer horns. See Holmes (2017: 236–7) on 'sympathy' and 'antipathy' within the natural world as principle organizing human knowledge and human use of the animal to its own benefit.
21. This and all citations hereafter of Dioscorides are from the edition by Wellmann (1907–1914).
22. As claimed by the author of a magical papyrus quoted by Laskaris (2005: 175): *Papyri Graecae Magicae* 12.401.444 (citation from the Teubner edition by Preisendanz 1973–1974), 403.
23. This leads to the wider anthropological remark that disgusting substances in human culture are always of animal (human, and non-human) provenance.
24. On disgust as historical product, as well as human experience 'resisting culture', see Miller (2009). See also Rumor (2016: 81–133) on her interpretation of part of the evidence as derivation from (and name misunderstanding of) Babylonian material on the part of the Greek readers; and more extensively Harris (2020: 4–7).
25. This citation of Hesiod is from the Loeb Classical Library edition by Most (2007). This citation of Semonides is from the Loeb Classical Library edition by Gerber (1999). This citation of Lucretius is from the Loeb Classical Library edition by Rouse (1924). This citation of Pseudo-Lucian is from the Loeb Classical Library edition by MacLeod (1967).
26. The gender polarization, however, was not exclusive: the papyri from Graeco-Roman Egypt also preserve recipes which include 'animal bile, fat, dung' among their ingredients, with no gender specifications (as in O. Tait. Bodl. II 2183, 4, in Gazza 1956: 75–6).

27. I thank Ianto Jocks for bringing these texts to my attention. These citations of Scribonius are from the Teubner edition by Sconocchia (1983).
28. This citation is from the Oxford University Press edition by Whittaker (1982).
29. On 'anthropotherapia' in ancient medicine see Ferraces Rodríguez (2006 and 2016) on late-antique sources elaborating on Pliny.
30. Other substances discussed are blood, milk, sweat, spit (ch. 7), ear wax (8), human hair and teeth (9), human blood (10), contact with dead corpses (11), human excretions such as scrapings from athletes' baths, male seminal fluid, meconium (infant first excrement) (13), urine (18), stillborn infants, menstrual discharge, burnt women's hair (20), woman's milk (21), spittle (22), menstrual discharge again (23).
31. Compare the same process with reference to animals above, 100–1.
32. On the relationship between theory and practice in Pliny's medical discussions as teaching act, see now Holmes (2017: esp. 233–6).
33. This and all citations hereafter are from the Collection des Universités de France edition by Jouanna (2003). An English translation by Jones (1923b) is also available in the Loeb Classical Library.
34. This citation is from the Loeb Classical edition by Potter (2012).
35. This citation of Plutarch's *Pericles* is from the Loeb Classical Library edition by Perrin (1916). This citation of the Hippocratic *Letters* is from the Brill edition by Smith (1990).
36. This and all citations hereafter are from the edition by van der Eijk (2000).
37. This citation of the Hippocratic treatise *On the Heart* is from the Loeb Classical Library edition by Potter (2010).
38. This and all citations hereafter are to the second volume of Kühn's edition, abbreviated as 'K2'.
39. The exception to this prevailing view is represented by Plutarch's inclusive argument on the rationality of animals: see Horky (2017) for an updated survey and discussion.
40. This citation is from the Corpus Medicorum Graecorum edition by Nutton (1979).
41. See von Staden (1995) for a reading framed within the Second Sophistic movement, and (2013: 134–9) on the forces at play in Galen's public vivisections.
42. This is the state of things according to Vegetius (*Digesta artis mulomedicinalis, Prologue* 1.7, on which see Goebel and Peters 2010: 590), and as lamented by the *Mulomedicina Chironis*, a fifth-century CE text which retorts that the scientific level of veterinary practice should not be considered, as it was, inferior to that of medicine (Bodson 2005).
43. This citation of Isidore's *Etymologies* is from the Oxford University Press edition by Lindsay (1911).
44. For an edition and English translation of Cato's *On Agriculture* and Varro's *On Agriculture*, see the Loeb Classical Library edition by Hooper and Ash (1934).
45. For an edition and English translation of Columella's *On Agriculture*, see the Loeb Classical Library volumes by Ash (1941) and Forster and Heffner (1954–1955).
46. For an English translation of Palladius' *On Agriculture*, see Fitch (2013). For an English translation of the *Geoponica*, see Dalby (2011).

47. For an edition, see Oder and Hopper (1924–1927).
48. That notion is already present in ancient science, most notably in the Aristotelian concept of a *scala naturae* where all living beings are classified as part of a *continuum*.
49. These citations are from the Loeb Classical Library edition by Lloyd-Jones (1994).
50. This and all citations hereafter of Sophocles' *Philoctetes* are from the Loeb Classical Library edition by Lloyd-Jones (1994).
51. For an English translation of Euripides' *Heracles*, see the Loeb Classical Library edition by Kovacs (1998).
52. Von Staden (2013) is a rare acknowledgement of the cultural complexity of scientific handling on animals in ancient cultures, under the heading of 'textualizing the animal', involving far more than the empirical knowledge or material gain that a scientist can extract from observing the animal.
53. Far from being merely the residue of a primitive mentality or a form of mythological thinking, however, the sense of communality through vulnerability between man and animal (with many variations) must be seen as universally human. In our more rigidly defined modern (Western) identities as human this feeling can only take refuge in the extreme – a meaningful example is offered by a niche, but thought-provoking contemporary subcultural phenomenon: 'therian communities', individuals who understand themselves as both human and non-human (www.therian-guide.com/index.php/4-psychological.html, accessed 16 October 2020), and who resist psychiatric categorization (on this kind of 'anomalous experience' see Grivell, Clegg and Roxburgh 2014).

CHAPTER FIVE

Objects

PATRICIA BAKER

INTRODUCTION

The archaeological remains of Roman medical implements no doubt bring to mind thoughts of gruesome surgical procedures that were painfully endured by patients without anaesthesia. Over the past century or so, artefacts related to surgical procedures, in particular, medical tools from the Roman era (first to third centuries CE), have received much attention from medical historians. When examining the instruments in comparison to Graeco-Roman medical texts, scholars have shown that the tools were manufactured in a meticulous manner and their uses in surgical treatment were sophisticated and carefully performed, quite unlike the butchering one might imagine (e.g. Bliquez 1981, 1994, 2014; Bliquez and Oleson 1994; Jackson 1990b, 1993, 1994a, 1995; Künzl 1983, 1996, 2002; Milne 1907; Molina 1981). Developments in material culture studies reveal archaeological remains are also indicators of social rules and behaviours that often remain unrecorded in the written record (Berger 2009; Hodder 1982; Hughes 2008; Moore 1982; Thomas 1996). Therefore, medical objects can be examined beyond their primary surgical functions to expand our awareness of ancient theories about the body, its care and social attitudes towards treatment and the instruments used in healing events (e.g. Baker 2004, 2011). In this chapter, six unpublished medical tools are examined to explain how ancient understandings of medical procedures can be derived from material remains. As space is limited, the focus will mainly be on medical instruments with comparisons to studies of votive offerings that have been examined with similar techniques to those described below, and these, too, give us wider knowledge of ancient medical perceptions (e.g. Hughes 2008; Graham 2013, 2016).

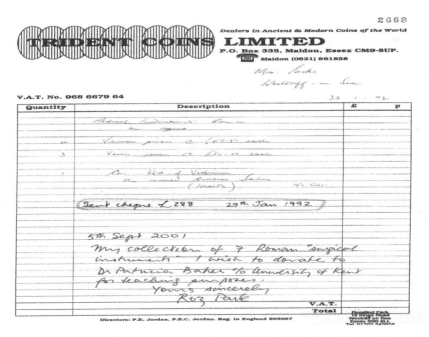

FIGURE 5.1: Scan of the original receipt from the Park Collection. ©Patty Baker.

In 2001, a friend and colleague, Roz Park, gave me a collection of seven objects she purchased in 1992 from an antique dealer, who specialized in ancient coins. These objects were classified by the dealer as Roman medical tools, but the receipt that came with the instruments provides no other information about them (see Figure 5.1). It is unclear if they were found in the archaeological record as part of a kit or as separate finds that were collected over time and sold together. In this chapter, they will be referred to as the Park Collection, but they will not be referenced as a kit or set because these terms imply that they were the equipment of single physician and found together in an excavation. Originally, seven items were sold by the dealer, but one was lost after I showed the implements during a talk on ancient medicine. The missing object was a thin rod of metal about 12.0–14.0 centimetres long. It had no definitive features that could be used to help identify its precise medical function(s).

The remaining six tools (see Figure 5.2a–f) are a useful teaching resource because they help to demonstrate Roman surgical procedures, as well as methods of archaeological interpretation. Besides teaching, the objects have always been of interest to me because two (see Figure 5.2e and 2f) of the six instruments are unlike any other medical implements I have seen in museum collections, artefact catalogues or site reports. There are a number of possibilities

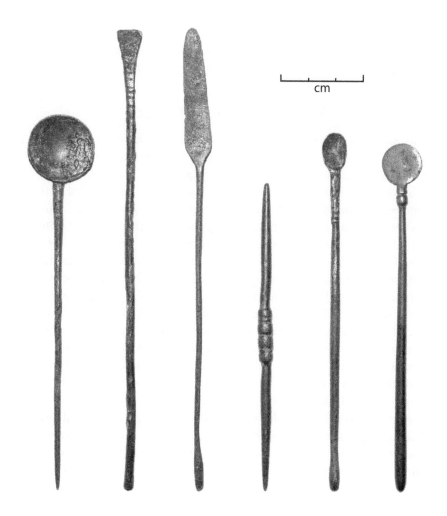

FIGURE 5.2: The tools in the Park Collection. From left to right 2a spoon, 2b stylus, 2c spatula probe, 2d handle, 2e small spoon probe, 2f disc probe. Photo by Lloyd Bosworth.

for their uniqueness: (1) the dealer misidentified them, and they are not medically related; (2) they had a surgical function, but similar tools have yet to be found or recognized in the archaeological record; (3) similar tools have been found but were not classified as medical, so I and other archaeologists might have missed them; (4) they date to a different time period; or (5) they are modern imitations thought to resemble Roman implements. To determine if any of these suggestions are likely, this chapter provides an opportunity to publish the Park Collection and examine what the unidentified objects might be. In order to undertake this survey, the objects will be compared with published studies of medical implements. Along with attempting to identify their surgical applications, other types of archaeological analyses will be drawn upon to demonstrate the multiple social meanings medical tools held.

THE OBJECTS OF STUDY

As with any study of artefacts, one of the first things an archaeologist will do once a find has been excavated, is to clean it, identify it and give it a number that is usually related to the site, the stratigraphic layer in which it was found, and the year it was excavated. The objects should then be recorded as part of the site report catalogue, each with a description that gives its basic function and notes of comparative examples of remains from other sites. This situation is the ideal archaeological process; however, many small finds were left unrecorded in earlier excavations because they were deemed insignificant in comparison to large finds and/or artefacts made of valuable metals, for example. Sometimes small finds were taken from sites or given away as souvenirs without a record of their archaeological provenance being taken. In some instances, these collections were bequeathed to museums or found themselves in teaching collections; while others, like the Park Collection, were acquired and sold by antiquities dealers without properly recorded contextual information. Nonetheless, even when data is lacking, it is still possible to study various aspects of the implements to help determine their main uses.

The first tool in the Park Collection is a spoon (see Figure 5.2a) and measures 13.2 centimetres long, and its bowl is 2.4 centimetres in diameter. The bowl has signs of wear on both its left and right sides as well as indications of metal deterioration that may have formed by another object resting on top of it when it was in the ground, as discussed below. It was made of copper alloy and has a green patina. The shape and size of the object conforms to other spoons unearthed in Roman excavations. Spoons are occasionally found with medical tools and could serve various functions, such as measuring medical ingredients, preparing medicines and administering them to patients. They could also have had other non-medical purposes such as those related to food preparation and dining (Milne 1907: 78–9).

Object number two (see Figure 5.2b) is a Roman writing implement, or stylus, consisting of a triangulated head and a straight, thin handle. In most cases, styli have pointed ends, but in this instance the end is rounded, suggesting it had broken. The copper alloy article measures 16.4 centimetres and has a green patina. It is decorated with eight horizontal lines that are incised below the head of the tool where it joins the handle. This is classified as a writing tool because it is comparable to other implements of this type. One can imagine that a literate doctor may have used it if they wished to make notes about a patient's condition. It is also possible that the artefact could have been utilized as a probe or a small cautery if a physician required these implements and did not have them in their kit. Milne (1907: 72) also reports that Galen (*On the Composition of Drugs according to Places* 5.5, K12.865) said that teeth could be extracted using a stylus.[1]

A spatula probe or *spathomele* is commonly found on its own and in kits of surgical tools. The probe in the Park Collection has a blade-shaped spatula on one end and it terminates in a small bulbous shape, or olivary probe, on the opposite end (see Figure 5.2c). It measures 16.5 centimetres long; the spatula is 4.8 centimetres long and 1.0 centimetre wide, which, according to Milne (1907: 60), is the average length of these tools. It is unadorned, with the exception of two small horizontal lines placed on one side of the handle just below the spatula. It has a green patina and slight wear on both the left and right sides of the spatula blade. Medically, the spatula could be used as a tongue depressor, cautery or blunt dissector. The olivary end could have been used as a probe or small cautery, for example. The tool also had pharmacological applications, such as measuring and mixing ingredients and applying ointments to a wound. Outside medical treatments, it might have been used for mixing paints and applying make-up (Milne 1907: 58–61).

A handle with a decoration in its centre is the fourth item in the collection (see Figure 5.2d). Decorative features similar to the one on the handle were regularly added to the handles of medical implements, likely to help the physician grip the tool, discussed in detail below. The functional ends of the artefact seem to have broken off at some point. However, breakage is uncertain because both ends are rounded. The rounding might indicate that the tool was either reworked after it was broken or that the object was originally intended to have two simple ends. Broken handles like this are fairly common finds, and some show signs of being reworked for another function. The rounded ends could have been used as a cautery, probe or ointment applicator. It could have non-surgical uses such as make-up application. The green, copper alloy handle measures 10.8 centimetres long and the decoration is about 1.8 centimetres in length.

A small spoon is the fifth artefact in the collection (see Figure 5.2e). The shape of the spoon bowl does not correspond to other objects identified as medical paraphernalia that I could find. There is a brownish green patina on the bowl and the top of the handle with a green patina on the handle. Some linear decorations were placed on the object where the spoon meets the top of the handle. It measures 12.6 centimetres in length, and the spoon bowl is 1.0 centimetre long and 0.9 centimetre wide. Usually small spoons, also known as *ligulae*, have thin handles that terminate in a point, rather than an olivary end like this instrument (see Figure 5.3). Although *ligulae* have been found with much smaller spoon bowls than this object, most have a round, flat head measuring about 0.4–0.7 centimetre in diameter. The heads are also angled rather than straight. Some of their various uses include cleaning the ears and removing medical ingredients from vials (Milne 1907: 68–9, 77–9). *Ligulae* were found in the archaeological record as single finds or as part of medical kits. In comparison, the tool in the Park Collection has a larger straight head and might have been used to remove medical ingredients from vials. It is also possible that it is an ear *specillum*, which was a probe with a large scoop used for removing objects from the ear, as mentioned by the seventh-century CE writer Paul of Aegina (6.88).[2] According to Milne (1907: 68–9; see also Bliquez 2014: 134–5), these objects might have terminated in an olivary end, like the one in the Park Collection. A potential archaeological comparison is a 'three cornered spoon' from Syria, which appears somewhat similar in design to the tool in the collection, though it is about 0.75 centimetre longer. However, the comparison is based on a drawing of an object in a private collection (Künzl 1983: 122–3, fig. 97, no. 7), which I have not seen in person.

The final artefact in the Park Collection is also unique (Figure 5.2f). It measures 12.5 centimetres long and has a simple handle that terminates in a rounded end. It has a flat, round disc measuring 1.5 centimetres in diameter on its functional end. A tiny decorative bulb was placed beneath the disc where it joins the handle. The handle of the tool has a greenish-grey patina and the disc is shiny on its outer edges. It may be that this was intended to be a *ligula*, but

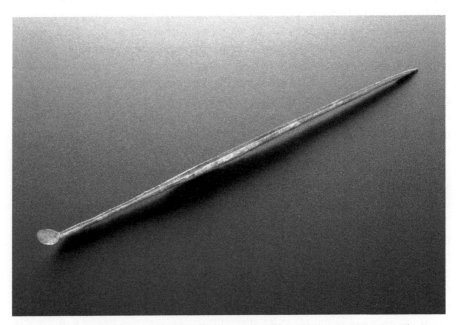

FIGURE 5.3: Roman bronze ligula, date uncertain. The Science Museum, London, object number A86272. Courtesy of Wellcome Images.

the head is too large to use to clean the ear and it is not angled. Another possibility, though admittedly unlikely, is that it is the flattened head of a *meningophylax*, an object that Celsus (*On Medicine* 8.3.8) described that was placed between the cranial bone and brain to protect the brain when a chisel was used to remove bone during trepanation.[3] Celsus described it as a plate of bronze that was smooth and slightly concave on one side. However, since the tool was curved it is possible that the disc probe was not the object. Nonetheless, Lawrence Bliquez (2014: 190–1) references other writers who described using flat objects in delicate procedures involving bone surgery. However, Bliquez agrees that tools of this name were more likely to be convex spatulae. The tool in the Park Collection also looks similar to a possible cautery from Colophon (Bliquez 2014: 403 fig. 35). Since there are no other similar artefacts or clear descriptions of the disc probe, only suggestions can be made for its intended function. It is plausible that it was used like a spatula probe to mix and apply ointments, it might have been a small cautery, or even a small mirror since Roman mirrors were made of polished metals.

Only four of these objects are identifiable as Roman medical objects, and many other types of tools have been found in the archaeological record. Detailed studies of these tools have been undertaken (e.g. Bliquez 1981, 1988; Jackson 1990b, 1994a; Künzl 1983, 1996; Milne 1907), the most recent is Bliquez's *The Tools of Asclepius: Surgical Implements in Greek and Roman Times* (2014). Thus, to familiarize the reader with other forms of Roman medical implements, only a brief review of the thorough work already undertaken is given here. Scholars tend to organize the objects into classifications that either have surgical or toilet functions. Although artefact classifications are helpful for arranging materials in reports, they are, for the most part, based on modern ordering systems that hold meanings and associations familiar to us, rather than those held by the Romans. Medical tools can serve various purposes that cross categorical boundaries, making the single classifications of implements restrictive to multiple interpretations.

The similarity between basic modern and ancient surgical objects is striking, so when archaeologists began finding them in the archaeological record in the eighteenth and nineteenth centuries, they based their identifications on comparisons with surgical implements with which they were familiar. It is possible, however, that the Romans may not have used, identified, classified or understood their tools in the same manner as the archaeologists, especially since the ancient names of medical tools mentioned by Graeco-Roman medical writers appear in a variety of descriptions of surgical, pharmaceutical and personal hygiene procedures (see Bliquez 2014 and Milne 1907). Giving instruments modern classifications and/or functions also means that we are likely to apply our own biases to how we interpret the care and uses of the tools. For example, the leaf-shaped probe in the Park Collection was possibly used as a tongue depressor. Today, tongue depressors are made of wood or plastic and are disposed of after one use because they are associated with bacteria and germs that can be passed to another person if reused. It can be argued that it would be environmentally sound to reuse tongue depressors if they were sterilized but, given that they are cheaply made and are disposable medical waste, we see their removal as a safe and justifiable practice in relation to our conceptions of how diseases are spread. Yet, the Romans reused their tools. They may have cleaned them after use on a patient, but the objects were not sterilized. They did not treat their instruments in the manners we do because they believed that diseases were mainly spread through bad air rather than germs (Nutton 1983). Thus, it must be remembered that seemingly innocuous categories and functions can carry biases that inform archaeological interpretations of object perception and use.

Besides comparing objects with modern examples to determine their functions, scholars also match medical artefacts to descriptions in Graeco-Roman medical texts, as stated (e.g. Bliquez 2014; Milne 1907). However, ancient medical writers rarely gave full descriptions of the objects they used and tended to mention them by name only. I have explained this problem elsewhere (Baker 2013), using the example of a medical probe, which is relevant in this chapter because object three is also a probe. The Greek term for a probe is *hupaleiptron*, and it is derived from the word *hupaleiphō*, and translates to 'to spread on thinly' or 'to anoint'. Unfortunately, no surviving texts, as far as I am aware, have any illustrations of this object, or full details about its shape. Thus, we assume an object like the spatula probe, which seems appropriate for anointing someone, was the tool mentioned in the texts. Although it is highly likely that this implement is identified correctly in relation to its name, caution is advised since there exists the possibility that the writer might have meant another tool. Some tools might be misidentified and others might be overlooked in the archaeological record if their descriptions are incomplete and/or unclear. With these caveats about the problems of archaeological categorization in mind, the general instrument types are now described.

Probes were made in various shapes ranging in size from about 6.0 to 15.0 centimetres. There are three common types: spatula probes, spoon probes, and *ligulae* or ear probes, mentioned briefly above. *Ligulae*, as described, had two designs: those with flat ends and those with small round spoon-scoped ends (Bliquez 2014: 126, 144–5; Jackson 1994b: 181; Künzl 1983: 27–8; Milne 1907: 63). The spoon probes (see Figure 5.4), like the spatula probe, had a leaf-shaped spoon instead of a spatula blade and they terminated in an olivary end. They could be used to remove ointments and medicinal ingredients from vials, or may have even been used to clean wounds.

Along with probes, forceps, too, are regularly found in the archaeological record because they were used by physicians and as personal toilet objects,

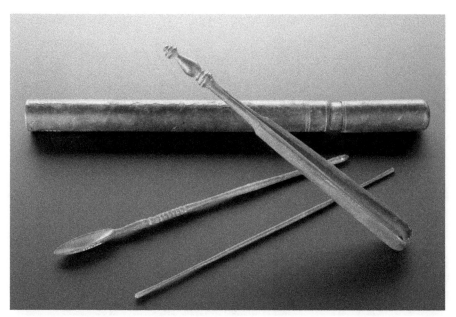

FIGURE 5.4: Reproductions of Roman medical implements from Pompeii: Forceps in the foreground, double simple probe, a spoon probe and a cylindrical container. These reproductions were made in the early twentieth century. The Science Museum, London, object number A156172. Courtesy of Wellcome Images.

similarly to tweezers (see Figure 5.4). They range in scale from roughly 6.0 to 10.0 centimetres. The simplest ones were made of one piece of metal that was folded at the centre. They acted as extensions of fingers and were used for depilation, the removal of objects from the skin, and in surgery. They could also have been used to clamp skin together or possibly keep it open. Their ends can be straight, turned inwards, or toothed. Bliquez (1988: 50–1) argued that the size of the object determined its classification as an either personal or surgical instrument: anything under 6.0 centimetres was personal. It was likely the case that forceps found on chatelaines were personal toilet items, but this does not eliminate the possibility that an ancient physician could have used them, particularly for delicate work. An individual could have also owned objects over six centimetres as part of their toilet kits.

The Romans also made stronger forceps with two separate handles that were crossed and bolted in the centre. These were crafted out of copper alloy or iron and were used in bone and dental surgery (Milne 1907: 135, 136–8). Slimmer versions of this type of forceps were used in the removal of tonsils, uvulae and haemorrhoids (Jackson 1994b).

Scalpels are necessary for many surgical procedures and are regularly identified by medical historians (see Figure 5.5). They have copper alloy handles

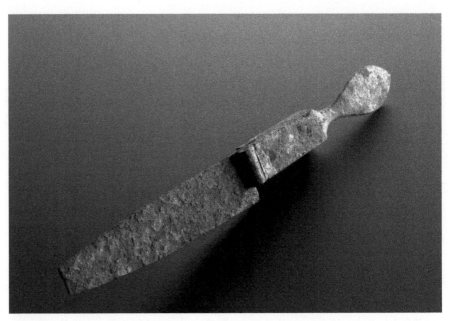

FIGURE 5.5: Roman scalpel, dated first–third centuries CE. The Science Museum, London, object number A129089. Courtesy of Wellcome Images.

that are usually rectangular, though some are hexagonal and cylindrical. One end of the handle has a leaf-shaped blunt blade that was used for blunt dissections. The other end has a slit for a steel blade made of naturally occurring steel, which has a tendency to rust, meaning they usually do not survive (e.g. Bliquez 2014: 72; Künzl 1983: 15–16; Milne 1907: 27). The blades were used for sharp incisions and came in several of shapes for different types of procedures.

Another sharp implement, the needle, like the scalpel, has a copper alloy handle with a needle that was inserted into a slot. It is usually only the handle that remains, though sometimes the needles have been found attached to them. They were used for piercing the skin and pustules (Milne 1907: 69–70). They were also used for couching cataracts (Jackson 1996; Milne 1907: 71).

Aside from these, additional types of instruments are known from the medical literature and from depictions on images, yet they are rarely, if ever, found in excavations. Cupping and bleeding, for example, were recommended for treating various illnesses to help balance the humours. Although tools, such as scalpels, for making incisions for bleeding are common, the cupping vessels are rare, despite the regularity in which the treatment is mentioned. There are a few reasons for this. Those made of copper alloy were hollow and may have been crushed under the weight of the soil where they were deposited, making them unidentifiable. Celsus also said (*On Medicine* 2.11.1; 2.5; 2.2.5–6;

3.21.9–10; 5.27.2) that they were made of other materials that break easily: horn, pottery and glass.

The shapes of most Roman-style medical implements could be used on anyone, but some objects were specifically made for the treatment of either a male or female. Catheters, for example, were designed specifically for the shape of male and female genitalia. These were tubes with an open end at their bottom, and a smooth rounded end at the top that was inserted into the urinary tract. A hole was placed on the side, beneath the rounded end, to allow for the flow of urine to empty out of the hole at the bottom of the object. Those shaped for the male urethra were S-shaped and longer than those for women, which were shorter and slightly curved at the top (Milne 1907: 143–5). The metal rods might have been crushed or misidentified as tubes. Moreover, the procedure was likely performed by a specialist, so this could also explain why they are rarely recognized by archaeologists.

Some implements might not have been correctly identified because they have designs similar to tools used in other types of work. For instance, implements used for bone surgery, such as saws, drills and files are easily confused with objects used for metal and woodworking. They also tend to be made of iron, so they are likely to deteriorate. Consequently, there are numerous reasons why less specialized, multi-functional tools are predominant in the archaeological record.

WHAT DOES THE TERM ROMAN MEAN?

Four of the six tools in the Park Collection are similar to those identified as Roman medical tools, but labelling them 'Roman' not only classifies the time period in which they were used, it also leads to assumptions about who used them and how they were used, no matter where they were found within the Roman Empire. Aside from function, archaeologists in the late nineteenth and early twentieth centuries generally classified objects by their date and the culture which supposedly used them. Explanations for changes within a society were argued by scholars to come about through influences by external forces either by invasion or colonization, and the indigenous population would have assumed the cultural traditions, including medical practices, of their occupiers without resistance (Johnson 1999: 15–20). For the Roman period, this process is referred to as Romanization. It is contentious because it ignores a two-way exchange of ideas and the possibility that the indigenous inhabitants may have rejected newly introduced material culture or ways of living. Recent research into Roman provincial life has challenged this traditional interpretation and has shown that the native inhabitants of the various provinces reacted differently to Roman occupation in many aspects of daily life: religion, art, technology and medicine (e.g. Baker 2001; Barrett 1989; Hingley 1997; Mattingly 2004, 2006:

14–17; Millett 1990; Woolf 1998). In some instances, people adopted the use of Roman objects and incorporated new ideas into their traditions; in other areas, there is an amalgamation of ideas and technologies; while in other examples, aspects of Roman life were rejected (e.g. Baker 2001; Webster 1997 a and b). Consequently, archaeologists and historians have found that lifestyles changed after Roman occupation, but these changes were heterogeneous across the empire, and ultimately led to different provincial identities that were both indigenous and Mediterranean/Roman. With something as intimate as the body and its care, anthropological studies demonstrate that it would be unlikely for people to trust newly introduced medical ideas that might not conform to their conceptions of healthcare and the body (e.g. Comelles 1997; Kleinman 1980; Saillant and Genest 2007).

In spite of the challenges to the concept of Romanization, there is an implicit supposition – or, at least, there is little to no challenge or discussion of this supposition – in reports of medical implements from the provinces that the tools indicate conformity to Graeco-Roman medical practices and technologies by the local inhabitants of the areas where the tools were uncovered (e.g. Jackson 199b; Milne 1907). Although the similarity in design of the tools across the empire adds to this conjecture, if the tools were manufactured and/or used in another province, there exists the possibility that their functions were different to those found in the Mediterranean regions. On a general level, Andrew Jones (2002: 90) has argued that artefact designs can be indicators that traditional technological knowledge of production was afforded to newly introduced objects. Basically, people may make new things in accordance with their own manufacturing practices that incorporate ideas about the materials and designs that work best for them. This indicates that, although objects are introduced and, in certain respects, reproduced, indigenous technologies and ideas may have been maintained in spite of appearances. At the same time, this provides an explanation for why some tools are dissimilar to the designs of medical instruments archaeologists expect to find, such as the two unusual objects in the Park Collection.

An example of this technological hybridization is identified in a set of medical instruments from a cremation burial in Stanway, Colchester, Britain (Crummy 2007; Jackson 2007). It dates to the mid-first century CE, just after Roman occupation. Along with the tools, pottery and metal vessels, a gaming board with playing pieces and bronze and iron rods with rings were also placed in the grave. The medical objects differ in design, material and size from the standard ones described above. The set contains two iron scalpels with fixed blades; a spatula probe made of copper alloy, which is similar to the one in the Park Collection; a copper alloy hook and an iron hook; a bronze object identified as a retractor, though its function is uncertain; copper alloy forceps; iron forceps; three iron needle handles; and an iron saw. Ralph Jackson (2007) and Philip

Crummy (2007) argue that the variant designs and materials used in their manufacture show that there was an exchange of medical ideas when the Romans invaded the area. The choice of using iron instead of copper alloy for some of the tools also indicates that local manufacturing traditions might have been maintained after Roman occupation, in line with Jones' argument above. Since these artefacts show a departure from Roman-style medical tools, they suggest the possibility that there exist other implements that have not and likely cannot be identified by the conventional means of textual comparison because there is little written material from the indigenous Roman provinces.

CONTEXT

The tools found at Stanway have a secure archaeological context. In contrast, the Park Collection does not have this information. However, a number of medical tools were properly recorded and they tend to be found in three types of deposition: burials, places for refuse disposal and locations used for votive offerings. Medical tools were also found in buildings in Pompeii that give a unique insight into where a physician might have lived and/or worked. For example, in the house of the Medico Nuovo II (area IX.9.3–5) the instruments were found in the south-east corner of the atrium of the house (Bliquez 1994: 84). It is possible that a physician might have worked in the atrium because it was naturally lit. Light was essential for surgical treatments, and ancient lamps did not emit enough strong light for a surgeon to perform certain procedures.

Another group of objects was found in the workshop of a residence by the Porta Stabiana (VIII.7.5–6). Houses in Pompeii and Herculaneum tended to have shops and workshops in their front rooms by the main entrance, and it might be that the tools found in the residence were sold and were, in addition, possibly made in the location. Bliquez (1994: 83–4) notes that the archaeologist who found the tools recorded that he also discovered a stove with an oven by the shop, which, as the archaeologist recorded, was 'to serve their needs'. There were other shops in the vicinity that manufactured and sold metalwork, making it likely that the tools were manufactured in this area of the city.

The provenances of the Pompeiian artefacts are unusual because they indicate where the instruments were likely used. In comparison, most medical implements were found in their final place of deposition, which probably does not indicate their original place of use or their initially intended function. Nonetheless, these spaces of deposition show how they were understood by those who used and came into contact with them at a particular period in their use-life.

Burials, particularly in the north-western Roman provinces, have been found to contain surgical tools. In comparison to the Mediterranean region, the Northern provinces appear to have had a tradition of burying the dead with objects, indicating that the implements were likely deposited because of a common cultural practice. In some instances, like Stanway, non-medical objects were found buried with the surgical equipment. Where possible, Ernst Künzl (1983) recorded associated artefacts in his catalogue of burials containing medical instruments. Some of these had few, if any, associated artefacts in them, but others included a variety of objects. For example, a large collection of finds was unearthed in a third-century CE inhumation burial at Dionysopolos in the Roman province of Moesia Inferior, in what is now Balcik, Bulgaria. The medical tools included two scalpels, two hooks and a cylindrical bronze container that had four probes in it. There were at least two other cylindrical containers and three scalpels mentioned in the site report. It is unclear whether the original archaeologists found the scalpels in the containers or if the containers were empty. Along with the medical tools, was a stone palate used for mixing medical ingredients. Other artefacts comprised two gold finger rings; a mirror made of 'white metal'; two spoons; fittings; a scale of white metal; a krater with a relief from the Iphigenia saga, which appears to be Augustan in date (late first BCE/early first century CE); four round containers; three buckets; two keys; two cup handles; another handle; bronze feet; two lamps; kitchen fittings; three iron strigils; an iron knife; an iron frame; an iron rod; an iron ring; eight glass vessels; eight clay vessels; three bone rods and a spindle whorl (Künzl 1983: 110–11). The metal and pottery vessels might have been part of a funerary feast, or could have been used for medical preparations along with the spoons and scale. Strigils were used in bathing, and physicians sometimes recommended bathing as a method for treating certain ailments, so it is possible that these, too, were related to medical treatments (e.g. Galen, *On the Preservation of Health* 1.10; 3.4).[4] The bronze feet might have been part of a statuette, though it is also possible that they were simply feet to a vessel. Although it is unclear what type of feet these are, if they were part of a statuette they could have been used to invoke divine assistance to aid the physician and/ or patient. Interestingly, the iron rod and ring call to mind the rods from Stanway; however, no information about their size and shape is specified. If a comparative archaeological analysis of associated finds with medical tools were undertaken, it might be possible to see patterns with the types of artefacts deposited with them that could alert us to aspects of ancient medical practice that went unrecorded, such as praying to certain deities.

Besides burials, artefacts have also been found in spaces identified as places for rubbish disposal. It would be expected that objects deposited in them were thought to be damaged. An example of this comes from the Schutthügel, a deposit from site clearance that lay just outside the legionary fortress wall at Vindonissa, Switzerland. The Romans often recycled metal objects, so finding metals in rubbish deposits suggests that the raw materials were not needed or that there were other reasons why the tools were thought to be rubbish.

Moreover, many probes and forceps from the deposit were found in good condition, meaning that they could have been reused. It is questionable, therefore, why they were found in a place for waste. It can be surmised that they were thought to have been polluted because they were associated with, or used on, someone who was ill or had died, which meant they could not have been reused or recycled (see Baker 2004). The fact that the deposit is on the outside of the fortress could also mean that the spot was a place used for making boundary offerings, though it seems unlikely in this instance. Nonetheless, the Romans did make offerings to chthonic deities at borders, and depositing objects associated with the body and its care in these spaces could be a request for the health of those living within the fortress (e.g. Bosman 1995; Webster 1997b; see Baker 2004).

Although the ritual status of the Schutthügel is doubtful, medical implements were also retrieved from places with direct evidence for votive deposition. Votive offerings of body parts were given to healing deities either to ask that a certain part of the body be healed or as an offering of thanks. These tend to be found in religious sanctuaries as well as in watery places such as springheads and rivers (e.g. Detys 1988). Besides using body parts to request healing, it is conceivable that tools associated with the body and a person, such as a personal toilet instrument, could also have been given to the deity to ask for assistance. Like the votive body parts, medical implements have also been found in water sources, including wells (Baker 2004, 2011; Salles 1985).

Throwing objects into wells seems to have been a conventional practice in the north-western provinces. For example, a well dedicated to the deity, Coventina, was discovered next to the fort of Brocolitta on Hadrian's Wall in Britannia. Numerous personal objects were cast into it: rings, bracelets, buckles, pins and shoe soles (Allason-Jones and McKay 1985). Although no medical implements were found, the collection of personal items evinces the fact that people were willing to part with objects that they associated with themselves. Thus, medical tools placed in streams and rivers could have been personal possessions used as an offering of thanks and/or request for help, possibly for health. For example, cataract needles and objects used to mark eye medicines, collyrium stamps, were found in rivers and springheads in the Gallic provinces, and four collyrium stamps were also deposited in wells (Baker 2011). There are examples of other objects found in ritual spaces that support the idea that medical tools had functions that extended beyond a 'practical' surgical/pharmaceutical use (Baker 2004). By looking beyond the purely mechanical, it is possible to argue that people saw objects associated with their body as a means of communication with a deity.

Depositional practices alert us to alternative meanings and uses for items originally thought to have straightforward mechanical functions; however, the find spot only shows one stage of the artefact's life. Their functions can change from the time of their production to when they become part of the archaeological record (Jones 2002: 83–102). It is unlikely that the full life of an object can be established, but comparisons with the provenances of other instruments, as discussed, can indicate a multiplicity of uses. Meaning of implements, however, are described in isolation, leading to the assumption that they had one use at a time, which is, of course, untrue because objects can be understood in several ways at once.

DECORATION AND MATERIALS

Although the provenance of the instruments in the Park Collection is unknown, the objects are decorated, and decorative features can also be examined to determine how artefacts were intended to be used or the significances they held. Some medical implements were decorated with the heads of deities, others had the symbols associated with particular gods on them, and some tools had metal inlays with floral and geometric patterns. The tools in the collection, however, have minimal decorative features only where the handle and functional ends were joined together, as previously described. The most intricate in the collection is the handle (see Figure 5.2d), which has four circular protrusions that wrap around its centre. The two circles on the outer edges of the decoration each measure about 3.0 millimetres wide. There are two inner protrusions, each measuring about 5.0 millimetres in width. A circular protrusion, about a millimetre in width, was placed between each of the smaller and larger protrusions. The entire feature measures roughly 1.8 centimetres long. This decorative attribute has been found on the centre of many other implement handles. For example, a spoon probe from a burial in Cologne has a similar design in its centre (Künzl 1983: 91, fig. 69, no. 2). They are also found on needle and scalpel handles, usually where they terminate (e.g. Bliquez 1994, plate 27, fig. 1). As mentioned above, it is likely that this helped keep the physician's hand from slipping when the object was wet with blood, pus and/or sweat.

The location of these decorative grips also indicates where and how the objects were intended to be held: either in the centre or at the ends of the handles. The shapes and designs of medical tools, although similar and fairly easy to place into recognizable categories, do vary considerably in size and decoration. The shape and size of a physician or surgeon's hands can determine how they held the object. Along with this, a grasp could be affected by the procedure being performed. Galen (*Avoiding Distress* 4–5) recorded that he made his own medical implements from wax and then took the samples to a metalsmith, indicating that he may have made these to suit his hand size or surgical needs, and quite possibly other surgeons did this as well.[5] Yet, size is only one factor in manufacturing shapes. How people move and operate tools is also learned through their cultural background (e.g. Gosselain 1992; Ingold 2001; Naji 2009).

Cultural variation in movement and the use of tools was witnessed by Mauss during World War I, about which he wrote a seminal paper (1979 [1936]) on the topic of bodily technique. In his study, he commented on how French and British soldiers moved and used tools differently from one another, particularly when marching, trench digging and the manner in which they held shovels. Moreover, he noticed that the tools used for digging the trenches were also made in shapes to accommodate the way they were meant to be grasped. Thus, when we see medical tools that are different from the standard designs identified by archaeologists, such as those at Stanway or the two unusual objects in the Collection, it is possible that their designs are also indicative of cultural variation in bodily technique. This is not something that is easy to identify, but the placement on the grips of the medical tools, may, if studied and compared, demonstrate how they were meant to be held. If designs were found to be common to certain areas in comparison to others, a case for different bodily technologies across the empire could be made.

Besides demonstrating how objects were held, decorations on medical tools also served other purposes. Some tools, like a set from a burial in Cologne, Germany, had silver decorative inlays. The two forceps and two scalpels had a straight line of silver that ran down the length of their handles. The silver line was decorated with circles. The hook had a spiral pattern that ran around the length of the handle (Künzl 1983: 89–90, fig. 68 nos. 1–5). It is possible that these were simply intended to be ornamental. Yet, decorations might have been used to attract patients, suggested by a story told by the Roman-period satirist Lucian (*The Ignorant Book Collector* 29), who said that he would rather trust a good surgeon with rusty tools than a charlatan with clean and shiny ones.[6]

Nonetheless, some decorative features on instruments appear to be more than ornamental. Bliquez pointed out that certain scalpel handles were designed to look like knotty wood. Although this would provide a gripping mechanism, Bliquez (1994: 104–6) argued that it was associated with the club of Hercules or the staff of Aesculapius because Hercules was likely invoked for strength and Aesculapius, healing. In some cases, scalpel handles have the head of Heracles on them, again indicating that the god might have been called upon for strength to undergo the procedure (Bliquez 1992, 1994: 119, nos. 40–1). Physicians who used these instruments and patients who came into contact with them may have believed that the symbolic features imbued the implements with extra powers, which were placed into the physician's hand when s/he performed a treatment.

Sixteen collyrium stamps from Gaul were also decorated with features including a rosette, a four-leaf clover, geometric designs, a pigeon-like bird, a caduceus (see Figure 5.6), an amphora shape, a sea-horse, sun or flower, moon and stars, and one with a man with a weapon, which might have been a crude

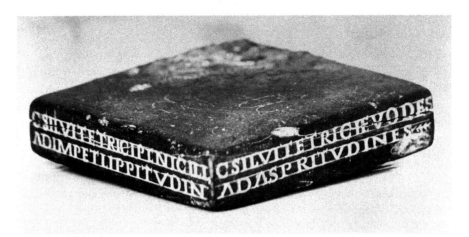

FIGURE 5.6: Roman collyrium stamp decorated with a caduceus design, second–third century CE. Wellcome Library, London, number 5395. Courtesy of Wellcome Images.

rendering of Heracles (Baker 2011: 174). Again, these could have been simple adornments, but it is also possible that these were used to summon extra powers in the medicines they marked. In fact, magical papyri and curse tablets sometimes have symbols on them. For example, one magical papyrus (*Papyri Graecae Magicae* 7.300) had instructions for the spell and magical words to be written around an image of an ibis. The image of the bird was essential for the spell's efficacy.[7]

Comparable to decorative features, the materials used to manufacture the objects were sometimes considered significant for medical purposes. Collyrium stamps were primarily made of green schist and steatite. The colour green was associated with the eyes and recommended for healing and clearing vision. It is quite possible that the use of green stones, and perhaps the properties of the stones themselves would have infused the medicines they marked with extra healing properties (Baker 2011).

On the other hand, sometimes the materials used in the manufacture of objects were chosen because they were best for the technological function of the item. Pliny the Elder (*Natural History* 36.157–8), for example, said that mortars for mixing medicines were best made of Phoenician siliceous slate or schist because nothing came off that would mix with the medicines.[8] Copper alloy was the main metal used for tools, possibly because it does not rust, it is easily recycled, and the metals used in it were widely available in the Roman Empire.

Most studies of the fabrics used in the production of medical tools have been made by eye, as it were, but there exist different types of metallurgical tests that can be performed to provide information on the exact metals used in an object's manufacture. I was able to have X-Ray Florescence undertaken on the Park

Collection. The department of Classical and Archaeological Studies at Kent owns a desktop X-Ray Florescence machine (Niton XL3t GOLDD XRF [X-Ray Florescence]). An x-ray beam is emitted from the machine onto a sample object. The beam has enough energy to affect the inner electrons of the atoms of the object x-rayed. In essence, it causes the electrons in the atoms of different metallurgical elements to become destabilized. When the electrons are knocked from their orbits, they leave a void, and the time taken for the electrons to fill the void is unique to each element. This timed movement is known as florescence. Thus, the fluorescent energy levels detected by the machine indicate the metallurgical elements of the objects tested. To obtain a reliable reading from the tools, a section of metal would be taken from the implement, ground-up and x-rayed. Not wishing to destroy the tools in the Park Collection, I was able to have sections of their surface, rather than interior, x-rayed. There is the potential for the test to pick up surface contamination from dirt, cleaning chemicals, metals in the air and chemicals on hands. However, it presented an opportunity to undertake a metallurgical study on instruments that would rarely, if ever, be given permission to do so if they were in a museum collection.

The common metals used by the Romans were gold, silver, copper, tin, lead, iron, zinc, mercury, arsenic and antimony. In Noricum (Austria), there are naturally occurring iron carbonates that contain manganese. When the ore is smelted, it creates a steel alloy (Cech 2008). Galen (*On Anatomical Procedures* 8.6, K2.682) noted that the best blades for scalpels came from the province.[9] Medical tools were largely made of copper alloys or bronzes, which contained copper and tin, though zinc and lead were sometimes added to them in varying quantities. Thus, tests were performed on the collection to determine if they were made with the metals one would expect to find in a Roman bronze. However, the test cannot indicate if the tools were genuine Roman objects, given that copper alloys are still made.

Each object was x-rayed in specific places (see Figure 5.7). Most metals were either undetected or had trace amounts that might have occurred from surface

TABLE 5.1: XRF readings for the spoon (see Figure 5.7, artefact 1). All numbers are percentages

Metal (elemental symbol)	1.a (back of the spoon bowl)	1.b (handle)	1.c (spoon bowl)
Al	1.498	11.869	2.986
Si	6.193	36.646	8.554
Fe	0.186	6.061	60.982
Cu	89.917	42.072	25.513
Zn	0.078	0.243	0.052
Sn	0.786	0.498	0.879
Pb	0.132	0.197	0.072

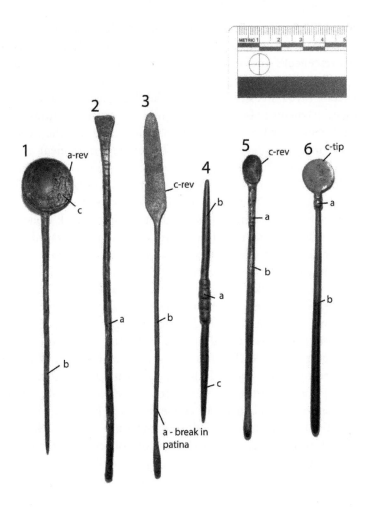

FIGURE 5.7: Park Collection showing where samples were taken for the XRF study. Photo and test by Lloyd Bosworth, Technician, University of Kent.

contamination. Therefore, tables for each implement are given that show the percentages of the main elements found in the tools (see Tables 5.1–6).

The spoon (Figure 5.7, artefact 1) mainly consisted of copper (Cu). However, the test showed high levels of aluminium (Al) and silicon (Si), which are modern metallurgical elements. It is possible that these metals formed part of a topical preservative that was used on the implement. Iron (Fe) was also found on the handle and in the spoon bowl, where there are signs of metal deterioration (Figure 5.7, artefact 1, part c), indicating that there is residue or rust from an iron object that might have been resting on it when it was buried.

Only one test was taken on the stylus handle. The metals found are consistent with what one would expect to find in a copper alloy: copper, tin (Sn) and lead (Pb).

The tests undertaken on the spatula probe revealed some surprising results, and demonstrate that scientific analysis can sometimes be inaccurate. The lower part of the handle (see Figure 5.7, artefact 3, part a) and the blade (see Figure 5.7, artefact 3, part c) have typical metals for Roman bronzes, along with traces of iron. However, the reading taken in the middle of the handle had a high level of hafnium, at 70.405 per cent. Hafnium is found in zirconium ores and has a melting point of 2,230 degrees Celsius or 4,051 degrees Fahrenheit. It is mainly used in the control rods of nuclear reactors. It is likely that the x-ray could not make contact with the thin handle and failed to read the copper and zinc found in the other sections. It may have read something on the table where the implement was placed. In spite of this one anomaly, the other two sections indicate possible Roman production.

The handle, like the spoon discussed above, appears to have a preservative on it because there is a reading of the silicon and phosphorus (Ph). However,

TABLE 5.2: XRF readings for the stylus (see Figure 5.7, artefact 2)

Metal (elemental symbol)	2.a (handle)
Cu	82.297
Sn	11.09
Pb	5.529

TABLE 5.3: XRF readings for the spatula probe (see Figure 5.7, artefact 3)

Metal	3.a (lower handle with a break in the patina)	3.b (middle handle)	3.c (reverse of the probe blade)
Fe	0.165	11.721	1.203
Cu	96.506	–	63.072
Zn	0.57	–	5.815
Sn	0.629	1.011	0.192
Hf (Hafnium)	–	70.405	–

TABLE 5.4: XRF readings for the handle (see Figure 5.7, artefact 4)

Metal	4.a (handle decoration)	4.b (handle)	4.c (handle)
Si	9.33	4.709	4.783
Ph	2.642	3.468	4.205
Fe	1.242	1.223	0.845
Cu	72.071	76.739	77.981
Zn	5.894	5.893	5.696
Sn	1.765	1.913	1.757
Pb	3.045	3.492	2.59

copper, zinc and tin have fairly consistent readings from the three areas where the x-rays were taken. The reading for lead is more variable. The machine also picked up traces of iron, though the percentages are quite low and could indicate a reading from the object on which the tool was resting.

X-rays taken for the small spoon probe revealed that the tool was likely to have been made of two separate objects. The area where the spoon and handle meet was made of brass rather than bronze. Brass has high levels of zinc added to copper, usually 33–39 per cent, which is close to the 31.683 per cent revealed in the test. It is possible that the metal used to solder the two objects together was brass. The Romans made brass, so they could have manufactured or reworked the tool. Silicon appears on both the handle and the bowl, possibly indicating that a preservative was used on it. With the exception of zinc, the readings for the other metals common to copper alloys only appear in trace amounts.

The disc probe is the most valuable object in the collection, as the analysis showed that the disc and the decorative protrusion between the disc and the handle were silver (Ag). It was suggested by my colleague that this was a Roman coin that was attached to the handle either during the Roman period or after it (Bosworth 2016; personal conversation). However, it is somewhat small for a silver Roman coin. Since the objects were purchased from a coin dealer, another suggestion is that the dealer made the addition, as there is no Roman equivalent of this tool that could be found. However, as suggested above, it could have been a small mirror since silver creates a reflective surface.

TABLE 5.5: XRF readings for the small spoon probe (see Figure 5.7, artefact 5)

Metal	5.a (location where the spoon and handle meet)	5.b (handle)	5.c (spoon bowl)
Cu	66.851	76.98	81.794
Zn	31.683	12.467	6.94
Sn	0.799	0.424	0.539
Pb	0.358	–	–
Si		4.654	5.745

TABLE 5.6: XRF readings for the disc probe (see Figure 5.7, artefact 6)

Metal	6.a (join of handle and disc)	6.b (handle)	6.c (disc)
Si	3.962	6.959	1.236
Cu	80.223	74.086	52.738
Zn	9.307	10.104	–
Ag	0.21	–	43.646
Sn	1.652	2.056	

The metallurgical analysis, although having its flaws, was able to show that the tools were all made of copper alloys with metals commonly used in the Roman period. There was no uniformity in the mixtures of the metals, probably because the person or people who made them might have used melted metals from recycled objects, which would have had their own alloys, or the metalsmith(s) created their own alloys with the raw materials that were available. For the two unusual tools, the metals on the handles indicate that they were likely to have been Roman objects.

If more studies of this kind were made on Roman implements, especially those that were found as sets, it would help to determine if kits were made at the same time and of the same composition of metals.

CONCLUSION

The objects in the Park Collection are likely to have been Roman artefacts, but it is uncertain if they were part of a set of tools or a collection of objects that originated from different places. Having gone through the various questions an archaeologist should consider when assessing material finds, it was possible to show the multiplicity of functions and meanings medical tools can hold, including some that may seem unconventional to what survives in the medical literature. Although no firm conclusions can be drawn about the ancient uses of the tools in the Park Collection, it is likely that they, too, were multi-functional. Interestingly, their use-life continues to this day: first, as part of a private collection and now as a teaching aid, quite different from what their original use was probably intended to be.

NOTES

1. This citation is from the twelfth volume of Kühn's edition, abbreviated as 'K12'.
2. This citation is from the Corpus Medicorum Graecorum edition by Heiberg (1921–1924).
3. This and all citations hereafter are from the Loeb Classical Library edition by Spencer (1931–1935).
4. These citations are from the Loeb Classical Library edition by Johnston (2018).
5. This citation is from the Collection des Universités de France edition by Boudon-Millot et al (2010).
6. This citation is from the Loeb Classical Library edition by Harmon (1921).
7. This citation is from the Teubner edition by Preizendanz (1973–1974). For an English translation, see Betz (1992).
8. This citation is from the Loeb Classical Library edition by Eichholz (1962).
9. This citation is from the second volume of Kühn edition, abbreviated as 'K2'.

CHAPTER SIX

Experiences

REBECCA FLEMMING

INTRODUCTION

As Roy Porter (1985: 175; see also Condrau 2007) pointed out, over thirty years ago, 'it takes two to make a medical encounter – the sick person as well as the doctor', so medical history must embrace both patient and practitioner. It must take the patient's view, explore the historical experience of illness and medicine, of wider concerns with health and well-being, as well as the physician's perspective; and, indeed, encompass interactions between the two, both direct and indirect (see Figure 6.1). A cultural history of medicine has particular obligations in this regard; even a cultural history of medicine in antiquity, which faces some daunting evidential challenges in carrying out these duties.

The most acute of these challenges is the scarcity of first-person accounts belonging to patients themselves, or their families or other carers, a problem which is confronted head on in a recent volume aiming precisely at recovering the view of the ancient patient (Petridou and Thumiger, eds, 2015). In the end, as the thoughtful epilogue by Michael Stolberg (2015: 500–1) reflects, the collected essays find it hard to break the dominance over writing on disease and cure exerted by learned physicians in the Greek and Roman worlds. They adopt a patient-focused approach to these texts, pursuing the stories of individual suffering and agency, of personal negotiation and healing, that are embedded in them, rather than the general medical theories or tales of professional triumph, which these cases are intended to illustrate. Valuable contributions are thus made to the history of the ancient patient and ancient medicine more generally, but the actual experience of being ill in antiquity, engaging medical services of some kind, working back towards health, remains underexplored.

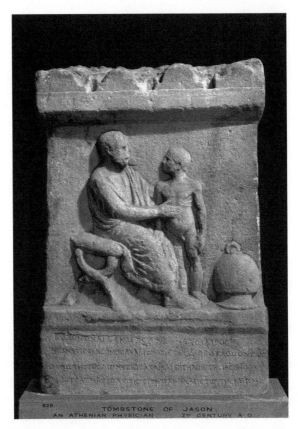

FIGURE 6.1: Marble tombstone of a physician (*iatros*) named Jason (and also called Decimus), from Roman imperial Athens. He dominates this medical encounter, as represented by the smaller size and nakedness of the patient he is examining. An oversize cupping-vessel, ubiquitous symbol of the medical art, sits on the right. For the funerary inscription at the bottom see IG 2 2 4513. 80 x 56 x 9 cm. British Museum, London, museum number: 1865,0103.3 © Trustees of the British Museum.

This study attempts to fill that gap. The surviving instances where ancient patients do speak for themselves, talk about the ailments that beset them, their family and friends, about their response to those situations, and the ways they were resolved will be gathered up and scrutinized, scattered and fragmentary as they are: eschewing medical treatises. This material is predominantly from the Roman Empire of the late first to early third century CE, and, in its richest form, from the male elite of that world. The letters and life-writing of senators and emperors, orators and littérateurs will be buttressed by papyrus documents from Roman Egypt which contain less privileged voices, of women and the more middling sort. But there is no competition between these two sets of evidence in terms of the detail provided, the self-conscious reflection on the issues; that needs to be admitted at the outset. It should not be assumed that 'experience' is a shared historical and political category. Cultural norms regarding behaviour in illness and care of the body more generally, possibilities for agency in these and other respects, vary according to gender and status.

This project also requires some more specific historical framing. The wider scholarship on classical medicine sets up some particular expectations about the overlap between lay and specialist understandings of the body, illness and cure in antiquity, indeed of the overlap between lay and specialist more generally (Nutton 1986; Porter 1986; Nutton 2013). This was a world where learned literate medicine had, from its Hippocratic beginnings in the late fifth century BCE onwards, built itself around traditional notions of balance and moderation, hierarchy and order, had explained and rationalized rather than rejected many existing assumptions and approaches, reworked and reinterpreted previous practice as much as adding new items to the therapeutic repertoire (Lloyd 1983). Specialist medical vocabulary was slow to develop, limited in scope, and always accessible to the educated (Lloyd 1983: 146–67; Langslow 2000). Debates on medical themes were conducted not just by physicians and philosophers but also amongst the intellectual elite more broadly, at symposia and dinner parties, in their houses and the more explicitly public spaces of ancient cities, in the literary culture which accompanied these social settings.

These points, and several others, can be illustrated by a frequently cited story told by the Roman imperial scholar Aulus Gellius in his erudite miscellany, the *Attic Nights* (Holford-Strevens 2003). As a young man, in the mid-second century CE, Gellius studied in Greece and on one occasion fell ill while staying at a villa in Attica. 'There I was confined to bed, having been gripped by flux of the bowels and a consuming fever' (*Attic Nights* 18.10.2).[1] His main teacher at Athens, the Platonist Lucius Calvenus Taurus, came to visit accompanied by some of his followers, and, finding the local physician (*medicus*) who had been called in also present at the bedside discussed the case with him. The doctor caused consternation when, having described Gellius' symptoms, he invited the philosopher to confirm his assessment that his patient was now on the mend by touching his 'vein' (*phleps* in Greek, *vena* in Latin), when Taurus and his entourage all knew he should have said 'artery' (*arteria*). Taurus stilled the disquiet by suggesting that the *medicus* had merely spoken loosely, using 'vein' as the inclusive term as was common in general parlance, rather than in ignorance. Of course, the physician was aware that only arteries move, that it is their pulsation which reveals the type and course of a fever. After his recovery Gellius took this criticism to heart, considering it shameful not just for a *medicus* but any cultured and educated man to lack such basic knowledge of his body. So, he began to read books on the medical art: nothing too specialist, but those suitable for his instruction, and he learnt much in the process. Both veins and arteries are vessels containing blood mixed with 'natural breath' (*naturalis spiritus*, that is a Latin version of the Greek innate *pneuma*, warm air which becomes integrated into somatic functioning), but blood dominates in the former, breath in the latter. 'The pulse (*sphugmos*) is the stretching and relaxing motion in the heart and in the artery, which is natural not voluntary', he says, then provides an equivalent Greek definition, using the more technical language of diastole and systole (*Attic Nights* 18.10.10–11).

Gellius' description of his illness is brief and impersonal, it consists of generic symptoms, not a name, and how he felt about them is not mentioned, rather the point is to set up the educational dialogue that took place around him. It is a learning experience he wishes to record. Still, he acquired considerable, though not too detailed, medical knowledge as a result. He could now participate in these bedside conversations himself, or, indeed, talk knowledgeably to any doctor who was ministering to him; though, if he did he does not say so. Gellius' own health does not arise again in the *Attic Nights*, and while visits to the sick certainly do, his role in these, and all other occasions of intellectual sociality he attends, is as silent observer, as pedagogic conduit to a wider audience. So, for example, later in Rome, he goes to see an anonymous sick man with the philosopher Favorinus (*Attic Nights* 16.3; Holford-Strevens 2003: 98–130). His companion first discussed the man's condition in Greek with the physicians – *medici* – present, then announced that it was hardly surprising that, though their patient was customarily fond of his food, a therapeutic three-day fast had blunted his appetite. The philosopher cited the writings of the great Hellenistic physician Erasistratus in support, and explanation, of this view. Afterwards, Gellius was reading Erasistratus' *Divisions* and came upon the passage in question, which he quotes in Greek, adding a further titbit on matters of appetite from the same book.

Still, that medical knowledge was shared is clear, as also the public nature of medicine more broadly, with patients and practitioners performing before an audience. Another point stressed in the recent scholarship comes through too, the physicians play a subordinate role in these vignettes, at least in relation to bedside visitors if not the actual invalid. The narrower gap between lay and specialist understanding in antiquity ties in with the larger absence of medical professionalization.[2] The lack of regulation and institutional organization left physicians with few status resources of their own in societies structured according to traditional aristocratic values, and made competition with other providers of health and healing services more even and open. Doctors had to establish their authority to intervene in the lives and bodies of those concerned about their fitness and functioning, just as purifiers, magicians, gymnastic trainers, midwives and astrologers did, to name a few of these other purveyors of somatic assistance: only the gods had their curative powers taken for granted. The ancient 'medical marketplace', as it has been called, was diverse and pluralistic (Nutton 1992; Jenner and Wallis 2007). Ancient patients, in most places, had choices, between physicians and much more widely, non-exclusive choices, in a world of medical 'promiscuity', to borrow another term from early modern history (Cook 1986: 29). These choices were greatest for the wealthy and those located in vast metropolises such as Rome, but even the butcher in Acanthus, a more modest city in northern Greece, and others like him who appear as patients in the Hippocratic *Epidemics* had options (*Epidemics* 5.52 and 7.71; Jouanna 1999: 112–25).[3]

So, as in other pre-modern societies, the idea is that lay people in antiquity experienced and interpreted their bodies and diseases in roughly the same terms as are found in contemporary medical treatises. There will surely be a different emphasis to the descriptions in first person accounts, and a more biographical, or at least personal, perspective on the meaning of any somatic travails. The specific aims and context of the writing itself must always be taken into account, but a basic conceptual unity underlies everything. The expectation is also that a variety of approaches to managing health and dealing with illness will be on display, including plenty of self-help. Patient choice, the negotiation of relationships with different curative practices and practitioners should also be revealed in action, at least to some extent. Though here, as elsewhere, cultural ideals and social norms will have a key role in shaping what is said, but this too is illuminating.

THE ELITE PATIENT SPEAKS

The two men who provide the most expansive ancient first-person accounts of their bodies and illnesses, treatments and cures, together with those of their friends and family, have much else in common too. Marcus Cornelius Fronto and Publius Aelius Aristides were both key cultural figures, significant participants in the wider public life of the Roman Empire in the mid- to late-second century CE. Both of elite provincial origins, Fronto from North Africa, Aristides from Asia Minor, and both oratorical superstars, in Latin and Greek respectively; issues of ill-health shaped their careers, in overlapping and divergent ways. Serious and sustained illness shattered Aristides' sense of self, forcing a radical rebuild, centred on his personal relationship with the most prominent healing deity of the classical world, Asclepius, while Fronto was able to accommodate chronic pain and debility within his identity as a member of the Roman political and literary elite. Glen Bowersock (1969: 71–5) labelled the pair of them hypochondriacs, leading representatives of the second-century CE turn to the body and its ailments, others have read the somatic focus of their discourses rather differently (Perkins 1995: 195–9).

Fronto, the senior of the two by a couple of decades, travelled to the imperial capital in search of education and opportunity as a young man, and quickly made his mark in its courts and literary salons, beginning a rapid ascent of the *cursus honorum*, the prescribed order of offices in a senatorial career (Champlin 1980). When his recurring difficulties of ill-health began is uncertain. Debilitating joint pain is a constant feature of his surviving writing and of the reports of those who interacted with him, such as Aulus Gellius (Holford-Strevens 2003: 131–9). Still, though bodily frailty certainly shaped his life in various ways, he remained in Rome, had a family, achieved the highest magistracies, becoming praetor in the late 120s CE and consul in 143, moved in circles close to imperial power, and dominated the literary scene until his death in 166 or 167. Appointed tutor to Marcus Aurelius, adopted son and heir of Antoninus Pius (together with Lucius Verus), soon after Pius' accession in 138 CE, Fronto's close relationship with his former pupil continued after he became emperor, with Verus, in 161 (see Figure 6.2). This association took epistolary

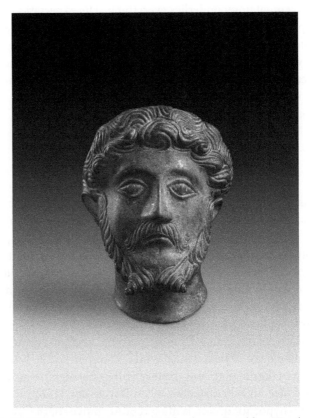

FIGURE 6.2: Half-life-size cast-bronze head found near Brackley (Northants) and now in the Ashmolean Museum in Oxford. The image closely resembles portraits of the emperor Marcus Aurelius on coinage, done in a Romano-Celtic style. 16 x 12 cm. Ashmolean Museum, Oxford, museum number: AN2011.46. © Ashmolean Museum, University of Oxford.

form, and it is many of his letters to Marcus, other members of the imperial family, assorted friends and acquaintances, and some of their letters to him, which are preserved, rather than his public oratory.[4] The collection is incomplete and problematic in various ways, but its 220 odd surviving items offer valuable insights into the elite experience of illness and treatment, of individual understandings and coping strategies in respect to health in the Roman Empire (Champlin 1980: 3). Or, at least, they offer insights into elite expression of that experience in the context of Roman friendship (*amicitia*), with its mutual investment in each other's health and wider obligations of reciprocity and presence.

According to the calculations of J. E. G. Whitehorne (1977: 416–18), Fronto refers to illness in one form or another in fifty-five letters, forty-three of which are about his own indisposition, while the fifty-three letters of Marcus on the same theme contain only sixteen which deal with his own condition, rather than Fronto's or that of various members of his family.[5] Fronto's most frequent complaint is pain (*dolor*) in his joints or other parts of his body. He variously specifies his neck, shoulders, elbows, hands and fingers, his back, groin and loins, knees, ankles, feet and toes (Whitehorne 1977: 415, n. 14). He often qualifies the pain, usually as severe (*gravis*) or very severe, sometimes violent (*vehementer*) and occasionally moderate (*modicus*), and speaks of it as having seized (*arreptus*) or troubled (*vexatus*) him, and as variously debilitating. These are very plain reports, lacking in medical detail, but performing a clear social function, or functions.

The first is to explain his inability to discharge his relational duties, as friend, tutor, senator in the circle of the emperor, as he would like, or, indeed, as his position demands. Fronto frequently wrote to Marcus Aurelius, whom he addressed as *dominus*, 'lord' or 'master', even as his pupil, in this vein. 'To my Lord. I cannot see you my Lord, till the day after tomorrow; for I am still incapacitated by pain in the elbow and neck . . .' (*Marcus Caesar* 5.44; Haines 1919: 218–19).[6] 'To my Lord. I am laid up with pain in the sole of my foot. That is why I have not paid you my respects these past days. Farewell, most excellent Lord. Greet my Lady' (*Marcus Caesar* 5.63; Haines 1919: 248–9). 'To my Lord. I have been troubled, my lord, in the night, with widespread pains in my shoulder and elbow, knee and ankle. So I have not been able to write this to you in my own hand' (*Marcus Caesar* 5.73; Haines 1919: 186–7). He was more fulsome in a letter to Pius accounting for his failure to attend the public ceremony marking the anniversary of his accession. 'But severe pain in my shoulder, and even more severe in my neck, so torments me that I am hardly able to bend, sit upright or turn around, so unmoving must I keep my neck. Still I discharged and renewed my vows among my *lares*, *penates* and household gods . . .' (*Antoninus Pius* 5; Haines 1919: 226–9). A slightly different, more summary, tone was adopted when explaining to the otherwise unknown

Praecidius Pompeianus why he had not fulfilled a promise to revise and send on one of his speeches. Fronto recounted that, 'Pain of the sinews (*dolor nervorum*) assailed me more violently than usual, and lingered longer and more vexatiously. And I cannot, when my limbs are being tortured, apply any effort to writing or reading texts . . .' (*Friends* 1.15; Haines 1920: 88–91).

The second role of these epistles is to invite an attentive and solicitous response to his pain and debility. Mutual concern about each other's health was a fundamental part of Roman friendship, but the regularity of Fronto's somatic failures put particular emphasis on this aspect of his relationship with Marcus, and developed it in a particular direction (Freisenbruch 2007). These letters were clearly integral to Fronto's self-medication, to his management of his condition. He adopted a number of strategies to deal with his *dolor nervorum*, a rather loose term but one which can also be found in Latin medical texts of the early imperial period (Celsus, *On Medicine* 1.9.1–2; 3.27.1–3; and 4.18.28; Scribonius Largus, *Composite Remedies* 256).[7] *Nervus* is here understood broadly, as encompassing sinews, tendons, ligaments and nerves, and *dolor nervorum* is associated with *podagra* (which includes modern 'gout' in its remit), *arthritis* and other painful joint problems. All these ailments were considered to arise most immediately from inflammation, swelling and general damage in the tendons and ligaments around the joints (see e.g. Anonymus Parisinus 48 and 50).[8] Also loosely in line with the basic tenets of the learned medicine of his time was a dietetic approach to his situation, a continual regulation and adjustment of his lifestyle to shore up his fragile health, punctuated by more focused therapeutic responses to specific outbreaks of pain.

There was a lot of moderation in Fronto's life, therefore, and he intensified his regimen on occasions, eating little and drinking only water, for example, in a sustained effort to increase the intervals between attacks in preparation for taking up the prestigious proconsular governorship of Asia in 157 CE (*Antoninus Pius* 8; Haines 1919: 236–9; Champlin 1980: 81–2). Severe episodes of joint pain generally kept him at home, out of harm's way, but certainly not secluded. Gellius visited the orator several times when he was 'suffering in his feet' (*pedes aeger*), finding him reclining on a 'Greek couch', surrounded by men noted for their learning, family, or fortune, and always ready for literary and linguistic debate (*Attic Nights* 2.26; 19.10; and 19.8).[9] Though Fronto himself never mentioned it, there also seem to have been some regular therapeutic ministrations in such cases. Marcus referred to massage and fomentation of the affected part, and other unspecified remedies. In one letter he found comfort in the hope that their application will by now have dulled the severe pain in the groin Fronto had reported to him, for, having recalled how much distress this pain causes his friend, Marcus was 'greatly upset' by the message (*Marcus Caesar* 5.34; Haines 1919: 224–5). Earlier, the young Caesar had expressed his wish to administer these treatments to his tutor's ailing foot himself but had to make do with statements of devotion and encouragement, and praying to the good gods that his 'dearest Fronto' might be, 'whole, sound and unimpaired in body, well and able to be with me' (*Marcus Caesar* 1.2; Haines 1919: 80–3). Regular engagement with the divine in support of each other's health, and that of each other's families, is a more widespread feature of the correspondence too (e.g. *Marcus Caesar* 5.21, 31, 40 and 49; Haines 1919: 192–3, 200–1, 211–12 and 248–9).

There is then an almost literally therapeutic dimension to these exchanges. Letter writing is one of Fronto's responses to being ill, and he receives reassurance, affirmation, love and care in return. Personal visits do some of the same work, perhaps even more so. 'Nothing . . . restores and aids a sick man as much as the affection of his friends', wrote the philosopher, poet and statesman Seneca the Younger almost a century earlier (*Moral Epistles* 78.4).[10] Cast as a didactic letter to his young friend Lucilius, this essay on bearing illness also claims to be grounded in its author's own experience.[11] Seneca's friends were assiduous, loquacious and encouraging attenders at his bedside during a particularly lengthy, taxing and disheartening bout of catarrh. The general principle that amicable visits have a key role in supporting patients is established, however, even if the rest of the story is more dubious. Fronto also picked up on another point in Seneca's discussion, about ill-health as a challenge to engagement, a demoralizing barrier to being a full and active member of society. His visitors come to listen and learn, rather than in any more dedicated caring capacity, which may itself be sustaining to him. They are impressed by Fronto's performances. He remains a leading contributor to literary life in the imperial capital. Chronic joint pain imposes some limitations, but illness and cultural function were compatible, could even be made to collaborate.

So far, no doctors or other medical attendants have been mentioned, Fronto's amicably sustained self-management has dominated. Physicians feature in Fronto's extant epistles only when his diseases depart from the routine of debilitating joint pain. Even then their appearance is low key. After the slaves carrying his sedan-chair carelessly crashed it into the entrance to the baths, injuring his knee, the *medici* advised bed-rest, while following three days of stomach complaints and flux they suggested bathing (*Marcus Caesar* 5.59 and 69; Haines 1919: 246–7 and 250–1). And, when an assault of what Fronto called *cholera* robbed him of voice, breath and then any perceptible pulse, rendering him insensible to the point that his family feared he had died, the *medici* barely managed to revive him (*Marcus Caesar* 5.55; Haines 1919: 240–3).[12] These physicians are entirely anonymous, it is unclear whether it was the same set every time, whether these were practitioners attached to his household, or those who customarily attended on him among other elite patients. There is certainly no hint that he might call in anyone new and different, either a particularly noted doctor or other kind of healer. There is no indication of any debate or dispute amongst this group, they speak with a single voice, and Fronto simply follows their recommendations. He does, however, consider that he has acquired sufficient understanding of medical matters to offer guidance to others, including to Lucius Verus on how to recover from extensive emergency venesection (*Emperor Verus* 2.6; Haines 1920: 84–7).

Marcus Aurelius, moreover, though he will later be described as an active, knowledgeable and enquiring patient by the great physician of the age, Galen of Pergamum, seems almost as uninterested in his doctors in this correspondence (Galen, *On Prognosis* 11; Mattern 2013: 187–223).[13] Illness appears in his letters mainly in relation to his family – his wife and, most especially, his children – and to Fronto, as Whitehorne emphasizes (1977: 417–18). He provided accounts of his own symptoms, and those of others, to his friend, and included his own recuperative moves in the reports, but everything is pretty basic, and no medical authority cited. Fevers and fluxes beset everyone at some point, and the countermeasures include rest and first abstaining from then gently returning to solid food, wine, bathing and exercise. 'I seem to have passed the night without fever, have willingly taken food, and am now feeling better' (*Marcus Caesar* 5.28; Haines 1919: 198–9). 'I have had a bath today and even walked a little' (*Marcus Caesar* 5.30; Haines 1919: 200–1). At one point, Marcus self-medicates his sore throat with honey-water, debating whether the verb *gargarizo* 'to gargle' is proper Latin or not; that is as technical as his involvement gets (*Marcus Caesar* 4.6; Haines 1919: 180–1). Still, there is a general sense that there were doctors around both himself and his family. Discussing a sustained period of ill-health, for instance, when he was affected by general weakness, chest pains, and an ulcer, maybe in the trachea (given its Greek name in the letter), Marcus stressed his obedience to the strictures of his *medici* (*Marcus Caesar* 4.8 and 5.26; Haines 1919: 184–7; and see also *Holidays* 1.1; Haines 1920: 2–3). Indeed, he insisted that obedience, as well as the strictures themselves, were part of the curative programme; which is, of course, to refigure doing what the doctor ordered, a conceptually problematic undertaking for a man of the Roman elite, as self-mastery. He has made himself follow instructions.

This point about self-management is articulated more programmatically in his *Meditations*, Marcus' notes to himself towards leading a good Stoic life, composed (in Greek) largely while on the military campaigns which occupied the latter years of his reign. Fronto probably died in 166 CE, and Verus certainly in 169 just as forces were being assembled to fight on the Danube frontier; after that Marcus would return to Rome only once before his own demise in 180. In the first book the emperor reprised all he was grateful for in respect of the exemplary conduct and attitudes, teaching and guidance, gifts and virtues of those who had a hand in his education and moral formation – family, tutors, mentors, friends and the gods. Pius is most extensively praised, paradigmatic in relation to his health as so much else:

Care of his body in moderation, not as one in love with living or over-
concerned with his personal appearance, though not neglectful of it either,
rather, so that by self-care he rarely required medical services, either drugs
or external applications.

— Marcus Aurelius, *Meditations* 1.16.5; see also 6.30.2[14]

Steadiness, remaining the same through good and bad fortune, 'in acute bouts
of pain, in the loss of a child, in protracted illness', was also something Marcus
aspired to (*Meditations* 1.8 and 1.16.7). And he cited with approval the
assertion of Epicurus, the founder of the rival Hellenistic philosophical school,
that, when sick, he did not allow his physicians to give themselves airs, 'as if
they were doing some great thing', since what was most important in such
circumstances occurred outside their remit, in the attitude, approach and
determination of his soul (*Meditations* 9.41).

How far Marcus lived up to these ideals he does not say, though other
evidence, such as Galen's, certainly raises questions. The epitome of Dio
Cassius' *Roman History*, originally composed in the early third century CE,
describes Marcus as 'frail' in body, poorly suited to the rigours of campaigning
(72(71).6.3).[15] These he endured only through a very abstemious diet and daily
doses of theriac, a globally protective, sustaining, and therapeutic drug made
famous by late Republican Rome's great enemy, Mithradates (Totelin 2004).
While the latter took it as a pre-emptive antidote to all poisons, Marcus' usage
was to shore up weakness of the stomach and chest. Galen also spoke of this
theriac. When the emperor departed with the armies he left the imperial
physician (*archiatros*) Demetrius in charge of its preparation and despatch to
the front, Demetrius died after a few years and Galen was selected to fill his
place (Galen, *On Antidotes* 1.1; Mattern 2013: 215–19).[16] His efforts met with
imperial approval and, on his return to Rome in 176 CE, Marcus asked Galen
about the recipe, taking an active and admiring interest in his treatment as any
good Galenic patient should (Mattern 2008, esp. 98–158). Nor was this the
sole medical support provided during campaigning. Galen narrowly avoided
enrolment in this provision, claiming that his patron deity Asclepius had
instructed otherwise after his name had been suggested by many of those
around the emperor (*On Prognosis* 9.5–7 and *On My Own Books* 3.1–6).[17]
Others went, however, while he was left in loose medical attendance on Marcus'
young son Commodus. They, or their successors, came back to Rome with the
emperor in 176, so that Galen could establish his superiority over them in
correctly diagnosing and curing an imperial stomach complaint they had
misread as an attack of fever (*On Prognosis* 11).

Galen, unsurprisingly, provides a full account of his success. The emperor
adjudicated between competing diagnoses offered at the bedside, seemingly
familiar with the process. He found the Pergamene physician's explanation

chimed with his own bodily sensations, and his suggested treatment similarly understandable and agreeable. Indeed, part of the prescription – the application of wool impregnated with warm nard ointment to the area over the mouth of the stomach – was what he would usually have done in such cases. However, while this episode and the one occasion on which Galen was called in to treat Commodus and found himself in dispute with the Methodic physicians attached to another member of the imperial family, Annia Faustina (*On Prognosis* 12), paint a picture of medical rivalries, debates between different medical schools and systems being played out at court, as in the homes of the sections of the senatorial elite who so admiringly engaged with Galen, there is nothing of this in Marcus' own words, or Fronto's.

Marcus did record having availed himself of one other medical resource, one which Fronto, not to mention Aelius Aristides, was also associated with. The emperor included on his list of things he was grateful to the gods for at the beginning of the *Meditations*, 'That through dreams I was given aids (*boēthēmata*) most particularly to prevent spitting blood and dizziness' (1.17.8). The orator was reported to have had a similar experience by Artemidorus of Daldis in his treatise on dream interpretation, another Greek literary product of the late-second or early-third century Roman empire (Bowersock 2004; Harris-McCoy 2012: 1–41). This work discusses, briefly, medical prescriptions sent by gods in dreams, a phenomenon most associated with the sanctuaries of Asclepius and the Graeco-Egyptian god Serapis, such as those at Pergamum and Alexandria (4.22; see also 2.44).[18] Many of the cures recorded are ridiculous Artemidorus asserted. The gods have a more straightforward approach to these matters than is attributed to them, and operate according to the principles of the medical art. A woman suffering from an inflamed breast dreamt she was being suckled by a sheep: she was cured by application of a plantain poultice to the affected part. For *arnoglosson*, the Greek for common or broadleaf plantain, literally means 'sheep-tongue'. Similarly, 'Fronto, who suffered from *arthritis*, having asked for a cure, dreamt he was walking in the suburbs (*proasteion*), and was much comforted by being anointed with *propolis*' ('bee-glue', but could also mean 'suburbs'). Both these materials – plantain and bee-glue – were standard items in the classical pharmacological repertoire (e.g. Dioscorides, *Materia Medica* 2.84; Galen, *On the Composition of Drugs according to Kind* 7.7, K13.976).[19]

Turning to Aelius Aristides is the best way to explore the wider context of these rather spare statements, to consider the details that have been omitted. For dreams and dream cures became central to his experience of his body, in sickness and health, as he was only too eager to explain and celebrate. Aristides also interacted with learned medicine and its practitioners, and participated in a broader array of religious activities in support of his well-being, but the relative importance of these aspects of his life was distinctive, the reverse of what has been observed so far for Fronto and Marcus Aurelius. Still there are numerous other points of both overlap and contrast, contact and divergence, between his career and those of all the other second-century CE figures discussed so far, especially Fronto.

A couple of decades younger than the North African orator, and even better educated, Aristides' ambitions took him to the great imperial metropolis only after he had established a considerable rhetorical reputation in the Greek East (Trapp 2016). But the trip to Rome in 143/4 CE was a disaster. His health, apparently always fragile, collapsed catastrophically and he was forced to return home, ill and dispirited. Back in Asia, Aristides received the first of a life-long series of dream visions from the healing god Asclepius, took up residence in his sanctuary at Pergamum, and dedicated himself to the deity and his own well-being as an indissoluble pair during a two-year stay he termed his 'kathedra' (literally, 'staying-still'). The strategy paid off, the god cared for him, and after a year of treatments began to encourage him back into oratory: he was able to re-enter public life in 147 CE. Still subject to occasional bouts of ill-health, but supported by Asclepius, Aristides enjoyed great success as an oratorical performer for the next few decades and was an active member of the local elite until his death in the early 180s. His surviving oeuvre includes many of his discourses and declamations, several hymns to gods and speeches in praise of sacred sites, and the autobiographical Sacred Tales (Hieroi Logoi), comprising a disjointed series of diseases, dreams and divine cures, personal and professional journeys, legal and political entanglements.[20] These accounts are, Aristides claimed, expanded and reworked versions of the dream diary Asclepius ordered him to keep from the outset, and which he was subsequently instructed to make public (Sacred Tales 2.3; Downie 2013). They offer a different kind of first-person narrative of illness, treatment and recovery from the letters, one which puts more emphasis on the relationship with the divine than other mortals, though they are present too, and was directed at a wider audience.

Aristides provided far more graphic descriptions of his illnesses and treatments than found in any correspondence. Having been increasingly troubled by ill-health on the journey to Rome, for instance, on the hundredth day after departure, Aristides arrived in the great metropolis:

Not long after that my innards swelled up, my sinews became chilled, shivering spread through my whole body, and my breath was laboured. The physicians prescribed purges, and I was purged for two days through drinking a preparation of squirting cucumber, until blood was discharged. Then fevers seized me, and now there were difficulties on all sides, and no hope of recovery whatsoever. Finally the physicians made a cut, beginning from my sternum all the way down to the bladder, and applied cupping vessels, which completely stopped my breath, and a numbing pain shot through me,

impossible to bear, and everything was mixed with blood and I became
excessively purged, and I felt as if my innards were cold and exposed, and
the trouble with my breathing increased. I did not know what to do, for in
the middle of eating or talking there would be an attack, and I was sure I was
going to choke. And the other weakness of my body worsened similarly.
Theriac drugs and all sorts of other things were administered.

— Aelius Aristides, *Sacred Tales* 2.62–4

Forced to retreat, a wider group of mortal medical practitioners failed him on
his return. Back in Smyrna, problems with his palate joined his other ills,
'physicians and gymnastic trainers' gathered, but did not recognize the disease
and could not help (*Sacred Tales* 2.69).[21] They agreed only that he should
transport himself to the local warm springs.

It was here that Asclepius appeared to him in a dream, commanding him to
walk barefoot, an order Aristides embraced, then took himself (and his foster-
father Zosimus) to the god's sanctuary at Pergamum so as to form a closer
relationship with the deity (*Sacred Tales* 2.7–9 and 70). Asclepius began almost
immediately to dispense 'cures' (*iamata*). First, as Aristides recalled, was some
balsam resin, to be applied in the baths, followed by many and various material
prescriptions (*Sacred Tales* 2.10). Also apparently positioned early in the
kathedra was a sequence of commands to have large amounts blood let from his
elbow ('sixty *litrai*'), and then from his forehead, interspersed with orders to
bathe in the river, all despite the weather and his weak and beleaguered
condition (*Sacred Tales* 2.45–9 and 51–3). He was still suffering from catarrhs,
chills and fevers, and problems of the palate and stomach. By following these
instructions, and having various predictive aspects of the dreams fulfilled at the
same time, Aristides was restored, strengthened and encouraged. One river
bath left him feeling 'relieved and refreshed', another made him warm all over
his body, with steam rising from his rosy skin as he and the friends who had
anxiously accompanied him sang a paean of praise to the god. He would have
recovered pretty swiftly if he had had stuck to his own interpretations of his
dreams rather than allowed himself to be misled by poor advice (*Sacred Tales*
2.73). He learnt from this experience, however, and moved more gradually
towards health.

For Aristides, like Fronto and Marcus Aurelius, describing symptoms was
more important than naming the disease, indeed, whether there was a single
disease to be named is unclear. Symptoms are experienced directly, form part of
personal communication, while to speak of diseases is something different: it
has its uses at a more general and abstract level of discourse and action. Aristides'
accumulation of ills also serves a particular purpose in highlighting the power
of Asclepius and how much the god had invested in this particular project of
salvation (*sōtēria*). The failings of human medicine operate similarly to increase

divine achievement. Still, Aristides' engagement with mortal medical practitioners is richer and more active than that recorded by either Fronto or Marcus. Gymnastic trainers and physicians were summoned at Smyrna, there were debates between doctors at his bedside, and, though he was mostly attended by anonymous groups of *iatroi*, some named individuals also feature. Theodotus seems to have been his regular physician while at the *Asclepeion*, appearing in his dreams as well as outside them, and his more occasional visitors included Satyrus, known from other sources as one of Galen's teachers, who spent time in Pergamum with the senator Rufinus when he was overseeing the construction of the new temple of Zeus Asclepius (Mattern 2013: 39–42; Petridou 2016: 306–12).

The encounter with the physician Satyrus, 'A sophist and of no humble birth, so it was said', is instructive (*Sacred Tales* 3.8). While in Pergamum he visited Aristides who was lying on his bed, and felt his chest and abdomen. When he discovered how many purges of blood the patient had endured he told him to desist, his body could not take any more, and gave him a light, simple plaster to place over his gullet and stomach instead. Aristides determined to keep on with the bloodletting, in obedience to Asclepius, but not to ignore Satyrus' prescription either, for the god has not forbidden it. Having suffered a setback on a subsequent trip to the springs at Lebedus, Aristides decided to try the poultice. It seemed immediately cold and disagreeable, but he persevered, and soon developed a terrible chest cold and cough. 'the god showed it was *phthoē* (consumption)', and the next day he felt pressure on his temples, general befuddlement, and his jaw locked. After attaining some relief, Zosimus was despatched to consult the god at nearby Colophon, and Aristides himself had a dream which he interpreted as signifying that a series of sacrifices should be offered to the divine. These he performed in thanks for help received and ongoing, but also, implicitly in recompense for having strayed with Satyrus' plaster. He had not trusted entirely to the god's power and beneficence. Still, as this and other episodes make clear, Asclepius' therapeutic instructions generally overlap with what learned doctors might have prescribed. Venesection was, after all, the quintessential medical remedy of the time, while bathing and abstaining from bathing, eating certain foods or not, and various forms of exercise, not to mention various medicaments, were all basic items in the physician's curative repertoire. The god simply tended to the extreme in his treatments, exceeding the injunctions and capacity of mortal healers, inevitably out-competing them, but on their terms.

It has been argued that the key difference between Asclepius and human physicians lies in their relationship with their patients, not in the content of their cures. Or, at least, that Aristides exchanged self-mastery for submission to divine command, surrendered the agency that is to be maintained in all dealings with mortal practitioners and became totally dependent on the god. He became, as it were, a patient in the strong sense of the word, signifying not simply a sufferer, a sick person, but a passive object of medical intervention, here of a divine kind. Except, as more recent scholarship has pointed out, such a conclusion is simplistic. While Aristides certainly saw his relationship with Asclepius as the most important in his life, he was a very active and authoritative participant in his own cures (Petridou 2015 and 2016). Indeed, his narrative of recovery and healing, of divine support and favour, clearly serves to rebuild and enliven his oratorical career, to substantiate competitive claims to professional prestige and status (Petsalis-Diomidis 2010; Downie 2013).

Aristides, Fronto and Marcus Aurelius, do all fit together, therefore, in the Roman empire of the second century CE. While emperor and orator seem to have operated in the intersecting realms of learned medicine and traditional Roman religion, of elite self-management and sociality in relation to health and disease, without displaying much interest in serious medical knowledge, or the real possibilities of the medical marketplace, they both received more specific divine assistance, through dreams. That latter was Aristides' main form of bodily support, but learned physicians and other religious activities also played important roles in his life, as he reworked traditional models of autonomy and social relations networks to suit his particular situation. Indeed, his interactions with doctors bear more resemblance to those described in Galen than the generic references in exchanges between Fronto and Marcus. Adding Aulus Gellius to the mix puts more weight on these interactions too. Though for him the bedside was less a site of debate between practitioners than of discussions between the attending doctor and the patient's friends, in which the latter have the epistemic edge. Still, it is Gellius who makes elite interest in medical learning most explicit, who moves beyond a loosely shared vocabulary and concepts towards more detailed knowledge of the human body and its workings, gained from engagement with medical texts. The overlap between lay and specialist understandings has been more widely on display, but in rather a weak and diffuse way.

This picture is essentially confirmed: expanded, with some shift of emphasis, but not changed, by the other sets of surviving (non-Christian) correspondence from the Roman world.[22] That is those belonging to Pliny the Younger and Cicero, from a little under a century and about two centuries earlier respectively. Neither had much to say about their own ailments, both were more forthcoming about the illness and treatment of friends, family and household dependents. When they did mention their own suffering it was with wider social relations, political and ethical issues in mind. 'For ten days I have been severely afflicted in the guts', Cicero wrote to his friend Fabius Gallus in 46 BCE (*Letters to Friends* 210: 7.26).[23] He did not have a fever, however, so retiring to his Tusculan villa, resting and fasting, now had him on the mend. The cause was not, in this instance, overindulgence, rather his attendance at a largely vegetarian dinner constructed in obedience to the new sumptuary laws had resulted, almost immediately, in violent *diarrhoia* and had him fearing *dusenteria* (both terms are in Greek). As well as drawing attention to the dangers of plain living, Cicero chided Gallus for neither visiting nor writing to him despite knowing he was sick. It was a fever which delayed Pliny at Pergamum on his way to take up the governorship of Bithynia, so he explained in a letter to the emperor Trajan, but he fortunately arrived in time to celebrate Trajan's birthday in the province (*Letters* 10.17).[24] Fever also allowed Pliny the opportunity for exemplary self-control, greater rigour than his doctors, a point he made to a young protégé when sick, while eye-trouble provided him with the occasion for taking advice and a present from a senior political figure, his fellow consul Cornutus Tertullus (*Letters* 7.1 and 7.21; see also 7.26).

THE FEMALE PATIENT SPEAKS

Letters and other documents preserved on papyrus from Roman Egypt bring a wider social group into view. Exchanged between more ordinary folk as well as the wealthy, those with some property and possessions but not much, by men and women, and between those who found writing a struggle as well as the practised and fluent, this correspondence contains matters of health and illness, care and cure within its remit. Hopes, wishes and prayers for good health are part of ancient epistolary protocol, customarily expressed in the opening formula, and the topic variously appears in the body of the letters too, together with other concerns, the record of items despatched and received, greetings to whole households, news of people on the move and other relevant developments. A message composed in a 'clumsy hand', with weak orthography and syntax, and delivered to Philadelphia in the early second century CE is typical in its contents:

> Thermouthis to Valerias her mother, very many greetings and always good health.
>
> I received from Valerius the basket with 20 pairs of loaves. Send me the blankets at the current price, and nice wool, 4 fleeces. Give these to Valerius. At the moment I am 7 month pregnant. And I salute Artemis and little Nikarous and Valerius my lord – I long for him in my mind – and Dionysia and Demetrious many times and little Taesis many times and everyone in the house. And how is my father? Please, send me news because he was ill when he left me. I salute nurse. Rodine salutes you. I have set her to the handiwork; again I need her, but I am happy.
>
> —SB 5.7572[25]

Pregnancy, advanced pregnancy and imminent birth, are among the more regular self-reports of physical condition in correspondence which more usually

speaks about the health of others, such as Thermouthis' father (see Figure 6.3).
These reports required action, movement was to follow, usually of female
relatives, sometimes of the expectant mother herself, so that the birth would be
properly attended and supported (*BGU* 1.261; *P.Oxf.* 19; *O.Florida* 14: Bagnall
and Cribiore, nos. 74, 148 and 48). Occasionally material supplies were
requested too (*P.Mich.* 8.508: Bagnall and Cribiore, no. 290. The information
provided was minimal, however, the tone casual, and the only reference to a
midwife (*maia*) or any other medical practitioner occurs in a legal dossier. Still,
it is a transcription of the account given by the widow Petronilla of her efforts,
when her husband died during her pregnancy, to follow the legal procedure
prescribed to ensure her baby's status as her deceased husband's heir (*P.Gen.*

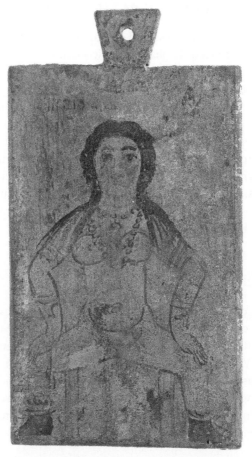

FIGURE 6.3: Painted wood mummy label or tablet showing a woman seated on a
birthing stool. Found in the Roman period cemetery at Hawara in the Fayum (Egypt)
at the head of a female mummy. National Museum of Scotland, Edinburgh, museum
reference A.1911.210.4 G. © National Museums Scotland.

2.103: Rowlandson 1998, no. 224). She had been inspected by the honest woman officially appointed to watch over her belly, together with a midwife (*maia*), confirming her pregnancy, though precise adherence to the rules surrounding the birth itself had not been possible. Shared understanding of the importance of timing in all this, the idea that while the seven- or nine-month child can be born alive, the eight-month child will not survive, is also articulated in the letters, as well as in medical and philosophical discourse, and more widely across the ancient world. The death of Herennia after giving birth to an eight-month child, also dead, was sadly reported to her father by her sister Thaubas in 64 CE (*P.Fouad.* 1.75; see also *SB* 16.12606: Bagnall and Cribiore, nos. 228 and 227; Hanson 1987).

While birth required travel, it seems that visiting the sick over the kinds of distances these letters covered was not deemed practical in this social milieu. The utility of announcing personal ailments was thus reduced, while the need for news about absent family and friends increased. Updates might be demanded of the ill as well as those around them, and there were exceptions to this first-person reticence. Specific help could be requested – a rest for a painful elbow (*O.Claud.* 1.174), for instance – and illness might explain non-attendance at a wedding (*P.Oxy.* 46.3313) or failure to despatch goods owed, and sometimes the sympathy card was played, over-played even. 'Why are you writing to me "I am sick"?', demanded Soeris of Aline, 'I was told that you are not ill: you make me awfully worried. But see, I have been sick in my eyes for four months' (*P.Brem.* 64: Bagnall and Cribiore, no. 42). The terminology is loose and imprecise here as elsewhere, eyes and elbows are as specific as these communications get. People are either well or not, that matters, the finer points not so much. While Roman physicians certainly engaged in epistolary consultations and prescriptions, which presumably required detailed descriptions of symptoms, this is not reflected in the papyrus evidence (Hanson 2010; Totelin 2020). There are more medical exchanges, mostly concerned with materials or recipes, but while it is possible to identify some correspondents as doctors, none is clearly and unambiguously a patient. The experience of disease is not part of these letters.

CONCLUSIONS

In the Roman world the diseases most frequently experienced were fevers and fluxes with eye-problems also common. Seriously sore throats, catarrh and chest complaints also featured, along with chronic joint pain and the impressive accumulation of ills that buffeted Aelius Aristides. The first-person reports and records discussed so far fit in to the wider patterns of the ancient pathenocoenosis – the ancient disease community – reconstructed from a more complete collation of textual sources combined with the results of an expanding array of palaeopathological and phylogenetic techniques (Grmek 1989; Mitchell 2011). In modern terms this was a world dominated by malarial fevers, acute infections of the digestive and respiratory systems, and the ongoing effects of physical injury and hardship. Infant mortality was very high (Woods 2007).

Elite patients have spoken about their health and illness in ways that overlap with ancient medical writings in other respects too, this was clearly a shared conceptual and epidemiological environment. But that overlap has been less substantial than was expected, largely consisting in a mixture of underlying assumptions and loose vocabulary rather than anything more sustained or profound. Aulus Gellius offered a different perspective, demonstrating a more systematic lay approach to mastering specialist medical knowledge engendered within the philosophically inclined elite circles he moved in. This is, therefore, a group exception to the rule, not individual whimsy, but still, the implication has often been that Gellius is representative of the educated upper echelons of Roman imperial society as a whole, which appears not to be the case. Furthermore, diseases have been rarely named by patients. Diagnostic labelling of this kind seems to have served little purpose, at least in the contexts of sufferers' self-presentation which have been the focus here. Symptoms and sensations, pains and incapacities have been foregrounded in these accounts.

In response to these illnesses the Roman sick had recourse to dietetic self-management and material self-medication, to family and friends, to mostly anonymous groups of physicians (and sometimes gymnastic trainers), and to the gods. The religious modes of engagement were varied. Gaining support for personal and familial health could be woven into everyday ritual practice, might be the focus of vows and prayers to the traditional deities of Rome and the local gods of Roman Egypt, or more specific efforts could be made in this respect. In the Roman imperial period this most commonly consisted in asking the divine for curative instructions sent in dreams.[26] Paradigmatically this would occur in a sanctuary, such as that of Asclepius at Pergamum, a sacred place set up to facilitate and sustain such activity, but it could happen anywhere. Nor did Asclepius have a monopoly. Aelius Aristides received his first dream instructions when at Smyrna, and though his relationship with Asclepius was certainly special, it was not exclusive, he received help and guidance from a number of deities in a variety of locations.

There is nothing surprising in any of this. This set of options, overlapping options unevenly distributed by wealth and status, is roughly as expected. It is perhaps a bit more limited than some evocations of ancient medical pluralism would suggest, there has been little 'medical promiscuity' on display, but the evidence has been quite limited too. More noteworthy, however, is the lack of a patient perspective on medical competition. There seems little contact with Galen's narratives of bedside arguments, public disputation, and rancorous rhetoric, amongst the community of learned physicians. Still, though Galen undoubtedly encouraged and exaggerated such activities and relationships, there is no reason to think he invented them. Rather, this was a more niche market than is often assumed, at least in so far as the acquisition of medical services were concerned. Such debates provide quite a distant background for the more mundane experience of illness and cure, of being treated by doctors, which predominated even amongst the Roman elite. Medical pragmatism perhaps best captures the ancient patient's view.

NOTES

1. Translations are my own unless specified. I have used the Oxford Classical Texts edition of Gellius, edited by Marshall (1968); details of this and the Loeb Classical Library edition and translation by Rolfe (1927) can be found in the source list.
2. Though William V. Harris (2016: esp. 29–3) has recently argued that there was at least weak medical professionalization in the ancient world.
3. The Loeb Classical Library volume containing *Epidemics 5* and *7* is edited and translated by Smith (1994).
4. There is some overlap between his letters and his speeches, and some oratorical fragments have been found; but, while he did 'publish' his speeches, there is no indication he intended his correspondence to reach a wider audience.
5. Whitehorne calculates that this is about forty per cent and sixty-five per cent of their extant epistolary output respectively. Many letters, of course, cover multiple topics.
6. I provide a traditional reference – and I have used van den Hout's edition (1988) – and one to the accessible Loeb Classical Library editions and translations of the correspondence by Haines (1919–1920). The letters are organized by correspondent and chronology.
7. The Loeb Classical Library edition and translation of Celsus is by Spencer (1935–1938). There is a Teubner edition of Scribonius Largus is from by Sconocchia (1983); and a Collection des Universités de France edition with French translation by Jouanna-Bouchet (2016).
8. *Anonymus Parisinus* has been edited by Garofalo and translated into English by Fuchs (1997).
9. The formula '*pedes aeger*' (and variants) is often translated as 'gout', but that is undoubtedly too precise an identification of the ailment concerned; on the other hand, it is clear that the phrase does designate something more specific and identifiable than simply 'foot disease'. It is a reasonably standard term in Latin literature, see e.g. Sallust, *The War with Catiline* 59.4. Text and translation of this work can be found in the Loeb Classical Library series, by Ramsey and Rolfe (2013).
10. I have used the Oxford Classical Texts edition by Reynolds (1965); there is an edition and translation in the Loeb Classical Library by Gummere (1920).
11. The degree of fictionalization in the *Moral Epistles* is debated, but all agree there is some, and many would argue that – whether or not Seneca and Lucilius ever actually exchanged letters – the collection as its stands is essentially a philosophical dialogue in epistolary form (see Griffin 1992: 416–19). So this is quite different from Fronto's extant correspondence.

12. This seems not to be either the *cholera* of ancient or modern medicine (which do overlap), but something more vaguely bile (*cholē*) based.
13. Text and translation of *On Prognosis* appears in the Corpus Medicorum Graecorum series (V 8,1) by Nutton (1979).
14. I have used the edition of Farquharson (1944), there is a text and translation in the Loeb Classical Library by Haines (1920). This, of course, fits very well with Michel Foucault's description of Roman 'cultivation of the self' more broadly, see *The History of Sexuality* Vol. 3: *The Care of the Self*, trans. Robert Hurley (London: Penguin, 1990), 37–68.
15. There is a Loeb Classical Library edition and translation by Cary (1927).
16. *On Antidotes* is in the fourteenth volume of Kühn's edition.
17. For *On My Own Books* see the Collection des Universités de France edition by Boudon-Millot (2007); there is also an English translation by Singer (1997)
18. There is an Oxford University Press edition and translation by Harris-McCoy (2012).
19. The Greek text of Dioscorides has been edited by Wellmann (1907–1914), and there is an English translation by Beck (2011). Galen's *On the Composition of Drugs according to Kind* is in the twelfth and thirteenth volume of Kühn's edition.
20. The six (one fragmentary) *Sacred Tales* are traditionally *Orations* 47–52 in his collected works. I have used the edition by Keil (1898); there is an English translation by Behr (1981).
21. On rivalry between physicians and gymnastic trainers see Galen, *Thrasybulus: Is Health a part of Medicine or Gymnastics* (there is a Corpus Medicorum Graecorum edition by Helmreich 1893 and an English translation by Singer 1997) and Philostratus, *Gymnasticus* (there is a Loeb Classical Library edition and translation by Rusten and König 2014).
22. There are a number of rich collections of Christian letters extant, but that is beyond the scope of this chapter.
23. See the Loeb Classical Library edition and translation by Shackleton Bailey (2001).
24. I have used the Oxford Classical Texts edition by Mynors (1963), there is also a Loeb Classical Library edition and translation by Radice (1969).
25. Translation: Bagnall and Cribiore (2008), no. 157. Details of this edition and other papyrological publications can be found in the source list, in the papyri section. See also the *Checklist of Editions of Greek, Latin, Demotic, and Coptic Papyri, Ostraca, and Tablets* published by the American Society of Papyrologists (http://papyri.info/docs/checklist, accessed 16 October 2020).
26. In contrast to the style of healing provided by Asclepius in classical Greece, which usually occurred within the dream (though instructions were sometimes delivered).

CHAPTER SEVEN

Brain

DAVID LEITH

INTRODUCTION

The ancient discourse on the mind and its functions largely revolves around the concept of the 'soul', which is the conventional translation for the Greek term *psuchē* and the Latin *anima*. At its simplest, the *psuchē* can be regarded as what renders things alive. What it actually is, however, and how exactly it contributes to an animal's continuing to be alive, were enormously controversial and widely debated issues. One approach to understanding the soul's nature better was to examine in detail the basic capacities of which it was thought to be in control. These often included capacities such as thinking, perceiving, moving, feeling emotion, but also what might be regarded as more basic functions such as reproduction, appetite, nutrition and growth, and so on. All these could in some senses be considered aspects of the same underlying entity, and therefore to belong to the same field of inquiry. Hence various physiological processes within the body that were of obvious relevance to the doctor in maintaining or restoring health could also be seen as potentially applicable to the question of the nature of the soul. At the same time, mental or 'psychic' disorders such as madness fell under the doctor's purview in such a way that a better understanding of the soul could be felt to have implications for treatment (see the recent studies in Harris 2013 and Thumiger 2017). Since doctors generally approached such issues from the perspective of concern for human health, the questions they formulated often had to do with the way in which the soul might interact with the body, and vice versa (e.g. Hankinson 1991a). So, as we shall see, issues to do with the bodily *locations* of psychic and physiological processes frequently came to the forefront. Similarly, the *substance* or *medium* by which such processes might be discharged was also very much a focus for doctors' inquiries.

Within all this, the brain occupied a central, though by no means uncontested, position. Plato, for example, had divided up the soul into rational and irrational parts, maintaining that the divine, rational part must be located in the head, while the irrational part was subdivided into the 'spirited' portion assigned to the chest, and the 'desiderative' to the abdomen (for a general introduction to Plato's psychology, see Lorenz 2008). In his *Timaeus* especially, the brain and marrow had a close relationship with the soul and its functions.[1] But Greek thinking had long associated cognition with the area of the chest and especially the heart, and this was to have a profound impact on theoretical inquiries. Aristotle, for instance, believed that the brain's purpose was principally as a cooling agent, tempering the excessive heat generated by the heart (see e.g. Aristotle, *Parts of Animals* 2.7, 652a 25–653a 21) (see Figure 7.1).[2] For him, the heart was the central organ or principle of most of the soul's basic capacities, the nutritive, the locomotive and perceptive (see e.g. Johansen 2012). So sensations, for example, were ultimately transmitted to the heart as the common sensorium, and the heart stood at the centre of the bodily apparatus – tendons, ligaments, etc – that controlled its movements. Other prominent philosophical traditions were in this respect more or less in line with Aristotle, not least Stoicism, whose adherents located the governing part of the soul (Greek: *hēgemonikon*) in the heart, and Epicureanism, which assigned the soul's rational part to the thorax in general (Annas 1992). In some ways, this philosophical discourse laid down the basic framework within which medical practitioners engaged with these central issues of the body and its interactions with the soul. Thus, Galen's theory of the mind and the brain's functioning explicitly sought to place itself in relation to the major philosophical, as well as medical, authorities influential in his own day; and much the same can be said of his rationalist predecessors in the Hellenistic and early Roman eras. In what follows, I want to focus in particular on what doctors had to say about the brain as an organ within the body, and how this picture fitted into broader debates about the mind, the soul and basic psychic functions. I shall also look at the ways in which these medical investigations unfolded through time, in particular how successive generations of doctors negotiated the authorities of the past, and how such preoccupations shaped their conceptual frameworks and determined their inquiries.

(IR)RELEVANCE TO MEDICINE

Yet it is important to observe that by no means all ancient physicians wished to pursue these sorts of inquiries, and developed sophisticated arguments for why they should avoid them. There was a strong tradition within Graeco-Roman

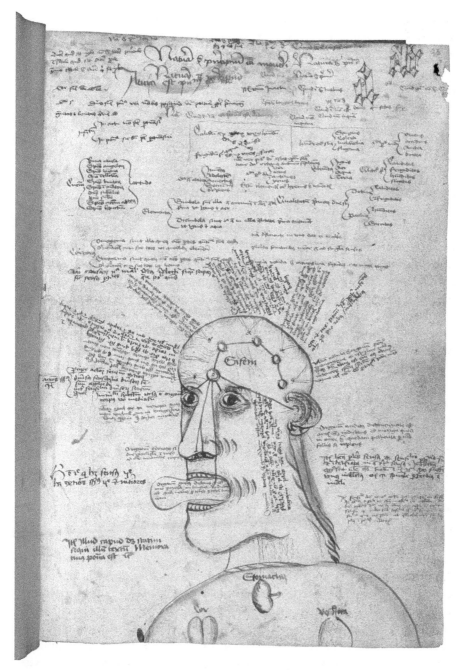

FIGURE 7.1: Medieval diagram of the brain and senses. This illustration is found in a
manuscript which contains several Aristotelian treatises, including *On the Soul*.
Wellcome MS 55, fol. 93r. Courtesy of the Wellcome Library.

medical circles of classifying questions to do with the soul and its functions as beyond the legitimate scope of the medical art. The sole aim of medicine was often taken to be the maintenance of bodily health and curing of illness. It was a commonplace that, while medicine dealt with the body, it was rather philosophy's job to take care of the soul. Some doctors reflected deeply on medicine's relationship to philosophy, and asserted its disciplinary subordination: medicine was a specialized discipline which partially overlapped with and built upon philosophical inquiries in natural science, but such philosophical foundations were not properly part of medicine itself. This was apparently a viewpoint adopted by the Hellenistic physicians Herophilus of Chalcedon and Erasistratus of Ceos (further discussed below), who believed that the inquiry into the fundamental physical elements (such as earth, air, fire and water) was a subject proper to philosophy, but not to medicine, since it did not contribute to human health (Leith 2015a). This was not a matter of disputing the philosophers' findings or methods, but merely of setting the correct disciplinary boundaries. Herophilus was well known for his slogan, 'Let the apparent things be primary, even though (/if) they are not primary', which stipulated that, within medicine, the most basic level at which the human body should be analysed is the level of perception, but with the acknowledgement that in reality there is a more basic level, i.e. the subsensible level of the ultimate elements; this, however, does not properly belong to the medical art (Galen, *On the Therapeutic Method* 2.5; Anonymus Londinensis, column xxi, lines 20–3, edition: Manetti 2011: 45–6).[3] The study of the soul was another topic which this tradition considered extrinsic to medicine. For example, a papyrus text written in the first century CE, the so-called Anonymus Londinensis papyrus, outlined the scope of its medical study by appealing to Herophilus' slogan regarding the elements, and similarly placed the study of the soul firmly outside medicine: 'the human being is composed of soul and body . . . Regarding the soul, I defer to others, but we must be concerned with the body, since medicine is especially focused on this' (Anonymus Londinensis, column xxi, lines 13–18).

Other, especially later, physicians advocated a more systematic ban on inquiries into obscure matters in general, which paradigmatically included that into the nature of the soul. The so-called Empiricists (*Empeirikoi*), founded in Alexandria by Philinus of Cos, a pupil of Herophilus, in the mid-third century BCE, maintained that effective treatment could only be reliably determined by observing remedies working repeatedly under the same circumstances. Attempts to understand the underlying processes at work, such as the hidden causes of disease, human anatomy and physiology, etc, were not just unreliable (witness all the competing theories devised by physicians), but also quite unnecessary. They claimed that their methodology dispensed entirely with the use of inferential reasoning: the efficacy of any remedy could only be established through experience, not through the development of some speculative account of how it interacted with the body (see e.g. Frede 1987). With all this, inquiry into a subject so obscure as the soul was hardly likely to be regarded as a relevant or useful pursuit for the Empiricist doctor.

The medical sect of the Methodists (*Methodikoi*), founded by Themison of Laodicea in the early first century BCE, similarly refused to get bogged down in inquiries into obscure matters, but their motivation in doing so was not primarily based on sceptical grounds as it was for the Empiricists (the evidence for medical Methodism is collected in Tecusan 2004). The Methodists identified two common features (Greek: *koinotētes*) which they believed could be identified in any disease. One was a state of constriction, in which the body is too constricted or compacted to allow the proper movement of bodily fluids; another was a state of laxity or looseness, in which fluids move too easily within the body and are excessively dissipated. These were easily identified by the Methodist physician, and moreover immediately indicated how the disease was to be treated: the state of constriction had to be countered by remedies which brought about a dissolution or relaxation of the body, such as a warm bath, while the state of laxity had to be countered by constricting treatments. Unlike the Empiricist approach, there was no need for repeated experiences of remedies working under the same conditions. However, in common with the Empiricists, the Methodists saw no place for inquiries into hidden matters, such as the soul or the mind, or the causes of diseases in general. For them, in a medical context at least, such inquiries were an irrelevant distraction which could happily be obviated by their Method (see van der Eijk 2005a). For example, one of the most successful Methodists, Soranus of Ephesus around 100 CE, repudiated other doctors for basing their treatment of the mental disorder phrenitis on prior assumptions about the location of the mind; for Soranus, treatment had to be based only on the manifest symptoms, which in phrenitis are evidently concentrated in the head (see the discussion preserved at Caelius Aurelianus, *On Acute Diseases* 1.8.53–6; for Soranus in general, Hanson and Green 1994).[4] Yet none of this, it is important to note, prevented Soranus from having strong interests in the subject of the soul; in fact, he wrote a treatise *On the Soul* in four books in which he set out various positive views on the soul's nature, including its corporeal nature and mortality, and its division into seven parts (the Christian author Tertullian made use of this book *c.* 200 CE: see esp. Tertullian, *On the Soul* 6.6, 8.3, 14.2, 38.3, with Podolak 2010 for recent discussion).[5] Evidently, for Soranus, this will not have had any bearing on medicine, but they were questions which were nevertheless of interest and could be answered. Once again, the study of the soul and mind, whatever else one might think about it, was a topic which did not properly belong to the medical art.

Nevertheless, as we shall see below, many doctors believed that medicine *should* investigate the nature of the soul and the mind, and indeed that medical expertise had a unique perspective which could furnish it with special authority in this field. Galen is a prominent example of this tendency within medicine, but he had precedents in physicians such as Asclepiades of Bithynia in the late second century BCE and the medical sect of the Pneumatists, who devised a medical system based on Stoic philosophy in the first century BCE. Yet much of their contribution in this area is expressed in polemical, defensive terms, justifying their right and duty to encroach on the territory of the philosophers, where the default position they expect to encounter is that they have little business in doing so. Galen's treatise *That the Capacities of the Soul Depend on the Mixtures of the Body* is a good example. Likewise, when the philosopher Antiochus of Ascalon reports Asclepiades' views on the soul, he describes him rather condescendingly as someone 'in medicine second to none, but who tried his hand also at philosophy' (Sextus Empiricus, *Against the Logicians* 1.201).[6] Greek and Roman medicine thus had a complex and contested relationship with the question of the mind and its interactions with the body, at times evincing complete indifference to the matter, at others making a significant and distinctive impact upon contemporary debates.

LOCATING THE MIND

Of those who maintained that the nature of the mind had some bearing on medicine, or who believed that medicine could have some impact on our understanding of its interaction with the body, two broad camps are often identified by scholars, both ancient and modern: 'cardiocentrists', who favoured the heart (see Figure 7.2) as the principal organ associated with various mental processes, and 'encephalocentrists', who favoured the brain. But such simple categories may disguise the complexity of the individual theories they are meant to categorize, or straightforwardly distort them (van der Eijk 2005b). Physicians throughout antiquity paid attention to physiological or pathological processes that involved the heart and brain, but our sources often too readily attribute to them comprehensive theories concerning the soul or mind. All sorts of unspoken assumptions may be built into the notions of cardiocentrism or encephalocentrism, and in the absence of much of the original writings of the relevant doctors, we are often very much in the dark about their real views and perspectives. Anachronism is common in ancient reports of the doctrines of earlier thinkers, and in fact much of the apparent simplicity in the ancient debate over the location of the mind derives precisely from the ways in which a succession of thinkers labelled the views of their predecessors, assigning candidates to either camp in a way which distorted their original interests. The labels 'cardiocentrist' and 'encephalocentrist' can of course still be useful shorthand, but it is important to be clear of the range of highly diverse and incommensurable theories that they may conceal.

In his *Parts of Animals*, Aristotle reflected on some of the considerations that

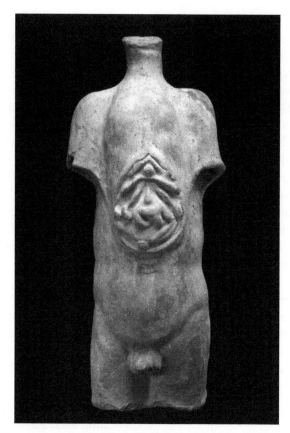

FIGURE 7.2: Terracotta votive male torso, Roman, date uncertain. This votive shows the internal organs of the abdomen, including the heart. The Science Museum London, object number A634998. Courtesy of Wellcome Images.

had persuaded Plato to identify the brain as the central organ of perception. Although he does not name his teacher explicitly, it is clear that Aristotle had Plato's *Timaeus* in mind when he stated that his predecessors

> are unable to discover the reason why some of the senses are placed in the head; but they see that the head is a somewhat unusual part, compared with the rest, so they put two and two together and argue that the brain is the seat of sensation.
>
> —Aristotle, *Parts of Animals* 2.10, 656a 26–8; translation Peck 1937: 175; compare Plato, *Timaeus* 74e–75c

Aristotle himself believed that all the senses were in fact ultimately connected with the heart, but this obvious proximity between the brain and sense-organs had already struck others as similarly significant. The (probably) early fifth century BCE thinker Alcmaeon of Croton, for example, had maintained that all the sense-organs are connected with the brain by means of certain channels (*poroi* in Greek), and later doxographers were to assert, perhaps on this basis, that he believed the brain to be the location of the ruling part of the soul. Aristotle's pupil Theophrastus (*c.* 371–*c.* 287 BCE) reports Alcmaeon's belief that 'one smells with the nostrils at the same time as respiration, by drawing the pneuma to the brain', and that 'all the senses are connected in some way to the brain, and for this reason they are incapacitated if it is disturbed or shifted, for it obstructs the channels through which the sensations take place' (Theophrastus, *On Sense-Perception* 25 and 26, with general discussion in Lloyd 1991).[7] Diogenes of Apollonia, working somewhat later in the fifth century, believed that air is responsible for thinking and for sense-perception, and worked out a detailed physiology explaining perception as due to the interactions of air between the sense-organs and the brain specifically:

> Diogenes attributes thinking and the senses, as also life, to air . . . The sense of smell is produced by the air round the brain . . . Hearing is produced whenever the air within the ears, being moved by the air outside, spreads toward the brain. Vision occurs when things are reflected on the pupil, and it, being mixed with the air within, produces a sensation . . . Taste occurs to the tongue by what is rare and gentle.
>
> —Theophrastus, *On Sense-Perception* 39–40;
> translation Kirk, Raven and Schofield

These ideas evidently had an important impact on contemporary physicians. Among surviving early medical texts, the Hippocratic treatise *On the Sacred Disease* assigns a range of basic functions to the brain, describing its role as a centre not only of perception, thought and bodily motion, but also of emotions and judgements, and it is due to malfunctions in the brain that madness and other mental disorders occur (see further Lo Presti 2008):

> Men ought to know that from the brain, and from the brain only, arise our pleasures, joys, laughter and jests, as well as our sorrows, pains, griefs and tears. Through it, in particular, we think, see, hear, and distinguish the ugly from the beautiful, the bad from the good, the pleasant from the unpleasant . . . It is the same thing which makes us mad or delirious, inspires us with dread and fear, whether by night or by day, brings us sleeplessness, . . .
>
> —*On the Sacred Disease* 14; translation Jones 1923b: 175[8]

The theory is worked out in considerable detail, especially in connection with the causes of epilepsy, and there are specific similarities to Alcmaeon's and Diogenes' views noted above. In particular, it is external air, flowing first to the brain through respiration, that enables the brain to discharge its various functions:

> I hold that the brain is the most powerful organ of the human body, for when it is healthy it is an interpreter to us of the phenomena caused by the air, as it is the air that gives it intelligence. Eyes, ears, tongue, hands and feet act in accordance with the discernment of the brain; in fact the whole body participates in intelligence in proportion to its participation in air. To consciousness the brain is the messenger. For when a man draws breath (pneuma) into himself, the air first reaches the brain, and so is dispersed through the rest of the body, though it leaves in the brain its quintessence, and all that it has of intelligence and sense.
>
> —*On the Sacred Disease* 16; translation Jones 1923b: 179

The author's interest in the brain here is of course stimulated by his aim of explaining the cause of epilepsy, which is attributed generally to phlegm blocking the proper motion of air through the brain to the appropriate parts of the body.

There was a sustained tradition in the fifth century BCE, then, which linked the brain closely with the functioning of the senses, but also with thought and emotion, and which moreover saw respiration and the inhalation of air as the mediating process by which these various functions were activated and maintained. However, there is little evidence of this tradition having any significant impact in medical circles in the fourth century BCE, though it was to be picked up again in certain respects later (see below). Rather, what information we have for theoretical medicine in the fourth century BCE seems to be generally more cardiocentric in its perspective, perhaps under a certain amount of Aristotelian influence. Two prominent physicians, Diocles of Carystus and Praxagoras of Cos, whose careers date probably to the mid- to later fourth century, appear to have been more interested in processes associated with the heart. The most important text for these physicians' views on issues to do with the mind is a much later treatise *On Acute and Chronic Diseases*, written apparently around the second century CE, by an unknown author referred to as the Anonymus Parisinus, and there are peculiar difficulties in assessing its reliability (van der Eijk 1999). One issue is that their views tend to be elided to a considerable extent, although we know that their theories were quite distinct, and it is not even clear whether Praxagoras, likely to be the later, even knew of Diocles' work (for Diocles, see van der Eijk 2000–2001; for Praxagoras' physiology, Lewis 2017). But the Anonymus Parisinus clearly attributes to both the idea that various capacities suffer impairment when there are blockages, in and around the heart, of the important airy substance in the body known as pneuma, which was thought responsible for mediating all sorts of bodily functions, such as sensation, thinking and motion, as we saw above in *On the Sacred Disease*. Here is the report on the cause of epilepsy:

> Praxagoras says that (epilepsy) arises in the thick artery (i.e. aorta) when phlegmatic humours collect in it. These bubble up and close off the passage of the psychic pneuma from the heart, and so agitate the body and cause spasm. When the bubbles subside again the affection stops. Diocles also thinks that there is an obstruction in the same area, and that the rest happens in the same way that Praxagoras says it occurs.
>
> —Anonymus Parisinus, *On Acute and Chronic Diseases*
> 3.1.1–2 = fragment 98 in the collection in van der Eijk 2000–2001,
> and fragment 25 in Lewis 2017

This and other doxographical sources additionally assert that each doctor located the soul or its basic functions, such as reason, in the heart (e.g. Anonymus Parisinus, *On Acute Diseases* 1.1.2–3 and 5.1; Athenaeus, *Deipnosophists* 15, 687d–688c; Tertullian, *On the Soul* 15).[9] The extent to which Diocles and Praxagoras actually went so far as to claim the heart as the seat of reason or of the soul, however, or whether such views were later elaborations or inferences from original comments about the causes of disorders that were regarded as 'mental', is not entirely clear, and certain aspects of their claimed beliefs have certainly been 'updated' using anachronistic theories and terminology (balanced discussion in van der Eijk 1999; van der Eijk 2001: xv–xvii; and Lewis 2017: 275–98). But there is a clear sense in which the heart, as opposed to the brain, is being privileged as a site of major functional significance in human physiology. An airy, pneumatic substance also seems to remain the most important medium for these central functions.

DISSECTION AND THE NERVOUS SYSTEM

Herophilus of Chalcedon (see Figure 7.3) was a Greek physician working in Alexandria in the early third century BCE. He is most famous for his anatomical discoveries, based at least in part on his dissection, and vivisection, of human beings. He gave a minutely detailed anatomical description of the human body, though only very meagre fragments from his *Anatomica* have survived, along with some general reports of individual findings, especially from Galen. Yet it is clear that his anatomy of the brain, with his distinction between its major features, including its four ventricles, marked a sea change in knowledge of its structure (von Staden 1989: 155–61 and 247–59). Of the four ventricles, he apparently assigned that in the cerebellum the greatest functional importance (von Staden 1989, testimony 138). Probably his most significant contribution, at least from a modern perspective, was his identification of the nervous system as

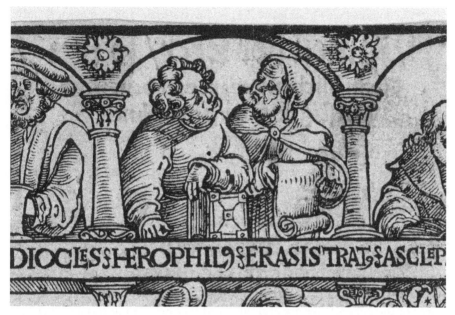

DIOCLES§HEROPHIL9§ERASISTRAT9§ASCLEP

FIGURE 7.3: Detail of a woodcut depicting the Hellenistic physicians Herophilus and Erasistratus, 1532. Herophilus and Erasistratus are both known for their anatomical work. The Wellcome Library, London. Courtesy of Wellcome Images.

a distinct structure within the human body, and his discovery that it is responsible for mediating sensation and voluntary motion (Solmsen 1961; von Staden 1989: 159–60). The pneuma drawn into the body through respiration was the medium by which these sensory and motor functions were transmitted through the nervous system (von Staden 1989: 257 and 2000: 89, with Leith 2020). His anatomical demonstration that the nerves have their origin in the brain (either directly, or indirectly via the spinal cord), together with these physiological findings, have been celebrated as a striking anticipation of the findings of modern neuroscience (hence it has seemed surprising that ancient philosophers and doctors failed to follow up properly on such an obvious scientific advancement).

Herophilus' younger contemporary Erasistratus of Ceos built on his discovery of the nervous system, developing a physiological theory that was founded on the interaction between three basic systems, the arterial, venous and nervous (Harris 1973: 195–233; Garofalo 1988: 22–58; Vallance 1990: 62–79; von Staden 2000: 92–6; Leith 2015b). Erasistratus, likewise drawing on his dissection and vivisection of both animals and humans, believed that each system had its own origin, unique fluid content, and distinct functions: the arterial system originated in the heart's left ventricle and naturally contained only 'vital' pneuma; the venous originated in the heart's right ventricle and naturally contained only blood; and the nervous system had its source apparently in the brain's meninges, and contained only what our sources call 'psychic' pneuma. The arterial system was responsible for basic physiological functions such as digestion, the venous system for transmitting nutriment as blood, and the nervous system for transmitting voluntary motion and perception, following Herophilus. We have more detailed knowledge of how Erasistratus believed pneuma mediated these functions than we do for Herophilus: pneuma inhaled in respiration was drawn firstly into the lungs, where it went through an initial process of refinement as it passed to the heart. From there, it was pumped by the heart throughout the arterial system, and some thereby sent via the carotid arteries to the meninges of the brain, where it underwent a second process of refinement. It was thus transformed into the form of pneuma required for transmitting sensation and voluntary motion as it spread throughout the entire nervous system. There are conflicting reports in our sources, with most testimonia privileging the brain's meninges (i.e. the *pia* and *dura mater*) as the origin of the nerves and the site of key processes, whereas Galen claims that Erasistratus changed his mind later in life, and named the brain itself as the source of the nerves.[10] We are also informed that Erasistratus thought that the brain matter, like that of other organs such as the liver and spleen, was a kind of fatty or fleshy substance distinct from the three systems of arteries, veins and nerves: he labelled this substance '*parenchuma* of nutriment' (from the Greek verb *parencheō*, to 'pour in alongside').

At some point later, all this complex physiological speculation, both medical and philosophical, came to be viewed through the conceptual lens of the so-called *hēgemonikon*, or 'ruling part' of the soul. This was in origin a Stoic concept, which envisaged the soul as having a single, localized command centre which oversaw and managed all its activities throughout the rest of the body. The fully developed theory is associated especially with the Stoic philosopher Chrysippus of Soli (*c.* 280/276–*c.* 208/204 BCE; for Chrysippus' psychology, see Tieleman 1996). Thus sensations had to be transmitted to the centre in order to be registered and to generate responses. Speech, conveying rational discourse, had to emanate from this command centre, as well as whatever was transmitted by the sperm in reproduction. This was all made possible, for the Stoics, by their view that the soul was made of pneuma, a unified, corporeal substance spread throughout the body and rendering it a cohesive and functional whole.

But there is little reason to suppose that Herophilus and Erasistratus had anything like such a conception of the soul, nor in particular the idea of its having a central command centre located in a particular place. As I have suggested above, there is good reason to believe that they never integrated any definite theory of the soul or its functioning at all into their medical system. Nevertheless, once the concept of the *hēgemonikon* had been put on the map, it seemed such an obvious one to later generations of doctors and philosophers that they believed their predecessors must have had an answer to the question of where it was located. Hence we find the widespread claim, prominently in the so-called *Placita* tradition of doxographical writings, that Herophilus located the command centre in the base of the brain, and that Erasistratus pinpointed it in the brain's membranes or meninges, i.e. the *dura* and *pia mater* (Aetius, *Placita* 4.5; see Mansfeld 1989 and 1990: 3092–108).[11] These reports have strongly contributed to the current and prevalent belief that Herophilus and Erasistratus had established, on grounds that we might recognize as scientific, that the brain has more or less the functions that we now attribute to it. But there are serious risks of anachronism in taking these reports concerning the *hēgemonikon* at face value: they imply all sorts of assumptions about the nature of the soul and the mind in particular that we have no reason to suppose Herophilus and Erasistratus entertained (for fuller discussion, see Leith 2020). One might insist that the idea of Herophilus and Erasistratus postulating a *hēgemonikon* in the area of the brain is not *too* distortive; after all, the brain, or its meninges, was undoubtedly a crucial site in the systems of both doctors, and they certainly believed that the pneuma, derived from respiration, once in the brain became the substance by which sensation and voluntary motion were mediated. But the idea of the brain as a command centre running the whole soul goes far beyond their attested interests, and distracts significantly from their evident attempt to explain human physiology as a unified and coherent body-wide system, spanning multiple organs and structures. Indeed, their interests seem to have been focused in particular on the body's *vessels*, and the connections and interactions between parts of the body that they enabled. There is no sign that they were interested in explaining more complex cognitive functions, such as thinking and emotions. Other core psychic functions had their origins in the – no less crucial – organ of the heart. The origin of the nerves in the brain or its meninges does not seem, for them, to have had comprehensive consequences for the understanding of the mind.

It may well also be significant that Herophilus' and Erasistratus' neurophysiology was generally speaking *not* taken by their medical and philosophical successors as evidence that the brain had a special psychic or mental role. The Stoics, or at least the vast majority of them, continued to hold that their *hēgemonikon* was located in the heart; the Epicureans were never dissuaded from locating the rational part of the soul in the area of the thorax; and later Aristotelians such as Alexander of Aphrodisias, in his *De Anima*, continued to maintain that the best evidence clearly favours the heart as a central organ for the soul's various faculties, nutritive/reproductive, perceptive and motive.

It was not just philosophers, but doctors too, who did not interpret Herophilus' discoveries as compelling evidence regarding the seat of the mind. After the third century BCE, and the introduction of the Stoic analysis, the concept of the *hēgemonikon* became central to the discourse on the soul. Asclepiades of Bithynia, the earliest major Greek medical authority to be based in Rome, around 100 BCE, developed a medical system derived from Epicurean atomism, positing imperceptible corpuscles as the basic elements of the universe (Vallance 1990; Casadei 1997; Leith 2009 and 2012). For him, health is preserved when these are allowed to move in a balanced and natural way within the human body, while disease occurs when they gather and obstruct each other in its different parts. He was also deeply influenced by the work of Herophilus and especially Erasistratus, and of course keen to criticize what he identified as their errors. They were evidently the principal medical authorities with whom he had to engage. Yet Asclepiades rejected outright the idea of a localized command centre, whether in the brain or the heart (see Polito 2006 for detailed discussion of Asclepiades' psychology). He pointed to the behaviour of bees and locusts, for example, which continue to defend themselves even after they have been decapitated. Similarly, crocodiles and tortoises will lash out after their hearts have been removed (Calcidius, *Commentary on Plato's Timaeus* 216; Tertullian, *On the Soul* 15).[12] For Asclepiades, the fact that the soul's functions could be discharged in the absence of these organs, even if only for a short time, showed that there is no command centre located in a specific part. He also denied that the nerves were responsible for transmitting sensation, believing that the soul, made of extremely fine, smooth and round corpuscles, and diffused throughout the body, received sense-stimuli directly (Leith 2009: 300–5). In fact, he was apparently the first doctor since the Hippocratic treatise *On Regimen* to develop a fully fledged theory of the soul.

Asclepiades' younger contemporary Athenaeus of Attaleia, a pupil of the famous Stoic philosopher Posidonius of Apamea, based his medical theory by contrast on the principles of Stoicism. The Stoic pneuma was for him the key to conceptualizing health: disease was brought about when this pneuma suffered excessively from the elemental qualities hot, cold, wet and dry, whether from external sources, such as the hot sun, or internally, from ingested drugs or poisons (Galen, *On Synectic Causes* 2).[13] Athenaeus was to follow the Stoic line on the question of the ruling part of the soul, locating it within the heart (see Galen, *On the Therapeutic Method* 13.21). It is not clear whether he felt that this was compatible with Herophilus' tracing of the origin of the nerves to the brain, but he may well have done, given that the Stoic Chrysippus, in the third century BCE, had certainly argued that the fact that the nerves originate in the brain need not show that the *hēgemonikon* must also be located there (see Galen, *On the Opinions of Hippocrates and Plato* 2.5.69–70, edition: de Lacy 1978–1984: 140).

'HIPPOCRATES' AND PLATO

It is striking, then, that what we regard as the groundbreaking work of Herophilus and Erasistratus on the brain and the nervous system did not lead to any straightforward conclusions that the brain must be the seat of the mind, either in the philosophical or medical traditions. Another perhaps surprising feature of the history of this debate is that there was indeed a prominent medical tradition which privileged the brain as the location of basic mental functions, but it was not obviously linked with the discovery of the nervous system. This was the tradition that Hippocrates had located the mind in the brain. This will have had its basis, in part, in the treatise *On the Sacred Disease*, discussed above, which could, in the Hellenistic period, be unproblematically attributed to Hippocrates (though of course we have no good reason to believe that he was indeed its author). During the third century BCE, probably in Alexandria, the Hippocratic Corpus started to be assembled, and a whole range of treatises were attributed to the historical figure Hippocrates of Cos, which in turn permitted inferences about his life to be made using details mentioned in those texts. An inventive biographical tradition grew up around him, incorporating various legends and stories, and a host of pseudepigraphic writings, such as epistolary exchanges between him and the Persian court, or the philosopher Democritus, as we shall see below. Interestingly, however, the tradition that Hippocrates placed the mind in the brain is principally grounded, not in explicit references to *On the Sacred Disease* or other treatises, but in assimilating Hippocrates' views to those of other philosophers, in particular Plato and Democritus, as prominent upholders of the brain as the higher psychic organ.

The so-called *Placita* tradition, which attributed to Herophilus and Erasistratus the views discussed above regarding the location of the *hēgemonikon*, likewise assigns one to Hippocrates, Plato and Democritus as a trio: 'Hippocrates, Democritus and Plato said that this (i.e. the *hēgemonikon*) is located in the brain' (Aetius, *Placita* 4.5.1). A pseudo-Galenic treatise, *Introduction or 'The Doctor'*, probably dating to the later second century CE, draws a similar picture of agreement between Hippocrates and Plato, and fills in some more detail:

> (The brain) is a simple body and for this reason the governing and most powerful of the parts in us. Therefore they entrust the *hēgemonikon* part of the soul to it, as do Plato and Hippocrates. It is surrounded by two membranes. One is next to it and adheres to it, called choroid, and it is more venous. The other lies on top of this one and is attached rather to the cranium in certain parts, and is more nervous.
>
> —Pseudo-Galen, *Introduction or 'The Doctor'* 11.2[14]

A report on the causes of phrenitis found in a treatise *On Acute and Chronic Diseases* by the so-called Anonymus Parisinus, referred to above, is more allusive, but evidently reflects the same tradition:

> Hippocrates says that the mind (*nous*) is placed in the brain, like a holy statue in the acropolis of the body, and that it uses as nutriment the blood in

the choroid membrane. When this (blood?) is corrupted by bile, it also deprives the nourished part of its own faculty. For if something's ordered and natural motion is thinking, its disordered and unnatural (motion) will be derangement.

—Anonymus Parisinus, *On Acute and Chronic Diseases*
1.1.4, edition Garofalo 1997: 2

In the extant Hippocratic Corpus, no such simile comparing the mind to a holy statue, or the body to an acropolis, is to be found. However, it clearly recalls, albeit inexactly, Plato's description in his *Timaeus* of the head as the body's acropolis, housing the rational soul (*Timaeus* 70a; see Mansfeld 1990: 3105 n. 202). It may be noted that the image attributed to Hippocrates brings out more clearly the notion of the mind's divinity, though not of its location as a vantage-point from which commands can be issued. Also striking is the reference to the choroid membrane in pseudo-Galen and the Anonymus Parisinus, as provider of blood as nutriment to the brain. This is a very rare means of describing the *pia mater* (normally, after Herophilus, called the 'thin membrane', *leptē meninx*), and again it is not to be found in the surviving treatises of the Hippocratic Corpus. These texts appear to be drawing on an earlier doxographical tradition, one which evidently took it that Hippocrates and Plato were basically on the same page as regards the soul's ruling part, and hence that various statements could be attributed to Hippocrates without the need for explicit confirmation in the Corpus itself. There is no suggestion of any divergence in their views here, implying deeper agreement on issues such as the distinction between the rational and irrational soul, and perhaps on the immortality and incorporeality of the soul as well.

A related association with Democritus is found in the collection of pseudepigraphic Hippocratic *Letters*, composed at some point in the Hellenistic period. In *Letter* 23, one of a series of letters concerned with the Abderite philosopher, Democritus himself writes to Hippocrates setting out his views on the nature of the human being, clearly promoting the significance of his ideas for Hippocratic thought (see Figure 7.4).[15] Specifically, Democritus tells Hippocrates that 'the brain stands guard at the summit of the body, entrusted with its safety, housed in nervous membranes, over which the natures of twin bones, fitted together by necessity, protect the brain as lord and sentinel of the mind (*dianoia*)' (Pseudo-Hippocratic *Letters* 23). The influence of the Platonic background becomes even clearer when Democritus comes to claim the heart as the 'nurse of anger', and the liver as 'the cause of appetite (*epithumiē*)' (Pseudo-Hippocratic *Letters* 23). In fact, the real Democritus appears to have believed that the soul, made up of a complex of spherical atoms, discharged its functions *as a whole*, and never made any functional distinctions between its parts, or located a ruling part in a specific organ. The account from the *Placita*

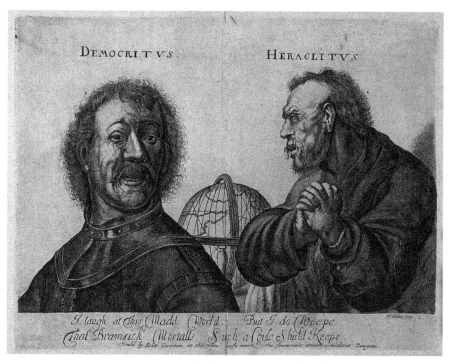

FIGURE 7.4: Democritus laughing and Heraclitus weeping. The story of the philosopher Democritus laughing incessantly is told in the Hippocratic *Letters*. Engraving by W. Hollar after J. van Vliet after Rembrandt, mid-seventeenth century. The caption reads 'I laugh at this madd world. But I do weepe that brainsick mortals such a coyle should keepe'. The Wellcome Library, London. Courtesy of Wellcome Images.

may be even more distortive in placing Democritus alongside Plato as an upholder of the brain as the seat of the mind than with the inclusion of Hippocrates. So Platonic psychology provided the dominant theory, and both Hippocrates and Democritus came to be assimilated to it. Of course, Plato famously had mentioned Hippocrates on two occasions in his dialogues, with Socrates at one point approving Hippocrates' holistic approach to understanding the body, adding some credibility to the assimilation (Plato, *Protagoras* 311b–c and especially *Phaedrus* 270c–e).[16] But what is interesting in this doxographical tradition is that, while *On the Sacred Disease* undoubtedly lies somewhere in the background, the emphasis is on situating Hippocrates within a better known, philosophical tradition on the mind.

So the potential sources of information about Hippocrates' views were extremely diffuse, and ideas drawn from various thinkers could plausibly be associated with his in different ways. But it is notable that there is little sign that

Herophilus and Erasistratus were implicated in this tradition. One might have expected that the medical discovery that the nervous system issues from the brain could have been retrojected onto Hippocrates and folded into the doxographical tradition on his encephalocentrism. This is certainly the strategy which Galen was to adopt, as we shall see shortly. But the tradition of a Platonic Hippocrates situating the mind in the brain was for a long time kept separate from the anatomical tradition stemming from Herophilus and Erasistratus' work, which traced the origin of the nerves, and their role in sensation and voluntary motion, to the brain or its meninges. We may note that, for Erasistratean doctors working in Galen's time, Hippocrates had no anatomical authority whatsoever. In one of his encounters with an Erasistratean named Martialis, for example, Galen records that

> when he (i.e. Martialis) learned that I praised Hippocrates, he announced that Hippocrates was not at all a subject of anatomical study for him, and he declared the superiority of Erasistratus in all areas of the art, but especially in this.
>
> —Galen, *On My Own Books* 1.9–10[17]

Looking back from the later Hellenistic and Roman periods, it appears to have been assumed that there were a limited set of possible views concerning the mind and its location. These views often tended to be simplified, boiled down to fundamental organs such as the brain or heart. Those with apparently similar views could then be lumped together, and their views elided, a process especially clear in the assimilation of Hippocrates' views to Platonic psychology. Medical theories connected with the mind were complex and varied, however, with some doctors refusing to grant it a specific location, others focusing on the heart, while others were reluctant to engage with the issue in detail at all, restricting themselves within a medical context to the functioning of the body as a whole organism. Different doctors had very different preoccupations and concerns when they touched on issues to do with the mind, and there is little sign of substantial areas of common ground between them, not even in connection with the discovery of the nervous system.

GALEN

All of this forms at least part of the background to Galen's medical education. Galen learned medicine and forged his career at a time when anatomy was very much in vogue. During his lengthy education, he spent much time travelling to various sites, including Smyrna, Corinth and Alexandria, trying to track down the most authoritative anatomists of the age (Galen, *On Anatomical Procedures* 1.1, K2.217–18).[18] His anatomical demonstrations in Rome were to contribute considerably to the notice taken in his career by the rich and powerful. It was also a time in which the Hippocratic Corpus was receiving renewed attention (Smith 1979: 234–40). The question of which texts within the Corpus were to be attributed to Hippocrates himself, which to his immediate circle, and which to other unrelated doctors, was under intense scrutiny. This also had obvious consequences for the question of what Hippocrates' genuine doctrines were, and Galen was highly critical of certain contemporaries, including his teachers, for what he regarded as their misinterpretations of the Hippocratic truth.

In a certain sense, Galen's medical project fundamentally sought to combine these two strands, Hippocrates and anatomy, into a philosophically coherent system, and the question of the soul and the mind was a key component of this. Herophilus' discovery of the nervous system and its origin in the brain was for Galen an indisputable scientific fact, and he himself was to make additional discoveries. But Galen believed that the discovery of the nervous system and its functions offered much more, including proof of one of the main planks of Plato's conception of the soul, namely that, as we have seen, the rational soul is located in the brain. Galen argues his position comprehensively in his work *On the Opinions of Hippocrates and Plato*, where the Stoic opposition are targeted mercilessly (Hankinson 1991b; Tieleman 1996; Gill 2010). As that title suggests, of course, the underlying motivation for this demonstration was to show, not only that Plato was correct, and could be proven scientifically to be so, but also that he had in fact been anticipated by Hippocrates. Hence Galen's goal was to merge the contemporary anatomical cutting edge on the one hand with the authority of Hippocrates on the other, who had a longstanding association with Plato in regard to the brain's psychic primacy. Galen himself presents this as an innovation on his part, and indeed we have no earlier surviving evidence for anyone arguing that Plato had learned his psychology from Hippocrates. But the close association of their views on these matters was already well established, as we have seen.

But what is particularly interesting is that Galen nowhere explicitly points to *On the Sacred Disease* as a Hippocratic source text for the view that the brain is the seat of the mind; he generally just takes it as read as a well-known Hippocratic view. In fact, Galen hardly acknowledges the existence of *On the Sacred Disease* at all, and never as authentically by Hippocrates (Jouanna 2003: cxiii–cxiv). Part of the reason for this is no doubt connected with the inaccurate anatomical descriptions found within the treatise, such as the description of the two large blood vessels in the body, one of which originates in the liver, the other in the spleen (*On the Sacred Disease* 3). One of Galen's main commitments was that Hippocrates had a detailed and accurate knowledge of human anatomy, and he wrote a treatise in six books to prove it, *On Hippocrates' Anatomy*, which unfortunately has not survived (Galen, *On My Own Books* 1.9–10). Another problem for Galen would have been the text's location in the brain, not only of rational functions, but also of the emotions, which he, Galen, was determined to locate in the heart, in line with Plato (Tieleman 1996: xxxii–xxxvi). Yet Galen may well have been relying on the apparently renowned tradition of Hippocrates' quasi-Platonic psychology, outlined above. Even if this tradition ultimately had its origins in *On the Sacred Disease*, Galen may have been able to take it for granted without appealing to that text explicitly. So we seem to have the paradoxical situation of Galen wishing to invoke Hippocrates' brain-centred psychology, while being apparently unwilling to make reference to specific passages in the Hippocratic Corpus for support.

Galen's own understanding of the brain and its function was far more sophisticated than anything found in the Hippocratic or Platonic corpora, based as it was on the developments introduced by Herophilus and Erasistratus, and the up-to-date anatomical traditions of his own day. His physiology of the brain focused on its ventricular cavities, especially the fourth ventricle (like Herophilus), as sites in which the (once again) all-important psychic pneuma was collected and distributed to the appropriate vessels, namely the sensory and motor nerves (Rocca 2003). Hence he rejected Erasistratus' focus on the brain's meninges. He developed a range of detailed experiments on the brain intended to demonstrate that loss of sensation and motor function results directly from incisions into the ventricles, concluding that this must be due to the escape of the requisite mediating pneuma; functions could be restored when the pneuma, as he believed, was allowed to replenish itself (Rocca 2003, especially chapters 5 and 6). The pneuma reached the brain's ventricles after being elaborated and refined in the retiform and choroid plexuses, complex vascular structures which receive pneuma from the lungs and heart via the arterial system. Some pneuma also goes directly to the brain's ventricles from the nostrils via the olfactory tracts (Rocca 2003: 219–37; Dean-Jones 2006).

Although Galen remained self-confessedly agnostic as to the precise nature and substance of the soul itself, his anatomical findings and the logical demonstrations built upon them left him convinced that the soul's rational functions (sensation and voluntary motion, but also thought, imagination, memory, recollection, knowledge, etc) must have their origin in the brain. In line with Plato's tripartition of the soul, he also located the non-rational 'spirited' part of the soul, and the emotions, in the heart, and the 'desiderative' soul, associated with appetites and desires, in the abdomen, specifically the liver in Galen's view. For these locations, Galen felt able to refer to a specific text in the Hippocratic Corpus, namely *Epidemics* 2, though it requires something of a leap of faith to read the relevant passages as advocating anything like the Platonic tripartition.[19] Just as the brain was the source of the nervous system, so the heart and liver were the sources of the arterial and venous systems respectively. Knowledge of the soul's tripartition, Galen felt, was important not only for medicine, since the doctor must understand the basic physiological processes which the soul governs in the different parts of the body, but also for ethics, in that it is crucial to understanding the conflict within the soul between its various rational and irrational parts. Not so, however, for topics such as the substance of the soul or its immortality, which are the domain only of theoretical philosophy and which, as we have noted, Galen also felt were beyond scientific demonstration. The fact, then, that anatomical knowledge was so important in establishing theses central to psychology, not only from a medical perspective, but also from a more straightforwardly philosophical and ethical one, perhaps in part explains Galen's unusual interests in the ethical sphere. Unlike any other known ancient physician, he published widely on ethical topics, and his treatise *The Capacities of the Soul Depend on the Mixtures of the Body*, for example, emphasizes the relevance of medical knowledge in such contexts (see further Singer et al 2013). With all this, Galen was not only claiming expertise in areas traditionally regarded as philosophical rather than medical, but also claiming an originally medical heritage for significant parts of the most authoritative philosophers' views. In regard to the brain and the structure of the soul, Galen forcefully argued that medical knowledge, especially anatomical, offered proof that some of the most influential psychological and ethical traditions, especially the Stoics', were simply wrong; but he also wanted to show that those which were thereby vindicated, in particular Plato's, had been anticipated by a physician, namely Hippocrates. Medicine, with its privileged authority on the body, was not a discipline subordinate to natural science, as Herophilus and Erasistratus apparently believed, but was key to determining whatever useful can be said about the soul and the mind at all.

CONCLUSIONS

Graeco-Roman medical interest in the brain, then, was motivated by a diverse range of interests, and generated an equally diverse range of observations and hypotheses. There was no unified medical tradition on the mind, but rather a range of competing and incompatible approaches to a huge variety of problems. From a modern perspective, the discovery of the nervous system was of course to have a decisive impact, and Herophilus' work on the brain is particularly celebrated as one of the most important aspects of his medical career. But in antiquity the picture was more complex, and his fame rested on much more than his groundbreaking anatomy. While there is little evidence of anyone denying his identification of the sensory and motor functions of the nervous system and its origin in the brain, it was not widely held to have far-reaching consequences for understanding the soul or mind in general, especially among philosophers. Even in Galen's hands, where the anatomy and physiology of the nervous system was crucial to demonstrating his view that the rational soul is located in the brain, its significance for him was at least partly to do with the picture he wished to paint of Hippocratic-Platonic harmony. The role of ancient authorities such as Hippocrates had a sustained and significant influence on the way that problems were formulated and approached. Often the focus was not just upon developing new theories, but also on reinterpreting, whether consciously or unconsciously, the writings of earlier authorities in light of the current state of knowledge. Within this, there was also a tendency to over-emphasize agreement between such authorities and to elide differences: the example of Plato and Hippocrates is a striking one in this particular field, well established long before Galen. Often this was used by individuals as a way of bolstering their own authority against rival, and therefore polarized, views. Given that much of the corpus of ancient medical writings is now lost to us, these tendencies can have a disproportionately distortive effect on our understanding of the complexity and variety of perspectives that were on offer.

NOTES

1. This and all citations hereafter are from the Loeb Classical Library edition by Bury (1929).
2. This and all citations hereafter are from the Loeb Classical Library edition by Peck and Forster (1937).
3. This and all citations hereafter of Galen's *On the Therapeutic Method* are to the Loeb Classical Library edition by Johnston and Horsley (2011).
4. This citation is from the Corpus Medicorum Graecorum edition by Bendz (1990–1993). For an English translation, see Drabkin (1950).
5. This and all citations hereafter are from the edition by Waszink (1947).
6. This citation is from the Teubner edition by Mutschmann (1914). For an English translation, see Bett (2005).
7. This and all citations hereafter are from the edition by Diels (1879). For Alcmaeon's location of the ruling part of the soul in the brain, see Aetius, *Placita* 4.17.1, which cites the same view concerning the mechanics of smelling as in Theophrastus, and Aetius, *Placita* 5.17.3.
8. This and all citations hereafter are from the Collection des Universités de France edition by Jouanna (2003). An English translation by Jones (1923b) is available in the Loeb Classical Library.
9. This citation of Athenaeus is from the Loeb Classical Library edition by Olson (2012).
10. For the meninges see e.g. Galen, *On the Use of Respiration* 5.1, K4.502; Galen, *On the Opinions of Hippocrates and Plato* 7.3.32–33, edition: de Lacy 1978–1984: 446; Aetius, *Placita* 4.5; for his change of mind, Galen, *On the Opinions of Hippocrates and Plato* 7.3.6–12, edition: de Lacy 1978–1984: 440–2; cf. Leith 2020.
11. This and all citations hereafter are from the edition by Diels (1979).
12. This citation of Calcidius is from the edition by Waszink (1975).
13. This citation of Galen's *On Synectic Causes* is from the Corpus Medicorum Graecorum edition by Lyons (1969).

14. This citation is from the Collection des Universités de France edition by Petit (2009).
15. This and all citations hereafter are from the Brill edition by Smith (1990).
16. This citation of Plato's *Protagoras* is from the Loeb Classical Library edition by Lamb (1924). This citation of Plato's *Phaedrus* is from the Loeb Classical Library edition by Fowler (1914).
17. This citation is from the Collection des Universités de France edition by Boudon-Millot (2007).
18. This citation is from the second volume of Kühn's edition abbreviated as 'K2'.
19. See *Epidemics* 2.5.16 (citation from the Loeb Classical Library edition by Smith 1994), on the heart, and *Epidemics* 2.4.1, on the liver; cf. Galen, *On the Opinions of Hippocrates and Plato* 6.8.45–7, 59–66 (edition: de Lacy 1978–1984: 416, 420).

Authority

LAURENCE TOTELIN

INTRODUCTION

The satirist Lucian of Samosata (second century CE), in his short diatribe *The Ignorant Book Collector*, compared the illiterate man who accumulated expensive books to various other impostors, and especially to the quack doctors, whose fancy instruments (see Figure 8.1) did not compensate for their lack of skill:

> Don't you know that the most ignorant among the doctors do exactly the same as you: they buy ivory cases, silver cupping glasses and gold-inlaid surgical knives, but when the time has come to use them, they do not even know how to handle them. They have to give place to one of the learned [doctors], whose lancet is well sharpened, even though it is rusty, and who immediately sets free the sufferer from their pain.
>
> —Lucian, *The Ignorant Book Collector* 29[1]

What distinguished a good doctor from a bad one in Lucian's view was the possession of knowledge; expensive equipment was a luxury that did not necessarily help the patient. Ancient medical texts insist on the importance of acquiring knowledge and wisdom before practising the art (see for instance the Hippocratic texts *The Law* 4 and *On Decorum* 1–2).[2] Determining the legitimacy of medical knowledge in the ancient world, however, was no simple matter. There were no formal medical qualifications; there were no official granting bodies that conferred the title of physician on people who had studied medicine. A physician learnt his or her trade through apprenticeship with an

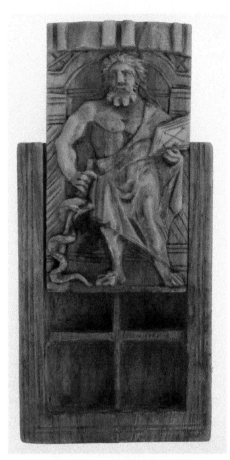

FIGURE 8.1: Ivory medicine box with six compartments, Roman, fifth century CE.
This case, which would have contained pharmacological preparations, has a sliding lid
with a representation of the god Asclepius holding a staff (with snake) in his right hand
and a book in his left hand. Treasure of the Cathedral of Chur, Switzerland.
© Rätisches Museum Chur.

established doctor, one who had authority (Nutton 2013: 70). That
apprenticeship could vary in length, and according to Galen (*On the Therapeutic
Method* 1.1), who may well have been exaggerating, Thessalus, a doctor of the
Methodist sect, promised to teach the art of medicine in six short months.[3] In
the first section of this chapter, I examine how ancient physicians (*iatroi* in
Greek) established their authority in such a context. I take the Hippocratic
Oath as my starting point, as it outlines the obligations of the new physician.[4]

The *Oath*, which is perhaps the most influential medical text produced in the
West, is preserved as part of the Hippocratic Corpus, a collection of some sixty
medical texts, ranging in date from the fifth century BCE to the first century CE.

While the name of Hippocrates, the famous physician of Cos, confers authority on this collection of texts, it is clear that he did not author all of them; it is even possible that he authored none of them. The link between authority and authorship in the transmission of medical knowledge is the topic of the second section of this chapter.

Most medical texts written in antiquity were composed by physicians. Physicians, however, were far from alone in practising healing in antiquity. Patients/consumers could also turn to root cutters, drug sellers, midwives, crowd gatherers, masseurs, witches, as well as the healing gods and their priests or priestesses – the list is far from exhaustive. The third section of this chapter is therefore devoted to the 'pluralism' of ancient medicine (Lloyd 2003: 41). Within that pluralistic landscape, patients had a central role to play, not only in finding the right healer, but also in caring for themselves. I turn to them in the final part of this chapter.

THE HIPPOCRATIC *OATH* AND THE ANCIENT PHYSICIAN'S AUTHORITY

The Hippocratic *Oath* (see Figure 8.2), probably composed in the late fifth or fourth century BCE, is without doubt one of the most famous medical texts of all times.[5] Nowadays, some medical schools, especially in the USA, still use a revised version for their students to swear at graduation or refer to the text in teaching (Dossabhoy et al 2018). In other words, the *Oath* is today one of the means through which some physicians establish their right to practice, their authority, by outlining their ethical principles. Two of the three famous prohibitions made in the *Oath* (the prohibition against giving deadly drugs; and that against giving women destructive pessaries – the third prohibition is that against cutting, especially for the stone) continue to inform ethical debates over euthanasia and abortion in the twenty-first century (see for instance Miles 2005). The interpretation of these prohibitions in the original *Oath*, however, is very much open to debate. In particular, one should ask whether these prohibitions are absolute or not (see e.g. Rütten and von Reppert-Bismarck 1996; Flemming 2005). Thus, were the people swearing the *Oath* supposed never to assist patients in suicide, or did they merely promise not to provide poison to people with murderous intent? Were they supposed never to carry out abortions, or simply abortions by means of pessaries, since the original version of the *Oath* specifies 'abortive pessaries'? Were they supposed to eschew all forms of surgery, or only the most complex ones? Certainly, at the time it was written, the principles of the *Oath* were far from universally accepted. The gynaecological treatises of the Hippocratic Corpus contain advice and various recipes on how to abort a foetus (see e.g. *On the Nature of the Child* 2); there are numerous ancient examples of medical suicide (examples in van Hooff

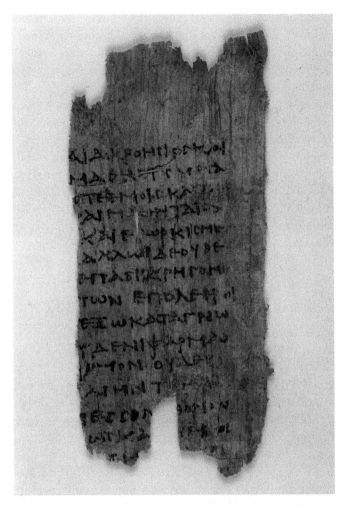

FIGURE 8.2: This papyrus, dated to the third century CE, is this earliest preserved copy of the Hippocratic Oath. It was found in Oxyrhynchus, a city in Middle Egypt where many Greek and Latin papyri were discovered. Instead of prohibiting abortive pessaries, it prohibits abortives more generally. Oxyrhynchus papyrus 2547, Wellcome Library Manuscript 5754. Courtesy of the Wellcome Library.

1990: 123–6);[6] and there is ample evidence that ancient physicians practised forms of surgery, as is indeed indicated in Lucian's passage which opens this chapter. Despite all the issues that surround its interpretation, the *Oath* is an excellent introduction to the question of how physicians acquired knowledge and authority in the ancient world.

The *Oath* starts with an invocation to the gods Apollo the Physician, Asclepius, Hygieia (Health) and Panacea, that is, the gods most associated with healing in the ancient world (Stafford 2004; Wickkiser 2008), but also to all other gods and goddesses, since they too had the power to heal when needed. While Hippocratic physicians are known for their mechanistic explanations of health and illness (seen respectively as balance and imbalance), they did not reject the authority of the gods in matters of healing. Ancient physicians regularly made dedications to Asclepius (Gorrini 2005); and they called themselves 'Asclepiads', the descendants of Asclepius (Edelstein and Edelstein 1945: 57). Thus, Plato in the *Protagoras* (311b) referred to Hippocrates of Cos as an Asclepiad.[7] In later antiquity, Galen on several occasions mentioned his devotion to Asclepius, the god who, in a dream, sent his father Nicias the message that he was meant for a career in medicine (*On the Order of My Own Books*, 4).[8]

After invoking the gods, the person who took the *Oath* swore to regard his teacher as equal to his parents (the gendering is male), to support this teacher in times of need, to consider his master's children as his own male siblings, and to teach them medicine for free and without written covenant, should they wish to learn it. What is described here is a typical ancient apprenticeship. In antiquity, apprenticeships involved a monetary transaction between apprentices (or their family) and masters: people did not learn the art of medicine for free unless they were the biological children of an established physician. Plato noted that Hippocrates of Cos took on paying students (*Protagoras* 311b–c). While the apprentice paid his master, he was also 'adopted' into his family, thus creating kinship links between people who were not blood relatives – a kinship that was inscribed in the name 'Asclepiads'. This intra-familial system of knowledge transmission gradually lost its prevalence in the ancient world, but never entirely disappeared: it is common to find families of physicians or other healers throughout antiquity (Nutton 1992: 19; Samama 2003: 62). One could also consider the ancient medical 'sects' (Greek *haireseis*), which first appeared in the Hellenistic period, to be analogous to very large families (see Leith 2016 for an introduction to these sects). It would have been natural for the son of an Empiricist, Methodist or Pneumatist to follow his father in his choice of sect. Galen obliquely alluded to this fact in the following passage:

> Doctors and philosophers admire other doctors and philosophers without having learnt their theories and practised their demonstrative method, which would allow them to distinguish between false arguments and true ones. It is simply the case that their father, or teacher, or friend or someone who was admired in their city happened to belong to the Empiricist sect, or Dogmatist or Methodist.
>
> —Galen, *On the Order of My Own Books* 1

In any case, throughout antiquity, finding the right master was important, as his name could be a guarantee of authority (Massar 2010)

The family-based system presented in the *Oath* aimed at preserving the medical *technē*, the medical art or craft, for the Hippocratic physicians was primarily an artisan. The word *technē* appears no fewer than four times in the short *Oath*, pointing to a strong desire on the part of its author to define medicine as a practical art, rather than a theoretical one (see von Staden 1996a: 411). *Technē*, a central notion in the philosophy of Plato and other classical philosophers, was distinct from *epistēmē*, knowledge, in that it required embodied practice (Cuomo 2007: 7–40). Medicine then had much in common with other *technai* such as pottery making, weaving, sculpting, farming, music playing and cookery.

Most *technai* in the classical world were transmitted orally; there is little written record on the transmission of the potter's art for instance. Medicine was no exception: it had been practised well before the adoption of the alphabet by the Greeks in the eighth century BCE, and the application of writing to philosophy in the sixth century BCE (for an introduction to Greek literacy, see Thomas 1992). Throughout antiquity, one could become a physician without being able to read and write, or with very limited literacy skills (Hanson 2010). On the other hand, physicians were among the first to make use of the prose written word to transmit their knowledge in the Greek world. The Hippocratic Corpus contains the earliest prose treatises fully preserved in Greek. (Some Presocratic philosophers wrote in prose, but only fragments of their works are preserved.) The Hippocratic *Oath* itself refers to a written covenant, which is necessary between a master and a new apprentice, but not between a master and members of his family (or quasi-family).

The act of writing allowed doctors to appropriate for themselves knowledge that may traditionally have belonged to other groups of healers, in particular in the case of the gynaecological texts, which constitute a significant portion of the Hippocratic Corpus (King 1998). Even so, literate physicians and philosophers expressed reservations as to the role that writing played in the transmission of medical knowledge. Plato, Aristotle and Xenophon all argued that one cannot learn medicine from books (Plato, *Phaedrus* 268c; Aristotle, *Nicomachean Ethics* 10.9, 1181b2–6; Xenophon, *Memorabilia* 4.2.10; see Totelin 2009: 246–7).[9] For the philosophers, writing was a poor substitute for the performative transmission of embodied practices. To these philosophical considerations, one could add more practical ones: texts in antiquity were copied by hand and were therefore subject to the vicissitudes of manuscript transmission. Unique copies of texts could get destroyed, as happened to Galen when several of his works were burnt in the Great Fire of Rome in 192 (*Avoiding Distress* 12–13).[10] Copyists could introduce mistakes when they reproduced a text. This is most noticeable in pharmacological texts such as recipes, where ingredients are omitted or are inadvertently substituted for others, and quantities are mistakenly given. Galen suggested writing recipes in verse to avoid errors, but also to help memory (see Totelin 2012b for references).

However much they criticized writing, physicians who were literate felt pride in their skill, to the point where it became common for them to be represented with their books on their funeral monuments (Hillert 1990: 94–7, 155–9). Thus, a sarcophagus from Ostia (near Rome) dating to the early fourth century CE bears a depiction of a doctor seated (the traditional position) reading an open scroll (see Figure 8.3). To his right is a cabinet that contains further book scrolls and a basin (perhaps to be used when bleeding patients). On top of the cabinet rests an open case of surgical instruments. The combination of those symbols (books and surgical instruments) signified the dual nature of the physician's art: theoretical and practical.

The type of medical practice advocated by the author of the *Oath* was one based on regimens: dietetic medicine, which is very prominent in the Hippocratic Corpus and in later medical texts. In the classical period, dietetic medicine, which encompassed food, sleep and dreams, exercise, sexual activity and other aspects of patients' lives, was relatively new and was still in search of recognition and authority. The comic playwright Aristophanes accused this type of medicine of being bookish and pedantic (*Frogs* 939–43; see Jouanna 2000);[11] Plato, in the *Republic* (406d–e), criticized dietetic medicine as being only affordable to the wealthy because it was time consuming.[12] A physician could easily abuse his position of authority when practising dietetic medicine, and that is perhaps why the *Oath* insisted that a doctor should keep his patient from harm, a principle repeated twice in this short text ('but from what is to their harm or injustice I will keep them'; 'I will go for the benefit of the ill, while being far from all voluntary and destructive injustice'). The famous exhortation 'do good or do not harm' (*primum non nocere*), however, is not to be found in the *Oath*, but rather in another Hippocratic text, *Epidemics* 1:

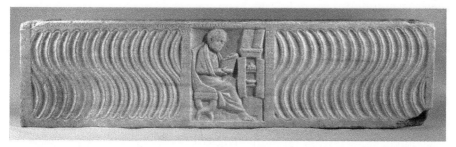

FIGURE 8.3: Marble sarcophagus of a physician from Ostia (near Rome), early fourth century CE. The physician is represented seated on a chair reading a papyrus scroll. Next to him is an open cupboard in which are stored further scrolls and a bowl. On top of the cupboard is a case containing surgical instruments. The Metropolitan Museum of Art, New York, accession number 48.76.1. Courtesy of the Metropolitan Museum of Art.

[The physician] must be able to tell the past circumstances, know the present ones and predict the future ones. He must attend to these. With regards to diseases, he must pay attention to two things, namely to help and at least to do no harm. The art involves three things: the disease, the patient and the physician. The physician is the servant of the art, and the sick must fight the disease with the physician.

—*Epidemics* 1.11[13]

This passage introduces us to a very important aspect of ancient medicine that is not discussed in the *Oath*: prognosis (see the 'classic' essay by Edelstein 1967: 65–85). Prognosis was the ability to predict the progression and outcome of the patient's illness, and as Vivian Nutton suggests (2013: 89), it 'incorporat[ed] what today would be termed obtaining the case history, diagnosis and prognosis'. As other passages of the Hippocratic Corpus make it clear, when physicians were skilled in the art of prognostication, they more easily gained the trust of patients – prognosis was a means to establish one's authority (*Prognostic* 1).[14] The converse was also true: a poor prognosticator would be derided by patients, as is expressed in the following passage from the Hippocratic treatise *Prorrhetic* 2:

I recommend you be as cautious as possible, not only in other areas of the medical *technē*, but also in such prognoses, knowing that when you succeed in making a prediction, you will be admired by the patient you are attending, but when you fail, you will not only be hated but perhaps even considered mad.

—*Prorrhetic* 2.2[15]

Several centuries later, Galen also placed great emphasis on prognosis, dedicating a treatise to examples of his own practice in the art: *On Prognosis*.[16] It is in this text that he recounted his first encounter with the emperor Marcus Aurelius (*On Prognosis* 11). Three doctors had already examined the emperor and taken his pulse and concluded that he was suffering from an incipient illness. The emperor, however, ordered Galen to examine him. Galen, through skilful pulse taking established that Marcus was suffering from indigestion and not from an incipient fever.

Good prognosis, then, was a means to establish one's authority while also avoiding doing harm to patients. This, however, raises the question of where the boundary between benefit and harm lies. Ancient physicians often accused their rivals of causing harm. Thus, the author of the Hippocratic text *On Diseases of Women* (1.34) criticized physicians (*iatroi*) for using astringents when swellings occur in the womb after childbirth.[17] The author of the Hippocratic treatise *On Joints* (chapter 42), for his part, berated those physicians (again, they are called *iatroi*), who attempted to straighten the spine of hunchbacked people by attaching them to a ladder, which was lifted off the ground by a system of pulleys, then dropped from a height.[18] This, he said, attracted gasping crowds but did not cure anyone. Further, the author of the Hippocratic tract *On Ancient Medicine* (chapter 9), when discussing the administration of food in illness, stated that 'I would praise strongly that physician who only makes small mistakes, for accuracy is seldom to be found'.[19] He then went on to compare the physician to the sailor, who can make mistakes when sailing on quiet seas without suffering consequences that are too severe, but whose ignorance is revealed in storms, when they lose their ships. Similarly, the bad doctors (and they were the majority) lose their patients to severe illnesses. He concluded that the 'punishment for each of them [the bad sailor and the bad doctor] follows swiftly'. Throughout antiquity, literate physicians continued to criticize their colleagues in writing, accusing them of being poor doctors. Galen wrote entire treatises refuting the theories and practices of his competitors (see for instance *Against Lycus; Against Julian*). In other words, physicians constructed their authority positively, by establishing their credentials, but also negatively, by deriding their rivals' lack of skills.

Good prognosis, then, led to good reputation, for which the *Oath* showed a deep concern. Indeed, the *Oath* closed with a promise of good repute for those who upheld it:

> If I render this oath fulfilled and if I do not blur and confound it making it to no effect, may it be granted to me to enjoy the benefits both of life and of *technē*, being held in good repute among all human beings for time eternal. If, however, I transgress and perjure myself the opposite of these.

It is the approval of fellow human beings, then, that motivated the swearer of the Hippocratic *Oath*, rather than any expectations of rewards in the afterlife (see von Staden 1996: 409).

To sum up, the *Oath* is an important introduction to several themes that are central to a study of authority in ancient medicine: family, *technē*, literacy and avoidance of harm. It is important to note, however, that it only gradually acquired its prominence. It is in the fourth century CE that we start to find firm evidence that it was sworn by new physicians, and certainly not by all of them; in fact, it might not have been sworn commonly until the sixteenth century (Nutton 1995b: 29). One did not need to swear the *Oath* to become accepted as a physician in the ancient world.

AUTHORSHIP AND AUTHORITY

The Hippocratic *Oath* is further relevant to a study of authority because its authorship is unknown. This text is preserved as part of the Hippocratic

Corpus, which as its name indicates is a collection of texts (around sixty) attributed to Hippocrates, the famous physician of Cos, active in the fifth century BCE. It is clear, however, that a single person could not have authored all these texts, as they sometimes contradict each other – not to mention the fact that they display pronounced stylistic differences. Since the Hellenistic period, and until recently, scholars have questioned which texts Hippocrates authored; which ones were penned by members of his family or circle; and which were unworthy of the great master (for a brief introduction, see Craik 2015: xx–xxiv; see also Smith 1979).

Until the twentieth century, the *Oath* was generally considered to be an authentic Hippocratic document, but the unusual character of the prohibitions included in this text led one prominent scholar, Ludwig Edelstein ([1943] 1967: 3–63), to argue that Pythagoreans had produced the text. Indeed, the followers of the philosopher Pythagoras (sixth century BCE) condemned any form of animal (and hence human) killing. This theory proved extremely influential outside the circle of historians of ancient medicine, for it informed the debates in *Roe* v. *Wade*, the landmark decision by the United States Supreme Court in 1973 that rendered unconstitutional state laws criminalizing or restricting access to abortion (410 US 113). Today, Edelstein's hypothesis has been discredited, and scholars have for the most part abandoned their quest to uncover the authentic Hippocratic treatises; nevertheless, the so-called 'Hippocratic question' still points to the complex link between authority and authorship in the transmission of medical knowledge in the ancient world.

Edelstein's theory was used in the *Roe* v. *Wade* case (Edelstein had passed away by 1973) to argue that one should not give too much credence to the *Oath* because it was a Pythagorean document. The case noted that the Pythagorean origin of the *Oath* 'is a satisfactory and acceptable explanation of the Hippocratic Oath's apparent rigidity. It enables us to understand, in historical context, a long-accepted and revered statement of medical ethics' (410 US 113, 131–2). This way of calling upon the authority (or lack thereof) of Hippocrates has a very long history. Indeed, throughout antiquity, and well beyond, medical authors invoked 'Hippocrates', or rather their own construction of Hippocrates, to justify their theories and practices. Most prominently, Galen often referred to the great master when he criticized his rivals and defended his own views, thereby positioning himself as a new Hippocrates. For instance, in the preface to his pharmacological treatise *On the Composition of Drugs according to Places*, he wrote:

And when they use the remedies which they have themselves written, many doctors not only act by chance, sometimes greatly, but they also cause a lot of damage, so that they make the condition incurable, in the same way as what happens to those who use these and many other remedies without method. As Hippocrates ordered, I have always attempted to act in the works of the art in order to offer help, as he has written: 'to help or at least not to harm'.

—*On the Composition of Drugs according to Places* 1, preface, K12.381; translation: Totelin 2012b, slightly modified[20]

In this paragraph, Galen contrasted his own practice, informed by the Hippocratic 'do no harm' principle, to that of physicians who work 'without method'. To Galen, Hippocrates was an authority figure, a concept defined as follows by Geoffrey Lloyd:

> By authority figures I mean those who are invoked as support or justification for a particular idea, theory or practice: it is not that such figures are necessarily held to be infallible or immune to criticism, though it is obvious that the more they are criticised, the less weight they carry for constructive purpose.
>
> —Lloyd 1996: 20

An authority figure is not necessarily an author, but to Galen, Hippocrates was the author of – the person who had written – the *Oath* and of many other Hippocratic treatises beside; and indeed, many of the writings collected in the Hippocratic Corpus display a well-developed authorial presence. That is, we find numerous instances of statements in the first person (using the pronouns 'I' or 'we') in the Hippocratic Corpus. Through these statements, the Hippocratic authors boasted about their own expertise in the field, criticized their rivals or referred to their own writings. Ancient Hippocratic 'authorship', however, is very different from modern authorship, in the sense that many Hippocratic treatises are compilatory in nature. These works are collections of descriptions of diseases, treatments and other medical information which were compiled together. It is common to find the same passages copied almost verbatim in two or more Hippocratic works (for an introduction to the compilatory method of the Hippocratic authors, see Langholf 2004). Pamela Long's definition of authorship is therefore particularly applicable to the Hippocratic authors:

> On the most basic level, authorship refers to the act or practice of creating something, such as a treatise, a painting, or a material invention. In the most mundane sense, an author of a written work is a writer, who must always do something more than copy another text verbatim; copying two or more texts and putting them together may suffice.
>
> —Long 2001: 7–8

Compiling material is not unique to the treatises of the Hippocratic Corpus; throughout antiquity physicians continued to re-use and 're-package' medical material in new formats. For instance, Galen's pharmacological treatise *On the Composition of Drugs according to Places* mentioned above is an extremely large compilation in ten books of recipes excerpted from older authorities (see Fabricius 1972) and organized by Galen in the head-to-toe order. Within that collection, Galen often quoted extremely long passages verbatim from his sources. However, ancient methods of quotation were less exacting than modern ones, and it can be difficult for the modern reader to determine where the quotations end and where Galen's own writing starts. Add to this the fact that Galen at times quoted material that had been written in the first person, that is, material that displays a strong authorial presence, and it becomes clear that the boundary between the authority of Galen and that of his sources is extremely blurred (see Totelin 2012b). What Galen, and many other medical authors before and after him, did would now be considered plagiarism, but as Pamela Long (2001: 10–12; see also Silk 1996) has convincingly argued, when we read ancient technical texts, we must distinguish between 'plagiarism' and 'intellectual property'. 'Intellectual property' was not much of a concern to ancient technical writers: they had no qualms about borrowing long passages from their sources. In fact, medical authors might have considered this borrowing good practice, as it showed them building upon the authority of past writers (Totelin 2012b).

Plagiarism, the misattribution of authorship, on the other hand, was a worry, as indicated by a famous anecdote told by Galen. The famous physician was browsing in the shopping area of Rome called the Sandalarium when he found a book entitled *Galen: The Doctor* which was not authentic (*On My Own Books*, preface).[21] This incident, Galen suggested, was not isolated: 'my books have been subject to all sorts of mutilations, whereby people in different countries publish different texts under their own names, with all sorts of cuts, additions, and alterations' (translation Singer 1997: 3). It is because of the mistreatments of his works that Galen had decided to compose an inventory of his writings. Galen's complaints introduce us to the agonistic character of the ancient medical marketplace, to which we now turn.

THE MEDICAL MARKETPLACE

We have encountered in this chapter several examples of ancient physicians' competitive behaviour: it is through competition that they acquired their clients and apprentices; and it is through competition that they constructed their authority. Such competition was not limited to that with other physicians; there were many other healers active in the ancient world, in what Vivian Nutton calls the 'medical marketplace' (1992; see also Jenner and Wallis 2007). It would be wrong, however, to see that competition as one where one group of healers tried entirely to surpass (and eradicate) another: most healers acknowledged that there were limits to their skills and expertise; and there are numerous examples of collaboration – sometimes reluctant, sometimes willing – between two types of healers.

The author of the *Oath* explicitly acknowledged the limits of his own *technē* and mentioned another category of healers beside the physicians: surgeons. Indeed, the person who swore the *Oath* promised not to cut, and certainly not to cut out stones, adding 'I will cede this to men who are practitioners of this activity'. In addition to the surgeons, the *Oath* might also allude to two other categories of healers: the herbalists and the midwives. For we know that poisonous plants and abortive pessaries, which are both mentioned in the *Oath*, were the province of the herbalists and the midwives respectively. Let us examine these two categories of healers in a little more detail; we will follow with a discussion of miracle healers active in the ancient medical marketplace.

The Hippocratic treatises contain numerous recipes, most of which are based on herbal ingredients (although mineral and animal ingredients are also represented). Unlike some later pharmacological treatises, they do not give much advice on how to procure ingredients. With one exception, the Hippocratic treatises do not mention the professionals involved in the gathering and selling of plants in antiquity. That exception is the late collection of Hippocratic *Letters*, an epistolary novella which tells the story of how Hippocrates encountered the philosopher Democritus, seemingly affected with a form of madness that made him laugh at everything.[22] In the sixteenth *Letter*, Hippocrates writes to Crateuas, the excellent root cutter (*rhizotomos*), the grandson of another root cutter named Crateuas, asking him for purging plants to treat Democritus. While this letter is fictional, it might reflect some of the reality of the collaboration between physicians and herbalists in the fifth and fourth centuries BCE.[23]

A more reliable source on the activities of people involved in gathering and selling plants is the philosopher Theophrastus (*c.* 371–*c.* 287 BCE), who in book nine of his *Enquiry into Plants* described the various rituals of those involved in gathering plants (e.g. 9.8.6–7) and named six root sellers (*pharmakopōlai*, see Samama 2006; Totelin 2016c): Thrasyas of Mantinea, his student Alexias, Eudemus, Eunomus of Chios, Aristophilus of Plataea and 'the Indian'.[24] These people knew how to become immune to the effects of hellebore (*Enquiry into Plants* 9.17.1–3); how to prepare drugs that enhance sexual potency (*Enquiry into Plants* 9.18.4 and 9); and how to provoke a painless death:

> Thrasyas of Mantinea said that he had discovered a drug that would cause an easy and painless death, by using the juices of hemlock, opium poppy and other such plants, prepared in such a way that it would be very portable and of a small weight of approximately one *drachma*. It had no cure whatsoever and it could be kept indefinitely without any alteration. He gathered the hemlock, not from any random place, but from Lousoi [in Arcadia] and

some other cold and thickly-shaded places; similarly, for other plants. He compounded many other drugs with many other ingredients. His student Alexias was also talented and no less skilled (*entechnos*) than his master. Indeed, he was also experienced in the medical art more generally.

—Theophrastus, *Enquiry into Plants* 9.16.8

Thrasyas, then, was able to deliver the deadly drugs that are prohibited in the Hippocratic *Oath*. He had a *technē* (he was *en-technos*) which Theophrastus defined as different from the medical one. His student Alexias, on the other hand, appears to have had broader medical skills, although we are not informed as to what they might have been.

Another story of a drug seller operating on the edge of what ancient physicians deemed acceptable is recounted by the historian Diodorus Siculus (first century BCE). Callō was a woman from Epidaurus (the location of one of the most important sanctuaries of Asclepius) who had an imperforate vagina. She married but could not have 'normal' sexual intercourse. She then developed an illness, which none of the doctors called to her help could address. Only a drug seller agreed to treat her:

> Later an inflammation occurred around her genitals, and as it gave rise to terrible pain, a number of physicians (*iatrōn*) were called. None of the others took upon themselves to treat her, but a certain drug seller who agreed to cure her cut the swollen area, whence male genitals fell out, namely testicles and an imperforate penis.
>
> —Diodorus Siculus 32.11; translation
> Totelin 2016c: 74, slightly modified[25]

The drug seller then went on to perforate the penis and, by means of a silver catheter, extract the fluids that caused the inflammation. For his treatment, he requested a double fee 'for he had taken on a sick woman and turned her into a healthy young man'. Callō changed her name into the masculine Callōn, gave up her wool work, changed her clothes and went on to live the life of a man.

In the story of Callō/n, the physicians refused to cut the genitals, perhaps because they felt that this was beyond their skills or perhaps because of some taboo on interfering with the genitals. In the Greek world, sexual intercourse brought with it pollution: people needed purification before entering sanctuaries after sex (see Parker 1983). It could be suggested that cutting the genitals would have been seen as much more polluting than sexual intercourse, and one possible reading of the Hippocratic *Oath*'s prohibition of cutting for the stone is that it reflects a form of 'self-censoring on the subject of cutting on male genitalia' (Miles 2005: 107).

While the link between cutting the genitals and pollution remains unclear, that between birth and death and pollution is certain. Being in contact with birth and death brought on pollution in the ancient world. This meant that many healers incurred the risk of pollution on a regular basis. That was particularly the case for midwives, who assisted in birth and often dealt with the death of infants and mothers in societies where peri-natal mortality was high (see Parkin 2013). It is perhaps because most of her patients survived in the face of high mortality that one of the earliest Greek midwives known by name, Phanostrate, was celebrated on her tombstone with the following verse epigram: 'Midwife (*maia*) and doctor (*iatros*) Phanostrate lies here // She caused pain to no-one and, having died, is missed by all' (*Carmina Epigraphica Graeca* 2.569; translation Lambert and Totelin 2017; see Samama 2003: 109–10). The claim that Phanostrate caused pain to no-one is reminiscent of the Hippocratic 'do no harm' principle and of the Hippocratic *Oath*.[26] Like Alexias the drug seller who was also skilled in medicine, Phanostrate was both a midwife and a physician. She might have treated all members of society, and not just women and infants.

On her tombstone, Phanostrate is represented as seated, holding the hand of another female character and surrounded by children. The imagery is typical of funerary steles and reveals little about Phanostrate's medical knowledge (see Demand 1995 for a slightly different argument). Later steles of female doctors, on the other hand, hint at knowledge acquired from books. Thus, the female doctor (Greek: *iatreinē*) Mousa, daughter of Agathocles, active in second- or first-century BCE Byzantium is shown on her tombstone holding a papyrus scroll in her hands (for the text of her epitaph, see Samama 2003: 413–4). Another female doctor (Latin: *medica*), active in second-century CE Metz, whose name is not preserved, also appears to be holding a book scroll. Literacy is given as one of the attributes of the good midwife in the portrait drawn by the medical author Soranus (first century CE, *Gynaecology* 1.2.2; on learned midwives, see Laes 2010).[27] Being literate, then, could be one of the ways in which midwives and female doctors constructed their authority in antiquity.

Another ancient female healer (the title she gave herself is unknown), Scribonia Attice, chose to be represented on her tomb in the act of practising her art: assisting a woman in childbirth (Ostia Antica, Necropolis of Isola Sacra, tomb 100). Scribonia looks towards us, while the labouring woman grips the handle of a birthing chair, and an attendant supports her. Scribonia was not the only healer in her family. She was buried with her husband, Marcus Ulpius Amerimnus, who is represented treating the leg of a patient next to a set of large-scale surgical instruments (see Figure 8.4). This couple established a profitable collaboration, which enabled them to afford a monumental tomb and the service of freedpeople (who are mentioned in the dedicatory inscription of the tomb, Helttula 2007: no. 133).

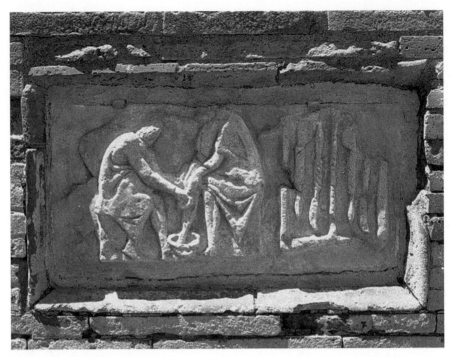

FIGURE 8.4: Relief sculpture representing the surgeon Ulpius Amerimnus from Ostia (near Rome), mid second century CE. Ulpius was buried with his wife Scribonia Attice, who is represented on another relief panel on the same tomb. Ulpius is shown attending to the leg of a patient. Next to them is an oversized case of surgical instruments. Ostia Antica, Necropolis of Isola Sacra 100. © Ministero per i beni culturali.

Galen provides us with another example of collaboration with midwives. He was called to help treat the wife of Boethus, a wealthy Roman of consular rank, who suffered from a female flux but 'was ashamed at first to tell this to the top doctors, of whom I was universally acknowledged to be one but put herself in the care of her usual midwives' (*On Prognosis* 8; translation Nutton 1979: 111). Galen worked alongside these midwives, describing the head midwife as 'excellent' yet presenting himself as a saviour who managed to find a way to heal his noble patient. After one month of Galen's treatment, Boethus' wife got better; he was rewarded with four hundred pieces, but became the object of other physicians' jealousy.

Galen stressed the fact that he had worked 'entirely according to the treatment prescribed by Hippocrates and the best of his medical successors'. Yet, his treatment earned him the title of 'wondermaker' (*paradoxopoios*). Galen appears to embrace that title, but it might have been meant as a jibe. While ancient physicians accepted that the god Asclepius, his acolytes and other divinities of the Graeco-Roman pantheon could perform exceptional cures (see above), they were highly suspicious of other miracle workers. A key text on this matter is the Hippocratic treatise *On the Sacred Disease*, in which the author recorded his views on the so-called 'sacred disease' (a disease characterized by fits). He asserted that this disease was no more sacred than any other, as it had a natural cause (an excess of phlegm), and criticized those who had first called it 'sacred':

> It seems to me that the people who first considered this disease sacred were like the magicians, purifiers, charlatans and quacks of today, who affect great piety and superior knowledge. These people, then, taking the divinity as a pretext and as a defence for their inability to offer any assistance, and in order not to show their complete ignorance, called this affliction 'sacred'. Adding suitable stories, they established a treatment which was safe for themselves: they made use of purifications and incantations and they ordered abstinence from baths and many foods.
>
> —*On the Sacred Disease* 2[28]

These people, the author argued, could hide behind the divinity if their treatments failed and the patient died, but could look very clever if they succeeded (see Laskaris 2002 for an analysis of this text). Medical authors throughout antiquity expressed reservations regarding quacks (see Boudon-Millot 2003; McNamara 2003), magicians (see Jouanna 2011; Petit 2017) and religious healers, but this certainly did not prevent some of those healers from rising to great fame. Among these, one could name Jesus of Nazareth, who cured the sick and raised the dead in the name of his god (see Ferngren 2009), or the wise Neopythagorean Apollonius of Tyana (first century CE), whose life was recounted by the sophist Philostratus (second–third century CE).[29]

Apollonius allegedly performed numerous feats of healing (Philostratus, *Life of Apollonius* 3.39 and 6.43): he cured a boy who had been affected with rabies for thirty days, a lame man who had been injured while lion hunting, a man who had lost his sight, one whose hand had been paralyzed and a woman who suffered excessively in labour:

> And a certain woman who had already experienced seven difficult labours was cured in the following way through the intermission of her husband. Apollonius ordered the man, whenever his wife should become pregnant, to carry into the room where she became pregnant a live hare, and to walk around her while at the same time releasing the hare. For the womb would be driven out together with the embryo, unless the hare was carried outside immediately.
>
> —Philostratus, *Life of Apollonius* 3.39

This passage is rather ambiguous, and it is difficult to know exactly what the outcome of Apollonius' cure was: did he cause an abortion and extrusion of the womb, or just an extrusion of the womb at the time when the pregnancy was at term? What is clear is that Apollonius 'healed' through a ritual which involved circling a patient, as well as a living hare, presumably chosen because of its reputation for high fertility. Galen and his Hippocratic predecessors would certainly have baulked at such a ritual, redolent of magic. Yet in some ways, this treatment does not differ that much from those recommended by a physician such as Galen. There are several examples of gynaecological remedies to be applied in hare's fur in the Hippocratic Corpus (e.g. *On the Nature of Woman* 97).[30] In choosing such a medium for the application of drugs, the Hippocratic physicians might have responded to the wishes of patients.

PATIENTS AND THE CONSTRUCTION OF AUTHORITY

So far, I have focused on healing practitioners and their methods to establish their authority. However, there are always at least two people in a medical encounter: the healer and the patient, to whom I now turn, starting as before with the Hippocratic *Oath*.

The Hippocratic *Oath* presents patients as passive recipients of care: they are the people who must be protected from the harm and injustice which a healer could cause. In particular, they must be protected from sexual abuse:

> Into as many houses as I may enter, I will go for the benefit of the ill, while being far from all voluntary and destructive injustice, especially from sexual acts both upon women's bodies and upon men's, both of the free and of the slaves.

The *Oath* taker further promised not to reveal what had been disclosed to him by his patients. In the context of classical Greek law, non-marital sex with a freeborn woman could led to heavy penalties, sometimes death (D. Cohen 1991); sexual relationships with free men were accepted, but only within some limited parameters (see e.g. Dover 1989; Davidson 2007); sexual intercourse with enslaved people were regulated by enslavers – slaves had very little sexual autonomy (E. Cohen 2014). The *Oath*, then, went beyond the laws of the Greek world in prohibiting sexual intercourse between a physician and some of his patients. In doing so it recognized sex as a way in which power can be yielded. It did not, however, acknowledge the fact that the physician, who was not always a freeborn, could himself be the object of unsolicited sexual advances and might not always have been a position to refuse them. That silence is perhaps natural in such a short text, but it points to a desire on the part of the *Oath*'s author to present patients as the weaker party in the medical encounter. In reality, patients – or at least some patients in some parts of the ancient world – might have exerted much power in the construction of medical authority. As argued by Melinda Letts (2015), in a medical market where no formal certifications existed, medical authority would have been a very fragile thing indeed. The theme of the disobedient patient, who refused to follow therapeutic recommendations, is a common one in ancient medical literature (see for instance the Hippocratic treatise, *On the Art* 7: 'It is much more probable that patients are unable to follow orders than that the doctors give the wrong instructions').[31] Galen argued that those freeborn physicians who pandered to their wealthy patients' every wishes behaved like slaves:

> In view of their inability to ensure anything valid (in therapy), they never request their patients to obey and follow their lead. Instead, they debase themselves to the status of the slaves of their patients. They obey and assist their patients in fulfilling their desires; their intention has never been to direct them towards what is most agreeable and useful because they are ignorant of any such knowledge. They satisfy the desires of their patients for the most pleasurable things, according to whatever the individual case may be, thus reaching the utmost depth of servility. In doing so they become wicked slaves whose services are useless, and indeed harmful.
>
> —Galen, *On Recognizing the Best Physician* 5; translation: Iskandar 1988: 77–9[32]

Galen's disdain for 'servile' physicians was the product of his privileged position in society: the son of a wealthy architect who had risen to the position of imperial physician, he could afford not to offer the most pleasant remedies to his patients. That privilege was not available to all, and most probably not to physicians who actually were slaves. But even the most honoured physicians could fall from grace in the ancient world, as the story of Archagathus, the first public physician employed by the city of Rome, shows:

> Cassius Hemina [Roman annalist historian active in the second century BCE], one of our most ancient authors, writes that the first physician to come to Rome was the Peloponnesian Archagathus, son of Lysanias, in the year 535 of the City [219 BCE], under the consulship of Lucius Aemilius and Marcus Livius. He was granted citizen rights, and a workshop was purchased with public funds for him at the Crossroads of Acilius. They say that he was a wound healer, and that his arrival was most welcome at first, but that soon, because of his cruelty in cutting and cauterizing, his name was changed to 'the butcher', and his art, together with all physicians, became objects of loathing.
>
> —Pliny, *Natural History* 29.12–13[33]

Since Pliny is our only source for this episode, it is impossible to determine whether Archagathus truly abused his position with his cruelty, or whether his treatments were sound but did not meet with the approval of his patients as they were too painful. Pliny himself had an agenda in telling the story. To him, professional medicine was an ill that had been imported from the Greek world: a very inferior form a healing to that practised in ideal Italian homes, where the head of the household, the *pater familias*, was responsible for the care of his wife, children and slaves (see Nutton 1993; von Staden 1996b). While Pliny's vision of traditional Roman healing most certainly did not reflect the realities of his day, it remains that much healing took place within the household in the Graeco-Roman world (see Draycott 2019). Ancient physicians acknowledged that reality by writing treatises addressed to literate laypeople, starting with the Hippocratic text *On Affections* (see Pérez Cañizares 2010). It was to the discerning patients, knowledgeable in matters of treatments, that healers in the ancient world had to present themselves as authorities.

CONCLUSIONS

It has become commonplace to refer to the ancient medical landscape as a marketplace, which was governed by the principle of competition. Within that market, healers had to compete for the attention of patients, who may themselves have been well versed in how to care for themselves and their relatives. Certainly, the level of choice available to patients must have varied depending on several factors, including wealth, social status, locality and level of literacy. Thus, a peasant in a remote locality would have had considerably less choice than a relatively wealthy person living in Athens, Alexandria or Rome. Elite medical authors, who typically made their living in the big metropolises of the ancient world, very regularly criticized their competitors. They established their authority both positively, by showing their competence, and negatively, by uncovering the incompetence of others.

While scholarship has very much focused on the agonistic, competitive, character of ancient medicine, it has perhaps not stressed enough another aspect: collaboration. In this chapter, I have discussed several examples of association between ancient healers. Physicians, herbalists, midwives and other healers might have worked together very reluctantly but they nevertheless did so. They did this because, in order for their skill to be acknowledged – in order for them to be recognized as authorities – it had to have well-defined boundaries. Thus, one of the most fundamental ancient medical texts, the Hippocratic *Oath*, is much preoccupied in defining the limits of the medical art. Healers could push those limits, sometimes encroaching on the territory of other healers, but they could not fully dispense with them. When they disregarded the limits of their art and refused to cooperate with others (or at the very least, to pass cases to others), healers risked harming their patients and their own reputation. Only the gods and a few miracle healers could operate beyond the confines of what the Greeks called *technē*, and the Romans *ars*.

NOTES

1. Unless stated otherwise, all translations in this chapter are the author's own. This citation of Lucian is from the Loeb Classical Library edition by Harmon (1921).
2. These citations of the Hippocratic texts *Law* and *Decorum* are from the Loeb Classical Library edition by Jones (1923b).
3. This citation is from the Loeb Classical Library edition by Johnston and Horsley (2011).
4. This and all citations hereafter are from the Collection des Universités de France edition by Jouanna (2018).
5. The bibliography on the *Oath* is immense. The study by Heinrich von Staden (1996a) is essential reading. See also Nutton 1995a; Jouanna 1999: 401–2; Craik 2015: 145–9. All translations of the *Oath* in this chapter are by von Staden.
6. This citation is from the Loeb Classical Library edition by Potter (2012).
7. This and all citations hereafter are from the Loeb Classical Library edition by Lamb (1924).
8. This and all citations hereafter are from the Collection des Universités de France edition by Boudon-Millot (2007). For an English translation, see Singer (1997): 23–34.
9. Citation of Plato's *Phaedrus* is from the Loeb Classical Library edition by Fowler (1914); of Aristotle's *Nicomachean Ethics* is from the Loeb Classical Library edition by Rackham (1926); of Xenophon's *Memorabilia* is from the Loeb Classical Library edition by Marchant, Todd and Henderson (2013).
10. This citation is from the Collection des Universités de France edition by Boudon-Millot et al (2010). For an English translation, see Nutton in Singer et al (2014): 77–99.
11. This citation is from the Loeb Classical Library edition by Henderson (2002).
12. This citation is from the Loeb Classical Library edition by Emlyn-Jones and Preddy (2013).
13. This citation is from the Loeb Classical Library edition by Jones (1923a).
14. This citation is from the Collection des Universités de France edition by Jouanna (2013). For an English translation, see Jones (1923b).
15. This citation is from the Loeb Classical Library edition by Potter (1995).
16. This and all citations hereafter are from the Corpus Medicorum Graecorum edition by Nutton (1979).
17. This citation is from the Loeb Classical Library edition by Potter (2018).
18. This citation is from the Loeb Classical Library edition by Withington (1928).
19. This citation is from the Collection des Universités de France edition by Jouanna (1990). For an English translation, see Jones (1923a).
20. This citation is from the twelfth volume of Kühn's edition, abbreviated as 'K12'.

21. This citation is from the Collection des Universités de France (2007). For an English translation, see Singer (1997): 3–22.

22. This citation is from the Brill edition by Smith (1990).

23. 'Crateuas' was the name of a drug seller (*pharmakopōlēs*) in a lost comic play by the Alexis (fourth century BCE). It was also the name of the later pharmacological author who corresponded with the King Mithradates VI.

24. This and all citations hereafter are to the Collection des Universités de France edition by Amigues (2006). For an English translation (at times incomplete), see Hort (1916).

25. This citation is from the Loeb Classical Library edition by Walton (1957).

26. There might also be allusions to Phanostrate's ability to bring on safe abortions in the epigram.

27. This citation is from the Corpus Medicorum Graecorum edition by Ilberg (1927). For an English translation, see Temkin (1956).

28. This citation is to the Collection des Universités de France edition by Jouanna (2003). For an English translation, see Jones (1923b).

29. The *Life of Apollonius* had been commissioned by the empress Julia Domna, at whose court Galen was active. Citations are from the Loeb Classical Library edition by Jones (2005).

30. This citation is from the Collection des Universités de France edition by Bourbon (2008). For an English translation, see Potter (2012).

31. This citation is from the Collection des Universités de France edition by Jouanna (1988). For an English translation, see Jones (1923b).

32. This citation is from the Corpus Medicorum Graecorum edition by Iskandar (1988). The original Greek of this text has been lost, but a medieval Arabic translation is available.

33. This citation is from the Loeb Classical Library edition by Jones (1963).

SOURCES

Aelius Aristides
Sacred Tales
Behr, Charles A., transl. (1981–1986), *The Complete Works of P. Aelius Aristides*. 2
    vols, Leiden: Brill.
Keil, Bruno, ed. (1898), *Aelii Aristidis Smyrnaei quae supersunt omnia*. Vol. II, Berlin:
    Weidmann.

Aeschylus
Prometheus Bound
Sommerstein, Alan H., ed. and transl. (2009), *Aeschylus. Persians. Seven against
    Thebes. Suppliants. Prometheus Bound. Edited and Translated by Alan H.
    Sommerstein*, Cambridge, MA: Harvard University Press.

Aetius
Placita
Diels, Hermann, ed. (1879), *Doxographi Graeci*, Berlin: G. Reimer.

Aetius of Amida
Medical Collection
Olivieri, A., ed. (1935–1950), *Aetiii Amideni Libri medicinales. Edidit A. Olivieri*. 2
    vols, Leipzig and Berlin: Teubner.

Anonymus Londinensis
Manetti, Daniela, ed. (2003), *Anonymus Londinensis. De medicina. Edidit Daniela
    Manetti*, Berlin: Teubner.

Anonymus Parisinus
Garofalo, Ivan and Brian Fuchs, eds and transls (1997), *Anonymi medici De morbis
    acutis et chroniis. Edited with Commentary by Ivan Garofalo. Translated into
    English by Brian Fuchs*, Leiden: Brill.

Apuleius
Apology
Hunink, Vincent, ed. and transl. (1997), *Apuleius of Madauros. Pro se de magia (Apologia). Edited with a Commentary by Vincent Hunink*, Amsterdam: Gieben.

Aristophanes
Frogs
Henderson, Jeffrey, ed. and transl. (2002), *Aristophanes. Frogs. Assemblywomen. Wealth. Edited and Translated by Jeffrey Henderson*, Cambridge, MA: Harvard University Press.

Aristotle
On Marvellous Things Heard
Hett, W. S., transl. (1936), *Aristotle. Minor Works: On Colours. On Things Heard. Physiognomics. On Plants. On Marvellous Things Heard. Mechanical Problems. On Indivisible Lines. The Situations and Names of Winds. On Melissus, Xenophanes, Gorgias. Translated by W. S. Hett*, Cambridge, MA: Harvard University Press.

Nicomachean Ethics
Rackham, H., transl. (1926), *Aristotle. Nicomachean Ethics. Translated by H. Rackham*, Cambridge, MA: Harvard University Press.

Parts of Animals
Peck, A. L. and E. S. Forster, transls (1937), *Aristotle. Parts of Animals. Movement of Animals. Progression of Animals. Translated by A. L. Peck and E. S. Forster*, Cambridge, MA: Harvard University Press.

Artemidorus
Harris-McCoy, Daniel E., ed. and transl. (2012), *Artemidorus. Oneirocritica: Text, Translation, and Commentary*, Oxford: Oxford University Press.

Athenaeus
Deipnosophists
Olson, S. Douglas, ed. and transl. (2012), *Athenaeus. The Learned Banqueters. Volume VIII. Book 15. Indexes. Edited and Translated by S. Douglas Olson*, Cambridge, MA: Harvard University Press.

Aulus Gellius
Attic Nights
Marshall, P. K., ed. (1968), *Aulus Gellius Noctes Atticae*. 2 vols, Oxford: Clarendon Press.
Rolfe, J. C., transl. (1927), *Gellius. Attic Nights. Translated by J. C. Rolfe*. 3 vols, Cambridge, MA: Harvard University Press.

Caelius Aurelianus
On Acute Diseases and *On Chronic Diseases*
Bendz, G., ed. and transl. (1990–1993), *Caelii Aureliani Celerum passionum libri III, Tardarum passionum libri V. Edidit G. Bendz, in linguam Germanicam transtulit I. Pape*, Berlin: Teubner.
Drabkin, I. E., ed. and transl. (1950), *Caelius Aurelianus. On Acute Diseases and On Chronic Diseases*, Chicago: University of Chicago Press.

Calcidius
Commentary on Plato's Timaeus
Waszink, J. H., ed. (1975), *Timaeus a Calcidio Translatus Commentarioque Instructus*,
   2nd edn, Leiden: Brill.

Carmina Epigraphica Graeca
Hansen, Peter A., ed. (1989), *Carmina Epigraphica Graeca Saeculorum VIII–V a. Chr.
   n.* Vol., Berlin: De Gruyter.

Cato
On Agriculture
Hooper, W. D. and Harrison Boyd Ash, transls (1934), *Cato. Varro. On Agriculture.
   Translated by W. D. Hooper and Harrison Boyd Ash*, Cambridge, MA: Harvard
   University Press.

Celsus
On Medicine
Spencer, W. G., transl. (1935–1938), *On Medicine. Translated by W. G. Spencer.* 3 vols,
   Cambridge, MA: Harvard University Press.

Cicero
Letters
Shackleton Bailey, D. R., ed. and transl. (2001), *Cicero. Letters to Friends. Volume II.
   Letters 114–280. Edited and Translated by D. R. Shackleton Bailey*, Cambridge,
   MA: Harvard University Press.

Columella
On Agriculture
Boyd Ash, Harrison, transl. (1941–1955), *Columella. On Agriculture. Translated by
   Harrison Boyd Ash.* 3 vols, Cambridge, MA: Harvard University Press.

Corpus Hippiatricorum Graecorum
Oder, Eugen and Karl Hoppe, eds (1924–1927), *Corpus Hippiatricorum Graecorum.*
   2 vols, Leipzig: Teubner.

Digest
Waston, Alan (1998), *The Digest of Justinian.* 2 vols, revised English language edn,
   Philadelphia: University of Philadelphia Press.

Dio Cassius
Roman History
Books 51–55: Cary, Earnest and Herbert B. Foster, transls (1917), *Dio Cassius. Roman
   History. Volume VI. Books 51–55. Translated by Earnest Cary and Herbert B. Foster*,
   Cambridge, MA: Harvard University Press.
Books 56–60: Cary, Earnest and Herbert B. Foster, transls (1924), *Dio Cassius. Roman
   History. Volume VII. Books 56–60. Translated by Earnest Cary and Herbert B.
   Foster*, Cambridge, MA: Harvard University Press.
Books 71–80: Cary, Earnest and Herbert B. Foster, transls (1927), *Dio Cassius. Roman
   History. Volume IX. Books 71–80. Translated by Earnest Cary and Herbert B.
   Foster*, Cambridge, MA: Harvard University Press.

Diocles
Fragments
van der Eijk, Philip J., ed. and transl. (2000–2001), *Diocles of Carystus. A Collection of the Fragments with Translation and Commentary.* 2 vols, Leiden: Brill.

Diodorus Siculus
Library of History
Walton, Francis R., transl. (1957), *Diodorus Siculus. Library of History. Volume XI. Fragments of Books 21–32. Translated by Francis R. Walton*, Cambridge, MA: Harvard University Press.

Dioscorides
Materia Medica
Wellmann, M. ed. (1907–1914), *Pedanii Dioscuridis Anazarbei De materia medica libri quinque. Edidit Max Wellmann.* 3 vols, Berlin: Weidmann.
Beck, Lily Y., transl. ([2005] 2011), *Pedanius Dioscorides of Anazarbus De Materia Medica. Translated by L.Y. Beck*, Hildesheim: Olms-Weidmann.

Erasistratus
Fragments
Garofalo, Ivan, ed. (1988), *Erasistrati fragmenta*, Pisa: Giardini.

Euripides
Heracles
Kovacs, David, ed. and transl. (1998), *Euripides. Suppliant Women. Electra. Heracles. Edited and Translated by David Kovacs*, Cambridge, MA: Harvard University Press.

Frontinus
On the Aqueducts of Rome
Rodgers, Robert H., ed. (2004), *Frontinus. De aquaeductu urbis Romae*, Cambridge: Cambridge University Press.

Fronto
Correspondence
Haines, C. R., transl. (1919–1920), *Fronto. Correspondence. Translated by C. R. Haines.* 2 vols, Cambridge, MA: Harvard University Press.
van den Hout, Michael P. J., ed. (1988), *M. Cornelii Frontonis Epistulae. Schedis tam editis quam ineditis Edmundi Hauleri; usus iterum edidit Michael P. J. van den Hout*, Leipzig: Teubner.

Galen and Pseudo-Galen
Opera omnia
Kühn, Karl Gottlob, ed. (1821–1833), *Claudii Galeni Opera omnia.* 22 vols, Leipzig: Cnobloch [henceforth abbreviated as 'K', followed by volume number].
Singer, Peter N., transl. (1997), *Galen. Selected Works*, Oxford: Oxford University Press.

Avoiding Distress
Boudon-Millot, Véronique, Jacques Jouanna and Antoine Pietrobelli, eds and transls (2010), *Galien. Œuvres. Tome IV. Ne pas se chagriner. Texte établi et traduit par Véronique Boudon-Millot et Jacques Jouanna, avec la contribution d'Antoine Pietrobelli*, Paris: Les Belles Lettres.

Singer, Peter N., Vivian Nutton, Daniel Davies and Piero Tassinari, transls (2014), *Galen. Psychological Writings: Avoiding Distress, Character Traits, The Diagnosis and Treatment of the Affections and Errors Peculiar to Each Person's Soul, The Capacities of the Soul Depend on the Mixtures of the Body. Edited by P. N. Singer. Translated with Introductions and Notes by Vivian Nutton, Daniel Davies and P. N. Singer. With the Collaboration of Piero Tassinari*, Cambridge: Cambridge University Press.

Causes of Pulses
K2

Commentary to Hippocrates' Epidemics VI
K17B

Introduction or 'the Doctor'
Petit, Caroline, ed. and transl. (2009), *Galien. Oeuvres. Tome II. Le médecin, Introduction. Texte établi et traduit par Caroline Petit*, Paris: Les Belles Lettres.

On Anatomical Procedures
K2

On Antidotes
K14

On Good and Bad Juices
Koch, Konrad, Georg Helmreich, K. Kalbfleisch and O. Hartlich, eds (1923), *Galeni De sanitate tuenda, edidit K. Koch. De alimentorum facultatibus, De bonis malisque sucis, edidit G. Helmreich. De victu attenuante, edidit K. Kalbfleisch. De ptisana, edidit O. Hartlich*, Leipzig and Berlin: Teubner.

On Mixtures
Helmreich, Georg, ed. (1904), *Galeni de temperamentis libri III*, Leipzig: Teubner.
Singer, Peter, N., trans. (1957), *Galen. Selected Works*, Oxford: Oxford World Classics.

On My Own Books and *On the Order of My Own Books*
Boudon-Millot, Véronique, ed. and transl. (2007), *Galien. Oeuvre. Tome 1. Introduction générale. Sur l'ordre de ses propres livres. Sur ses propres livres. Que l'excellent médecin est aussi philosophe. Texte établi, traduit et annoté par Véronique Boudon-Millot*, Paris: Les Belles Lettres.
Singer, Peter N., trans. (1997), *Galen. Selected Works*, Oxford: Oxford World Classics.

On Prognosis
Nutton, Vivian, ed. and transl. (1979), *Galeni De praecognitione. Edidit, in linguam Anglicam vertit, commentatus est Vivian Nutton*, Berlin: Teubner.

On Recognizing the Best Physician
Iskandar, A. Z., ed. and transl. (1988), *Galeni De optimo medico cognoscendo libelli. Versio Arabica, edidit, in linguam Anglicam vertit, commentatus est A. Z. Iskandar*, Berlin: Teubner.

On Synectic Causes
Lyons, Malcolm, ed. and transl. (1969), *Galeni De partibus artis medicativae, De causis contentivis, De diaeta in morbis acutis secundum Hippocratem libellorum versiones Arabicas edidit et in linguam Anglicam vertit Malcolm Lyons*, Berlin: Teubner.

On the Composition of Drugs according to Kind
K12 and K13

On the Composition of Drugs according to Places
K12

On the Opinions of Hippocrates and Plato
De Lacy, Philip, ed. and transl. (1978–1984), *Galeni De placitis Hippocratis et Platonis. Edidit, in linguam Anglicam vertit, commentatus est Philip De Lacy.* 3 vols, Berlin: Teubner.

On the Order of My Own Books
See under *On My Own Books*

On the Powers of Simple Drugs
K11 and K12

On the Preservation of Health
Johnston, Ian, ed. and transl. (2018), *Galen. Hygiene. Volume II. Books 5–6. Thrasybulus. On Exercise with a Small Ball. Edited and Translated by Ian Johnston*, Cambridge, MA: Harvard University Press.

On the Properties of Foodstuffs
Wilkins, John, ed. and transl. (2013), *Galien. Oeuvre. Tome V. Sur les facultés des aliments. Texte établi et traduit by John Wilkins*, Paris: Les Belles Lettres.
Powell, Owen, transl. (2003), *Galen. On the Properties of Foodstuffs. Introduction, Translation and Commentary. With a Foreword by John Wilkins*, Cambridge: Cambridge University Press.

On Theriac to Pamphilianus
K14

On Theriac to Piso
Boudon-Millot, Véronique, ed. and transl. (2016), *Galien. Oeuvres. Tome VI. Thériaque à Pison. Texte établi et traduit par Véronique Boudon-Millot*, Paris: Les Belles Lettres.
Leigh, Robert, ed. and transl. (2015), *On Theriac to Piso, Attributed to Galen. A Critical Edition with Translation and Commentary*, Leiden: Brill.

On the Therapeutic Method
Johnston, I. and G. H. R. Horsley, eds and transls (2011), *Galen. Method of Medicine. Edited and Translated by Ian Johnston and G. H. R. Horsley*. 3 vols, Cambridge, MA: Harvard University Press.

On the Use of Respiration
K4

On the Usefulness of Parts of the Body
Helmreich, Georg, ed. (1907–1909), *Galeni De usu partium libri XVII. Ad codicum fidem recensuit Georgius Helmreich*. 2 vols, Leipzig: Teubner.

The Capacities of the Soul Depend on the Mixtures of the Body
Singer, Peter N., Vivian Nutton, Daniel Davies and Piero Tassinari, transls (2014), *Galen. Psychological Writings: Avoiding Distress, Character Traits, The Diagnosis and Treatment of the Affections and Errors Peculiar to Each Person's Soul, The Capacities of the Soul Depend on the Mixtures of the Body. Edited by P. N. Singer. Translated with Introductions and Notes by Vivian Nutton, Daniel Davies and P. N. Singer. With the Collaboration of Piero Tassinari*, Cambridge: Cambridge University Press.

Thrasybulus: Is Health a Part of Medicine or Gymnastics
Helmreich, Georg, ed. (1893), *Claudii Galeni Pergameni Scripta Minora. Bd. III*, Leipzig: Teubner.
Singer, Peter N., transl. (1997), *Galen. Selected Works*, Oxford: Oxford World Classics.

Geoponica
Dalby, Andrew, transl. (2011), *Geoponica: Farm Work. A Modern Translation of the Roman and Byzantine Farming Handbook by Andrew Dalby*, Totnes: Prospect Books.

Herodian
History of the Empire
Whittaker, C. R., transl. (1970), *Herodian. History of the Empire. Volume II. Books 5–8. Translated by C. R. Whittaker*, Cambridge, MA: Harvard University Press.

Herodotus
The Histories
Godley, A. D., transl. (1920–1925), *Herodotus. The Persian Wars. Translated by A. D. Godley*. 4 vols, Cambridge, MA: Harvard University Press.

Herophilus
Fragments
von Staden, Heinrich, ed., transl. and comm. (1989), *Herophilus: The Art of Medicine in Early Alexandria*, Cambridge: Cambridge University Press.

Hesiod
Works and Days
Most, Glenn W., ed. and transl. (2007), *Hesiod. Theogony. Works and Days. Testimonia. Edited and Translated by Glenn W. Most*, Cambridge, MA: Harvard University Press.

Hippocrates and Hippocratic Corpus
Opera omnia
Littré, Émile, ed. and transl. (1839–1861), *Œuvres Complètes d'Hippocrate*. 10 vols, Paris: J. B. Baillière [henceforth abbreviated as 'L', followed by the volume number].

Aphorisms
Jones, W. H. S., transl. (1931), *Hippocrates. Heracleitus. Nature of Man. Regimen in
    Health. Humours. Aphorisms. Regimen 1–3. Dreams. Heracleitus: On the Universe.
    Translated by W. H. S. Jones*, Cambridge, MA: Harvard University Press.

Epidemics 1 and 3
Jones, W. H. S., transl. (1923a), *Hippocrates. Ancient Medicine. Airs, Waters, Places.
    Epidemics 1 and 3. The Oath. Precepts. Nutriment. Translated by W. H. S. Jones*,
    Cambridge, MA: Harvard University Press.

Epidemics 2, 4–7
Smith, Wesley D., ed. and transl. (1994), *Hippocrates. Epidemics 2, 4–7. Edited and
    Translated by Wesley D. Smith*, Cambridge, MA: Harvard University Press.

Epidemics 5 and 7
Grmek, Mirko D. and Jacques Jouanna, ed. and transl. (2000), *Hippocrate. Tome IV.
    3e partie. Epidémies V et VII. Notes de Mirko D. Grmek. Texte établi et traduit par
    Jacques Jouanna*, Paris: Les Belles Lettres.

Law
Jones, W. H. S., transl. (1923b), *Hippocrates. Prognostic. Regimen in Acute Diseases.
    The Sacred Disease. The Art. Breaths. Law. Decorum. Physician (Ch. 1). Dentition.
    Translated by W. H. S. Jones*, Cambridge, MA: Harvard University Press.

Letters
Smith, Wesley D., ed., and transl. (1990), *Hippocrates. Pseudepigraphic Writings:
    Letters, Embassy, Speech from the Altar, Decree. Edited and Translated with an
    Introduction by Wesley D. Smith*, Leiden: Brill.

Oath
Jouanna, Jacques, ed. and transl. (2018), *Hippocrate. Tome 1. 2e partie. Le serment.
    Les serments chrétiens. La loi. Texte établi et traduit par Jacques Jouanna*, Paris: Les
    Belles Lettres.
Jones, W. H. S., transl. (1923a), *Hippocrates. Ancient Medicine. Airs, Waters, Places.
    Epidemics 1 and 3. The Oath. Precepts. Nutriment. Translated by W. H. S. Jones*,
    Cambridge, MA: Harvard University Press.

On Airs, Waters and Places
Jouanna, Jacques, ed. and transl. (1996), *Hippocrate. Airs, Eaux, Lieux. Texte établi et
    traduit par Jacques Jouanna*, Paris: Les Belles Lettres.
Jones, W. H. S., transl. (1923a), *Hippocrates. Ancient Medicine. Airs, Waters, Places.
    Epidemics 1 and 3. The Oath. Precepts. Nutriments. Translated by W. H. S. Jones*,
    Cambridge, MA: Harvard University Press.

On Ancient Medicine
Jouanna, Jacques, ed. and transl. (1990), *Hippocrate. Tome II. 1ʳᵉ partie. L'ancienne
    médecine. Texte établi et traduit par Jacques Jouanna*, Paris: Les Belles Lettres.
Jones, W. H. S., transl. (1923a), *Hippocrates. Ancient Medicine. Airs, Waters, Places.
    Epidemics 1 and 3. The Oath. Precepts. Nutriments. Translated by W. H. S. Jones*,
    Cambridge, MA: Harvard University Press.

On Barrenness
Potter, Paul, ed. and transl. (2012), *Hippocrates. Generation. Nature of the Child.
Diseases 4. Nature of Women and Barrenness. Edited and Translated by Paul Potter*,
Cambridge, MA: Harvard University Press.

On Decorum
Jones, W. H. S., transl. (1923b), *Hippocrates. Prognostic. Regimen in Acute Diseases.
The Sacred Disease. The Art. Breaths. Law. Decorum. Physician (Ch. 1). Dentition.
Translated by W. H. S. Jones*, Cambridge, MA: Harvard University Press.

On Diseases 1
Potter, Paul, transl. (1988), *Hippocrates. Affections. Diseases 1. Diseases 2. Translated
by Paul Potter*, Cambridge, MA: Harvard University Press.

On Diseases of Women
Potter, Paul, ed. and transl. (2018), *Hippocrates. Diseases of Women 1–2. Edited and
Translated by Paul Potter*, Cambridge, MA: Harvard University Press.

On Fistulas
Potter, Paul, ed. and transl. (1995), *Hippocrates. Places in Man. Glands. Fleshes.
Prorrhetic 1–2. Physician. Use of Liquids. Ulcers. Haemorrhoids and Fistulas. Edited
and Translated by Paul Potter*, Cambridge, MA: Harvard University Press.

On Joints
Withington, E. T., transl. (1928), *Hippocrates. On Wounds in the Head. In the Surgery.
On Fractures. On Joints. Mochlicon. Translated by E. T. Withington*, Cambridge,
MA: Harvard University Press.

On Regimen
Joly, Robert, ed. and transl. (1967), *Hippocrate. Du régime. Texte établi et traduit par
Robert Joly*, Paris: Les Belles Lettres.
Jones, W. H. S., transl. (1931), *Hippocrates. Heracleitus. Nature of Man. Regimen
in Health. Humours. Aphorisms. Regimen 1–3. Dreams. Heracleitus: On the
Universe. Translated by W. H. S. Jones*, Cambridge, MA: Harvard University
Press.

On Regimen in Acute Diseases
L2

On the Art
Jouanna, Jacques, ed. and transl. (1988), *Hippocrate. Tome V. 1ʳᵉ partie. Des vents. De
l'art. Texte établi et traduit par Jacques Jouanna*, Paris: Les Belles Lettres.
Jones, W. H. S., transl. (1923b), *Hippocrates. Prognostic. Regimen in Acute Diseases.
The Sacred Disease. The Art. Breaths. Law. Decorum. Physician (Ch. 1). Dentition.
Translated by W. H. S. Jones*, Cambridge, MA: Harvard University Press.

On the Heart
Potter, Paul, ed. and transl. (2010), *Hippocrates. Coan Prenotions. Anatomical and
Minor Clinical Writings. Edited and Translated by Paul Potter*, Cambridge, MA:
Harvard University Press.

On the Nature of Man
Jones, W. H. S., transl. (1931), *Hippocrates. Heracleitus. Nature of Man. Regimen in Health. Humours. Aphorisms. Regimen 1–3. Dreams. Heracleitus: On the Universe. Translated by W. H. S. Jones*, Cambridge, MA: Harvard University Press.

On the Nature of the Child
Potter, Paul, ed. and transl. (2012), *Hippocrates. Generation. Nature of the Child. Diseases 4. Nature of Women and Barrenness. Edited and Translated by Paul Potter*, Cambridge, MA: Harvard University Press.

On the Nature of Woman
Potter, Paul, ed. and transl. (2012), *Hippocrates. Generation. Nature of the Child. Diseases 4. Nature of Women and Barrenness. Edited and Translated by Paul Potter*, Cambridge, MA: Harvard University Press.

On the Sacred Disease
Jouanna, Jacques, ed. and transl. (2003), *Hippocrate. Œuvres. Tome II. 3ᵉ partie. La maladie sacrée. Texte établi et traduit par Jacques Jouanna*, Paris: Les Belles Lettres.
Jones, W. H. S., transl. (1923b), *Hippocrates. Prognostic. Regimen in Acute Diseases. The Sacred Disease. The Art. Breaths. Law. Decorum. Physician (Ch. 1). Dentition. Translated by W. H. S. Jones*, Cambridge, MA: Harvard University Press.

Prognostic
Jouanna, Jacques, Anargyros Anastassiou and Caroline Magdeleine, eds and transls (2013), *Hippocrate. Tome III. 1e partie. Pronostic. Texte établi, traduit et annoté par Jacques Jouanna avec la collaboration d'Anargyros Anastassiou et Caroline Magdeleine*, Paris: Les Belles Lettres.
Jones, W. H. S., transl. (1923b), *Hippocrates. Prognostic. Regimen in Acute Diseases. The Sacred Disease. The Art. Breaths. Law. Decorum. Physician (Ch. 1). Dentition. Translated by W. H. S. Jones*, Cambridge, MA: Harvard University Press.

Prorrhetic
Potter, Paul, ed. and transl. (1995), *Hippocrates. Places in Man. Glands. Fleshes. Prorrhetic 1–2. Physician. Use of Liquids. Ulcers. Haemorrhoids and Fistulas. Edited and Translated by Paul Potter*, Cambridge, MA: Harvard University Press.

Homer
Iliad
Murray, A. T., transl. (1924), *Homer. Iliad. Volume I. Books 1–12. Translated by A. T. Murray. Revised by William F. Wyatt*, Cambridge, MA: Harvard University Press.

Odyssey
Murray, A. T., transl. (1919), *Homer. Odyssey. Volume I. Books 1–12. Translated by A. T. Murray. Revised by George E. Dimock*, Cambridge, MA: Harvard University Press.

Horace
Epistles
Fairclough, H. Rushton, transl. (1926), *Horace. Satires. Epistles. The Art of Poetry. Translated by H. Rushton Fairclough*, Cambridge, MA: Harvard University Press.

Inscriptiones Latinae Selectae
Dessau, Hermann, ed. (1906), *Inscriptiones Latinae Selectae. Vol. II. Pars II. Edidit Hermannus Dessau*, Berlin: Weidmann.

Isidore
Etymologies
Lindsay, Wallace Martin, ed. (1911), *Etymologiarvm sive Originvm libri XX. Recognovit brevique adnotatione critica instrvxit W. M. Lindsay*, Oxford: Oxford University Press.

Juvenal
Morton Braund, Susanna, ed. and transl. (2004), *Juvenal and Persius. Edited and Translated by Susanna Morton Braund*, Cambridge, MA: Harvard University Press.

Lucian and Pseudo-Lucian
Affairs of the Heart
MacLeod, M. D., transl. (1967), *Lucian. Soloecista. Lucius or The Ass. Amores. Halcyon. Demosthenes. Podagra. Ocypus. Cyniscus. Philopatris. Charidemus. Nero. Translated by M. D. MacLeod*, Cambridge, MA: Harvard University Press.

The Ignorant Book Collector
Harmon, A. M., transl. (1921), *Lucian. Volume III. The Dead Come to Life or The Fisherman. The Double Indictment or Trials by Jury. On Sacrifices. The Ignorant Book Collector. The Dream or Lucian's Career. The Parasite. The Lover of Lies. The Judgement of the Goddesses. On Salaried Posts in Great Houses. Translated by A. M. Harmon*, Cambridge, MA: Harvard University Press.

Lucretius
On the Nature of Things
Rouse, W. H. D., transl. (1924), *Lucretius. On the Nature of Things. Translated by W. H. D. Rouse. Revised by Martin F. Smith*, Cambridge, MA: Harvard University Press.

Marcus Aurelius
Meditations
Farquharson, A. S. L., ed., transl. and comm. (1944), *The Meditations of the Emperor Marcus Antoninus*. 2 vols, Oxford: Clarendon Press.
Haines, C. R., ed. and transl. (1916), *Marcus Aurelius. Edited and Translated by C. R. Haines*, Cambridge, MA: Harvard University Press.

Martial
Epigrams
Shackleton Bailey, D. R., ed. and transl. (1993), *Martial. Epigrams, Volume I. Spectacles, Books 1–5. Edited and Translated by D. R. Shackleton Bailey*, Cambridge, MA: Harvard University Press.

Mnesitheus
Fragments
Bertier, Janine, ed. and transl. (1972), *Mnésithée et Dieuchès*, Leiden: Brill.

Muscio
Rose, Valentin, ed., (1882), *Sorani Gynaeciorum vetus translatio latina nunc prima edita a Valentino Rose*, Leipzig: Teubner.

Nicander
Theriaka
Jacques, J. M., ed. and transl. (2002), *Nicandre de Colophon. Œuvres. Tome II. Les thériaques, Fragments iologiques antérieurs à Nicandre. Texte établi et traduit par J.-M. Jacques*, Paris: Les Belles Lettres.

Onasander
Illinois Greek Club, transl. (1928), *Aeneas Tacticus, Asclepiodotus, and Onasander. Translated by Illinois Greek Club*, Cambridge, MA: Harvard University Press.

Oribasius
Raeder, J., ed. (1928–1933), *Oribasii Collectionum medicarum reliquiae. Edidit J. Raeder*. 4 vols, Leipzig and Berlin: Teubner.

Palladius
On Agriculture
Fitch, John G., transl. (2013), *Palladius. Opus agriculturae: The Work of Farming. A New Translation from the Latin by John G. Fitch*, Totnes: Prospect.

Papyri and Ostraca
BGU
= *Aegyptische Urkunden aus den Königlichen (later Staatlichen) Museen zu Berlin, Griechische Urkunden*
(1895), *Aegyptische Urkunden aus den Koeniglichen Museen zu Berlin: Griechische Urkunden*. Vol. 1, Berlin: Weidmann.

O.Claud.
= *Mons Claudianus. Ostraca graeca et latina*
Bingen, J., A. Bülow-Jacobsen, W. E. H. Cockle, H. Cuvigny, L. Rubinstein and W. Van Rengen, eds (1992), *Mons Claudianus. Ostraca graeca et latina*. Vol. 1, Cairo: Institut Français d'Archéologie Orientale.

O.Florida
= *The Florida Ostraka*
Bagnall, R. G., ed. (1976), *The Florida Ostraka: Documents from the Roman Army in Upper Egypt*, Durham, NC: Duke University Press.

P.Brem.
= *Die Bremer Papyri*
Wilcken, U., ed. (1936), *Die Bremer Papyri*, Berlin: Verlag der Akademie der Wissenschaften.

P.Fouad
= *Les Papyrus Fouad*
Bataille, A., O. Guéraud, P. Jouguet, N. Lewis, H. Marrou, J. Scherer and W. G. Waddell, eds (1939), *Les Papyrus Fouad*. Vol. I, Cairo: Institut français d'archéologie orientale.

P.Gen.
= *Les Papyrus de Genève*
Wehrli, Claude, ed. (1986), *Les Papyrus de Genève*. Vol. II, Geneva: Bibliothèque publique et universitaire.

PGM
= *Papyri Graecae Magicae*
Preisendanz, Karl and Albert Henrichs, eds and transls (1973–1974), *Papyri Graecae magicae. Die griechischen Zauberpapyri. Herausgegeben und übersetzt von Karl Preisendanz. Zweite, verbesserte Auflage. Mit Ergänzungen von Karl Preisendanz. Durchgesehen und herausgegeben von Albert Henrichs.* 2 vols, Stuttgart: Teubner.
Betz, Dieter, transl. (1992), *The Greek Magical Papyri in Translation, Including the Demotic Spells. Vol. 1 Texts, with an Updated Bibliography. Edited by Hans Dieter Betz.* 2nd ed., Chicago: University of Chicago Press.

P.Mich.
= *Michigan Papyri*
Youtie, H. C. and J. G. Winter, eds (1951), *Michigan Papyri. VIII, Papyri and Ostraca from Karanis,* Ann Arbor: Michigan University Press.

P.Oxf.
= *Oxford Papyri*
Wegener, E. P., ed. (1942) (text) and (1948) (plates), *Some Oxford Papyri,* Leiden: Brill.

P.Oxy.
= *The Oxyrhynchus Papyri*
Rea, J. R., ed. (1978), *The Oxyrhynchus Papyri.* Vol. XLVI, London: Egypt Exploration Society.

SB
= *Sammelbuch griechischer Urkunden aus Aegypten*
(1934–1955), *Sammelbuch griechischer Urkunden aus Aegypten.* Vol. V, Heidelberg and Wiesbaden: Harrassowitz.

Paul of Aegina
Heiberg, J. L., ed. (1921–1924), *Paulus Aegineta. Edidit J. L. Heiberg.* 2 vols, Leipzig and Berlin: Teubner.

Pausanias
Description of Greece
Jones, W. H. S., ed. and transl. (1918–1935), *Pausanias. Description of Greece.* 4 vols, Cambridge, MA: Harvard University Press.

Philostratus
Life of Apollonius of Tyana
Jones, Christopher P., ed. and transl. (2005), *Philostratus. Life of Apollonius of Tyana. Edited and Translated by Christopher P. Jones.* 2 vols, Cambridge, MA: Cambridge University Press.

Philostratus of Athens
Gymnasticus
Rusten, Jeffrey and Jason König, eds and transls (2014), *Philostratus. Heroicus. Gymnasticus. Discourses 1 and 2. Edited and Translated by Jeffrey Rusten and Jason König,* Cambridge, MA: Harvard University Press.

Plato
Gorgias
Lamb, W. R. M., transl. (1925), *Plato. Lysis. Symposium. Gorgias. Translated by W. R. M. Lamb*, Cambridge, MA: Harvard University Press.

Menexenus
Bury, R. G., transl. (1929), *Plato. Timaeus. Critias. Cleitophon. Menexenus. Translated by R. G. Bury*, Cambridge, MA: Harvard University Press.

Phaedrus
Fowler, Harold North, transl. (1914), *Plato. Euthyphro. Apology. Crito. Phaedo. Phaedrus. Translated by Harold North Fowler*, Cambridge, MA: Harvard University Press.

Protagoras
Lamb, W. R. M., transl. (1924), *Plato. Laches. Protagoras. Meno. Euthydemus. Translated by W. R. M. Lamb*, Cambridge, MA: Harvard University Press.

Republic
Emlyn-Jones, William and William Preddy, eds and transls (2013), *Plato. Republic, Volume I. Books 1–5. Edited and Translated by Christopher Emlyn-Jones and William Preddy*, Cambridge, MA: Harvard University Press.

Timaeus
Bury, R. G., transl. (1929), *Timaeus. Critias. Cleitophon. Menexenus. Translated by R. G. Bury*, Cambridge, MA: Harvard University Press.

Pliny the Elder
Natural History
Books 20–23: Jones, W. H. S., transl. (1951), *Pliny. Natural History, Volume VI. Books 20–23. Translated by W. H. S. Jones*, Cambridge, MA: Harvard University Press.
Book 24–27: Jones, W. H. S., transl. (1956), *Pliny. Natural History. Volume VII. Books 24–27. Translated by W. H. S. Jones*, Cambridge, MA: Harvard University Press.
Book 28–32: Jones, W. H. S., transl. (1963), *Pliny. Natural History. Volume VIII. Books 28–32. Translated by W. H. S. Jones*, Cambridge, MA: Harvard University Press.
Books 33–35: Rackham, H., transl. (1952), *Pliny. Natural History, Volume IX. Books 33–35. Translated by H. Rackham*, Cambridge, MA: Harvard University Press.
Books 36–37: Eichholz, D. E., transl. (1962), *Pliny. Natural History, Volume X. Books 36–37. Translated by D. E. Eichholz*, Cambridge, MA: Harvard University Press.

Pliny the Younger
Letters
Mynors, R. A. B., ed. (1963), *C. Plini Caecili Secundi epistularum libri decem*, Oxford: Clarendon Press.
Radice, Betty, transl. (1969), *Pliny the Younger. Letters. Translated by Betty Radice.* 2 vols, Cambridge, MA: Harvard University Press.

Plutarch
How to Tell a Flatterer
Babbitt, Frank Cole, transl. (1927), *Plutarch. Moralia. Volume I. The Education of Children. How the Young Man Should Study Poetry. On Listening to Lectures. How to Tell a Flatterer from a Friend. How a Man May Become Aware of His Progress in Virtue. Translated by Frank Cole*, Cambridge, MA: Harvard University Press.

Pericles
Perrin, Bernadotte, transl. (1916), *Plutarch. Lives. Volume III. Pericles and Fabius Maximus. Nicias and Crassus. Translated by Bernadotte Perrin*, Cambridge, MA: Harvard University Press.

Roman Questions
Babbitt, Frank Cole, transl. (1936), *Plutarch. Moralia. Volume IV. Roman Questions. Greek Questions. Greek and Roman Parallel Stories. On the Fortune of the Romans. On the Fortune or the Virtue of Alexander. Were the Athenians More Famous in War or in Wisdom? Translated by Frank Cole Babbitt*, Cambridge, MA: Harvard University Press.

Praxagoras
Fragments
Lewis, Orly, ed. and transl. (2017), *Praxagoras of Cos on Arteries, Pulse and Pneuma*, Leiden: Brill.

Presocratic Philosophers
Fragments
Kirk, G. S., J. E. Raven and M. Schofield ([1973] 1983), *The Presocratic Philosophers*, Cambridge: Cambridge University Press.

Quintus Serenus
The Medical Book
Vollmer, Friedrich, ed. (1916), *Quinti Sereni Liber Medicinalis*, Leipzig: Teubner.

Sallust
The War with Catiline
Ramsey, John T. and J. C. Rolfe, ed. and transl. (2013), *Sallust. The War with Catiline. The War with Jugurtha. Edited by John T. Ramsey. Translated by J. C. Rolfe*, Cambridge, MA: Harvard University Press.

Scribonius Largus
Composite Remedies
Jouanna-Bouchet, Joëlle, ed. and transl. (2016), *Scribonius Largus. Compositions médicales. Texte établi et traduit par J. Jouanna-Bouchet*, Paris: Les Belles Lettres.
Sconocchia, Sergio, ed. (1983), *Scribonii Largi Compositiones. Edidit Sergio Sconocchia*, Leipzig: Teubner.

Semonides
Fragments
Gerber, Douglas E., ed. and transl. (1999), *Archilochus, Semonides, Hipponax. Greek Iambic Poetry: From the Seventh to the Fifth Centuries* BC. *Edited and Translated by Douglas E. Gerber*, Cambridge, MA: Harvard University Press.

Seneca the Younger
On Providence
Basore, John W., ed. and transl. (1928), *Moral Essays. Volume I. De providentia. De constantia. De ira. De clementia. Translated by John W. Basore*, Cambridge, MA: Harvard University Press.

Moral Letters
Gummere, Richard M., transl. (1920), *Seneca. Epistles, Volume II. Epistles 66–92. Translated by Richard M. Gummere*, Cambridge, MA: Harvard University Press.
Reynolds, L. D., ed. (1965), *L. Annaei Senecae ad Lucilium epistulae morales*. 2 vols, Oxford: Clarendon Press

Sextus Empiricus
Against the Logicians
Mutschmann, H., ed. (1914), *Sexti Empirici Opera. Vol. II. Adversus dogmaticos libros quinque (Adv. Mathem. VII–XI)*, Leipzig: Teubner.
Bett, Richard, transl. (2005), *Sextus Empiricus. Against the Logicians*, Cambridge: Cambridge University Press.

Sophocles
Philoctetes and *Women of Trachis*
Lloyd-Jones, Hugh, ed. and transl. (1994), *Sophocles. Antigone. The Women of Trachis. Philoctetes. Oedipus at Colonus. Edited and Translated by Hugh Lloyd-Jones*, Cambridge, MA: Harvard University Press.

Soranus
Gynecology
Ilberg, Johannes, ed. (1927), *Sorani Gynaeciorum libri IV. De signis fractuarum. De fasciis. Vita Hippocratis secundum Soranum. Edidit J. Ilberg*, Leipzig and Berlin: Teubner.
Temkin, Owsei, transl. (1956), *Soranus' Gynecology. Translated by Owsei Temkin, with the Assistance of Nicholson J. Eastman, Ludwig Edelstein, and Alan F. Guttmacher*, Baltimore, MD: Johns Hopkins Press.

Strabo
Geography
Jones, Horace Leonard, transl. (1917–1932), *Strabo. Geography. Translated by Horace Leonard Jones*. 8 vols, Cambridge, MA: Harvard University Press.

Suetonius
Lives of the Caesars
Rolfe, J. C. and K. R. Bradley, transl. (1914), *Suetonius. Lives of the Caesars, Volume I. Julius. Augustus. Tiberius. Gaius. Caligula. Translated by J. C. Rolfe. Introduction by K. R. Bradley*, Cambridge, MA: Harvard University Press.

Tacitus
Agricola and *Germania*
Hutton, M., W. Peterson, R. M. Ogilvie, E. H. Warmington and Michael Winterbottom, transls (1914), *Tacitus. Agricola, Germania. Dialogue on Oratory.*

Translated by M. Hutton, W. Peterson. Revised by R. M. Ogilvie, E. H. Warmington and Michael Winterbottom, Cambridge, MA: Harvard University Press.

Annals
Jackson, John, transl. (1937), Tacitus. Annals. Books 4–6, 11–12. Translated by John Jackson, Cambridge, MA: Harvard University Press.

Tatian
Whittaker, Molly, ed. and transl. (1982), Oratio ad Graecos and Fragments. Edited and Translated by Molly Whittaker, Oxford: Oxford University Press.

Tertullian
On the Soul
Waszink, J. H., ed. (1947), Q. Septimi Florentis Tertulliani De anima, Amsterdam: Meulenhoff.

Theophrastus
Enquiry into Plants
Amigues, Suzanne, ed. and transl. (2006), Théophraste. Recherches sur les plantes. Tome V. Livre IX. Texte établi et traduit par S. Amigues, Paris: Les Belles Lettres.
Hort, Arthur F., transl. (1916), Theophrastus. Enquiry into Plants, Volume II. Books 6–9. On Odours. Weather Signs. Translated by Arthur F. Hort, Cambridge, MA: Harvard University Press.

On Sense-Perception
Diels, Hermann, ed. (1879), Doxographi Graeci, Berlin: G. Reimer.

Thucydides
History of the Peloponnesian War
Smith, C. F., transl. (1919–1923), Thucydides. History of the Peloponnesian War. Translated by C. F. Smith. 4 vols, Cambridge, MA: Harvard University Press.

Varro
On Agriculture
Hooper, W. D. and Harrison Boyd Ash, transl. (1934), Cato. Varro. On Agriculture. Translated by W. D. Hooper, Harrison Boyd Ash, Cambridge, MA: Harvard University Press.

Vegetius
Epitome of Military Science
Reeve, M. D., ed. (2004), Vegetius. Epitome rei militaris. Edited by M. D. Reeve, Oxford: Clarendon Press.
Milner, N. P., transl. (1993), Vegetius. Epitome of Military Science. Translated with Notes and Introduction, Liverpool: Liverpool University Press.

Vitruvius
On Architecture
Granger, Frank (1931), Vitruvius. On Architecture. Volume I. Books 1–5. Translated by Frank Granger, Cambridge, MA: Harvard University Press.

Xenophon
Anabasis
Brownson, Carleton L. and John Dillery, transls (1998), *Xenophon. Anabasis. Translated by Carleton L. Brownson. Revised by John Dillery*, Cambridge, MA: Harvard University Press.

Memorabilia
Marchant, E. C., O. J. Todd and Jeffrey Henderson, eds and transls (2013), *Xenophon. Memorabilia. Oeconomicus. Symposium. Apology. Translated by E. C. Marchant, O. J. Todd. Revised by Jeffrey Henderson*, Cambridge, MA: Harvard University Press.

BIBLIOGRAPHY

Africa, Thomas W. (1961), 'The Opium Addiction of Marcus Aurelius', *Journal of the History of Ideas*, 22: 97–102.

Allason-Jones, Lindsay and Bruce McKay (1985), *Coventina's Well: A Shrine on Hadrian's Wall*, Gloucester: Alan Sutton Publishing.

Allen-Hornblower, Emily (2013), 'Sounds and Suffering in Sophocles' *Philoctetes* and Gide's *Philoctète*', *Studi Italiani di Filologia Classica*, 11 (1): 5–41.

Allen-Hornblower, Emily (2016), 'Moral Disgust in Sophocles' *Philoctetes*', in Donald Lateiner and Dimos Spatharas (eds), *The Ancient Emotion of Disgust, Emotions of the Past Series*, 69–86, Oxford: Oxford University Press.

Amigues, Suzanne (2008), 'Remèdes et poisons végétaux transmis à l'homme par l'animal', in Isabelle Boehm and Pascal Luccioni (eds), *Le médecin initié par l'animal*, 97–107, Lyon: Maison de l'Orient et de la Méditerranée – Jean Pouilloux.

Amundsen, Darrel W. and Carol Jean Diers (1969), 'The Age of Menarche in Classical Greece and Rome', *Human Biology*, 41 (1): 125–32.

Annas, Julia E. (1992), *Hellenistic Philosophy of Mind,* Berkeley, CA: University of California Press.

Arnott, Robert (2005), 'Disease and the Prehistory of the Aegean', in Helen King (ed.), *Health in Antiquity*, 12–31, London and New York: Routledge.

Arnott, Robert (2008), 'Chrysokamino: Occupational Health and the Earliest Medicine on Crete', in Yannis Tzedakis, Holley Martlew and Martin Jones (eds), *Archaeology Meets Science: Biomolecular and Site Investigations in Bronze Age Greece*, 108–20, Oxford: Oxbow Books.

Arnott, Robert, Stanley Finger and Christopher U. M. Smith, eds (2003), *Trepanation: History, Discovery, Theory*, Lisse: Swets & Zeitlinger.

Bagnall, Roger S. and Rafaella Cribiore (2008), *Women's Letters from Ancient Egypt:300 BC–AD 800*, Ann Arbor, MI: University of Michigan Press.

Baker, Patricia (2001), 'Medicine, Culture and Military Identity', in Gwyn Davies, Andrew Gardner and Kris Lockyear (eds), *TRAC 2000: The Theoretical Roman Archaeology Conference Proceedings 2000*, 51–70, Oxford: Oxbow Press.

Baker, Patricia (2004), 'Roman Medical Instruments: Archaeological Interpretations of their Possible "Non-functional" Uses', *Social History of Medicine*, 17: 3–21.

Baker, Patricia (2011), 'Collyrium Stamps: An Indicator of Regional Medical Practices in Roman Gaul', *European Journal of Archaeology*, 14 (1–2): 158–89.

Baker, Patricia (2013), *The Archaeology of Medicine in the Greco-Roman World*, Cambridge: Cambridge University Press.

Barbara, Sébastien (2008), 'Castoréum et basilic, deux substances animales de la pharmacopée ancienne', in Isabelle Boehm and Pascal Luccioni (eds), *Le médecin initié par l'animal*, 121–48, Lyon: Maison de l'Orient et de la Méditerranée – Jean Pouilloux.

Barrett, John C. (1989), 'Afterwards: Render unto Caesar', in John C. Barrett, Andrew P. Fitzpatrick and Lesley Macinnes (eds), *Barbarians and Romans in North-West Europe from the Later Republic to Late Antiquity*, 235–41, Oxford: British Archaeological Reports.

Bartoš, Hynek (2015), *Philosophy and Dietetics in the Hippocratic* On Regimen: *A Delicate Balance of Health*, Leiden: Brill.

Berger, Arthur A. (2009), *What Objects Mean: An Introduction to Material Culture*, Walnut Creek, CA: West Coast Press.

Bertier, Janine (1972), *Mnésithée et Dieuchès*, Leiden: Brill.

Bianucci, Raffaella, Adauto Araujo, Carsten M. Pusch and Andreas G. Nerlich (2015), 'The Identification of Malaria in Paleopathology: An in-Depth Assessment of the Strategies to Detect Malaria in Ancient Remains', *Acta Tropica*, 152: 162–80.

Bliquez, Lawrence (1981), 'Greek and Roman Medicine', *Archaeology*, 34 (2): 10–17.

Bliquez, Lawrence (1988), *Roman Surgical Instruments and Minor Objects Found in the University of Mississippi*, Göteborg: Paul Åstroms Förlag.

Bliquez, Lawrence (1992), 'The Hercules Motif on Greco-Roman Surgical Tools', in Antje Krug (ed.), *From Epidaurus to Salerno: Symposium Held at the European University Centre for Cultural Heritage, Ravello, April 1990*, 35–50, Rixensart, Belgium: PACT 34.

Bliquez, Lawrence (1994), *Roman Surgical Implements and Other Minor Objects in the National Archaeological Museum of Naples*, Mainz: Verlag Philipp von Zabern.

Bliquez, Lawrence (2014), *The Tools of Asclepius: Surgical Implements in Greek and Roman Times*, Leiden: Brill.

Bliquez, Lawrence and J. P. Oleson (1994), 'The Origins, Early History and Applications of the *Pyoulkos* (Syringe)', in Gilbert Argoud (ed.), *Science et vie intellectuelle à Alexandrie*, 83–103, Saint-Étienne: Publications de l'Université de Saint-Étienne.

Bodson, Liliane (2005), 'Tierheilkunde', in Karl-Heinz Leven (ed.), *Antike Medizin: Ein Lexikon*, 863–4, München: C.H. Beck.

Bosman, Arjen V. A. J. (1995), 'Velserbroek B6 Velsen1-Velsen2: Is there a Relationship between the Military Equipment from the Ritual Site and the Fortress of Velsen?' *Journal of Roman Military Equipment Studies*, 6: 89–98.

Boudon-Millot, Véronique (2003), 'Aux marges de la médecine rationnelle: Médecins et charlatans à Rome au temps de Galien (IIe s. de notre ère)', *Revue des Études Grecques*, 116: 109–31.

Boudon-Millot, Véronique (2010), 'Aux origines de la thériaque: La recette d'Andromaque', *Revue d'Histoire de la Pharmacie*, 367: 261–70.

Boudon-Millot, Véronique (2012), *Galien de Pergame: Un médecin grec à Rome*, Paris: Les Belles Lettres.

Bouffartigue, Jean (2008), 'L'automédication des animaux chez les auteurs antiques', in Isabelle Boehm and Pascal Luccioni (eds), *Le médecin initié par l'animal*, 79–96, Lyon: Maison de l'Orient et de la Méditerranée – Jean Pouilloux.

Bourbon, Florence (2008), 'Poulpe de mer et crabe de rivière dans la *Collection Hippocratique*', in Isabelle Boehm and Pascal Luccioni (eds), *La médecin initié par l'animal*, 109–19, Lyon: Maison de l'Orient et de la Méditerranée – Jean Pouilloux.

Bowersock, Glen W. (1969), *Greek Sophists in the Roman Empire*, Oxford: Clarendon.

Bowersock, Glen (2004), 'Artemidorus and the Second Sophistic', in Barbara Borg (ed.), *Paideia: The World of the Second Sophistic*, 53–63, Berlin: De Gruyter.

Braund, David (forthcoming), 'Milk and Mutilation', in *Scythians in Greek Culture*.

Braund, David and John Wilkins, eds (2000), *Athenaeus and His World*, Exeter: Exeter University Press.

Bruun, Christer (2012), 'La mancanza di prove di un effetto catastrofico della "Peste Antonina" (dal 166 D.C. in poi)', in Elio Lo Cascio (ed.), *L'impatto della 'Peste Antonina'*, 123–65, Bari: Edipuglia.

Byl, Simon (1999), 'La thérapeutique par le miel dans le Corpus Hippocraticum', in I. Garofalo et al (eds), *Aspetti della Terapia nel Corpus Hippocraticum*, 119–24, Florence: L. S. Olschki.

Campbell, Gordon (2008), 'And Bright Was the Flame of Their Friendship (Empedocles B130): Humans, Animals, Justice, and Friendship, in Lucretius and Empedocles', *Leeds International Classical Studies*, 7 (4): 1–23.

Casadei, Elena (1997), 'La dottrina corpuscolare di Asclepiade e i suoi rapporti con la tradizione atomista', *Elenchos*, 18 (1): 77–106.

Cech, Brigitte, ed. (2008), *Die Produktion von Ferrum Noricum am Hüttenberger Erzberg: Die Ergebnisse der interdisziplinären Forschungen auf der Fundstelle Semlach. Eisner in den Jahren 2003–2005*, Wien: Österreichische Gesellschaft für Archäologie.

Champlin, Edward (1980), *Fronto and Antonine Rome*, Cambridge, MA: Harvard University Press.

Chandezon, Christophe (2015), 'Animals, Meat and Alimentary By-Products: Patterns of Production and Consumption', in John Wilkins and Robin Nadeau (eds), *A Companion to Food in the Ancient World*, 135–47, Malden, MA: Wiley-Blackwell.

Chandezon, Christophe and Christine Homdoume, eds (2004), *Les Hommes et la terre dans la Méditerranée gréco-romaine*, Toulouse: Presses universitaires du Mirail.

Charpentier, Marie-Claude and Jordi Pàmias (2006), 'Les animaux et la crise de panique en Grèce antique', in Isabelle Boehm and Pascal Luccioni (eds), *Le médecin initié par l'animal*, 197–209, Lyon: Maison de l'Orient et de la Méditerranée – Jean Pouilloux.

Ciaraldi, Marina (2000), 'Drug Preparation in Evidence? An Unusual Plant and Bone Assemblage from the Pompeian Countryside, Italy', *Vegetation History and Archaeobotany*, 9(2): 91–8.

Clafin Kyri W. and Peter Scholliers, eds (2012), *Writing Food History: A Global Perspective*, London: Bloomsbury.

Clarke, Michael (1995), 'Between Lions and Man: Images of the Hero in the *Iliad*', *Greek, Roman and Byzantine Studies*, 36: 137–60.

Cohen, David (1991), *Law, Sexuality and Society*, Cambridge: Cambridge University Press.

Cohen, Edward E. (2014), 'Sexual Abuse and Sexual Rights: Slaves' Erotic Experience at Athens and Rome', in Thomas K. Hubbard (ed.), *A Companion to Greek and Roman Sexualities*, 184–98, Chichester: Wiley-Blackwell.

Cohn, Samuel K. (2012), 'Pandemics: Waves of Disease, Waves of Hate from the Plague of Athens to A.I.D.S', *Historical Research: The Bulletin of the Institute of Historical Research*, 85, no. 230: 535–55.

Cohn-Haft, Louis (1956), *The Public Physicians of Ancient Greece*, Northampton, MA: Smith College Studies in History.

Collins, Andrew W. (2012), 'Alexander the Great and the Office of *Edeatros*', *Historia*, 61(4): 414–20.

Comelles, Josep M. (1997), 'The Fear of (One's Own) History: On the Relations between Medical Anthropology, Medicine and History', *Dynamis*, 17: 37–68.

Condrau, Flurin (2007), 'The Patient's View Meets the Clinical Gaze', *Social History of Medicine*, 20: 525–40.

Cook, Harold (1986), *The Decline of the Old Medical Regime in Stuart London*, Ithaca, NY: Cornell University Press.

Cowen, David L. (1985), 'Expunctum est Mithridatium', *Pharmaceutical Historian*, 153: 2–3.

Craik, Elizabeth (2015), *The 'Hippocratic' Corpus: Content and Context*, London: Routledge.

Craik, Elizabeth (2017), 'Malaria and the Environment of Greece', in Orietta D. Cordovana and Gian Franco Chiai (eds), *Pollution and the Environment in Ancient Life and Thought*, 153–62, Stuttgart: Franz Steiner Verlag.

Craik, Elizabeth (2020), 'Malaria, Childbirth and the Cult of Artemis', in Laurence M. V. Totelin and Rebecca Flemming (eds), *Medicine and Markets in the Graeco-Roman World and Beyond: Essays on Ancient Medicine in Honour of Vivian Nutton*, 87–99, Swansea: Classical Press of Wales.

Croon, J. H. (1967), 'Hot Springs and Healing Gods', *Mnemosyne*, 40: 225–46.

Crummy, N. (2007), 'The Identities of the "Doctor" and the "Warrior"', in Philip Crummy, S. Benfield, N. Crummy, V. Rigby and D. Shimmin (eds), *Stanway: An Élite Burial Site at Camulodunum*, 444–7, London: Society for the Promotion of Roman Studies.

Crummy, Philip (2002), 'A Preliminary Account of the Doctor's Grave at Stanway, Colchester, England', in Patricia Baker and Gillian Carr (eds), *Practitioners, Practices and Patients: New Approaches to Medical Archaeology and Anthropology*, 44–57, Oxford: Oxbow Books.

Cuomo, Serafina (2007), *Technology and Culture in Greek and Roman Antiquity*, Cambridge: Cambridge University Press.

Curtis, Robert I. (1991), *Garum and Salsamenta: Production and Commerce in Materia Medica*, Leiden: Brill.

Dalby, Andrew (1996), *Siren Feasts: A History of Food and Gastronomy in Greece*, London: Routledge.

Dalby, Andrew (2003), *Food in the Ancient World from A to Z*, London: Routledge.

D'arms, John H. (1970), *Romans on the Bay of Naples: A Social and Cultural Study of the Villas and Their Owners from 150 BC to AD 40*, Cambridge, MA: Harvard University Press.

Davidson, James N. (1995), 'Don't Try this at Home: Pliny's Salpe, Salpe's *Paignia* and Magic', *The Classical Quarterly (New Series)*, 45 (2): 590–2.

Davidson, James N. (1997), *Courtesans and Fishcakes: The Consuming Passions of Classical Athens*, Chicago: University of Chicago Press.

Davidson, James (2007), *The Greeks and Greek Love: A Radical Reappraisal of Homosexuality in Ancient Greece*, London: Weidenfeld & Nicolson.

Deacy, Susan and Fiona McHardy (2015), 'Ajax, Cassandra and Athena: Retaliatory Warfare and Gender Violence at the Sack of Troy', in Geoff Lee, Helène Whittaker and Graham Wrightson (eds), *Ancient Warfare: Introducing Current Research Volume I*, 252–72, Newcastle: Cambridge Scholars Publishing.

Dean-Jones, Lesley A. (1994), *Women's Bodies in Classical Greek Science*, Oxford: Oxford University Press.

Dean-Jones, Lesley A. (2006), 'Galen on the Brain', *Apeiron*, 39: 289–92.

Debru, Armelle (1994), 'L'expérimentation chez Galien', in Hildgard Temporini and Wolfgang Haase (eds), *Aufstieg und Niedergang der Romischen Welt*. Band II 37.2, 1728–56, Berlin: De Gruyter.

Debru, Armelle (1995), 'Les démonstrations médicales à Rome au temps de Galien', in Philip J. van der Eijk, Herman F. J. Horstmanshoff and P. H. Schrijvers (eds), *Ancient Medicine in its Socio-Cultural Context. Papers Read at the Congress Held at Leiden University. 13–15 April 1992*, 69–82, Amsterdam: Rodopi Press.

Demand, Nancy (1994), *Birth, Death, and Motherhood in Classical Greece*, Baltimore, MD: Johns Hopkins University Press.

Demand, Nancy (1995), 'Monuments, Midwives and Gynecology', in Philip J. van der Eijk, Herman F. J. Horstmanshoff and P. H. Schrijvers (eds), *Ancient Medicine in its Socio-Cultural Context. Papers Read at the Congress Held at Leiden University. 13–15 April 1992*, 275–90, Amsterdam: Rodopi Press.

Desch, Franziska (2017), 'Reconsidering the Term *Dreckapotheke* for the Ancient Near-East', in Lennart Lehmhaus and Matteo Martelli (eds), *Collecting Recipes: Byzantine and Jewish Pharmacology in Dialogue*, 35–50, Berlin: De Gruyter.

Detys, S. (1988), 'Les ex-voto de guérison en Gaule', *Dossiers Histoire et Archéologie*, 123: 82–7.

Dossabhoy, Shernaz S., Jessica Feng and Manisha S. Desai (2018), 'The Use and Relevance of the Hippocratic Oath in 2015: A Survey of US Medical Schools', *Journal of Anesthesia History*, 4 (2): 139–46.

Dover, Kenneth J. (1989), *Greek Homosexuality: Updated and with a New Postscript*, Cambridge, MA: Harvard University Press.

Downie, Janet (2013), *At the Limits of Art: A Literary Study of Aelius Aristides'* Hieroi Logoi, Oxford: Oxford University Press.

Draycott, Jane (2019), *Roman Domestic Medical Practice in Central Italy: From the Middle Republic to the Early Empire*, London: Routledge.

Duncan-Jones, R. P. (1996), 'The Impact of the Antonine Plague', *Journal of Roman Archaeology*, 9: 108–36.

Edelstein, Ludwig (1967), *Ancient Medicine: Selected Papers of Ludwig Edelstein*, Baltimore, MD: Johns Hopkins University Press.

Edelstein, Emma J. and Ludwig Edelstein (1945), *Asclepius: A Collection and Interpretation of the Testimonies*. 2 vols, Baltimore, MD: Johns Hopkins University Press.

Elliott, Colin P. (2016), 'The Antonine Plague, Climate Change and Local Violence in Roman Egypt', *Past & Present*, 231 (1): 3–31.

Etkin, Nina L. (1988), 'Cultural Constructions of Efficacy', in S. van der Geest and S. Reynolds Whyte (eds), *The Context of Medicines in Developing Countries: Studies in Pharmaceutical Anthropology*, 299–326, Dordrecht: Kluwer Academic.

Etkin, Nina L. (2008), *Edible Medicines: An Ethnopharmacology of Food*, Tucson, AZ: University of Arizona Press.

Fabricius, Cajus (1972), *Galens Exzerpte aus älteren Pharmakologen*, Berlin and New York: De Gruyter.

Faure, Eric (2014), 'Malarial Pathocoenosis: Beneficial and Deleterious Interactions between Malaria and Other Human Diseases', *Frontiers in Physiology*, 5, no. 441: 1–13.

Fernando, Sumadhya D., Chaturaka Rodrigo and Senaka Rajapakse (2010), 'The "Hidden" Burden of Malaria: Cognitive Impairment Following Infection', *Malaria Journal*, 9, no. 366: 1–11.

Ferngren, Gary (2009), *Medicine and Health Care in Early Christianity*, Baltimore, MD: Johns Hopkins University Press.

Ferraces Rodríguez, Arsenio (2006), 'Antropoterapia de la Antigüedad Tardía', *Les Études Classiques*, 74: 219–52.

Ferraces Rodríguez, Arsenio (2016), *Curae quae ex hominibus atque animalibus fiunt*, Santiago de Compostela: Andavira Editora.

Flemming, Rebecca (2003), 'Empires of Knowledge: Medicine and Health in the Hellenistic World', in Andrew Erskine (ed.), *A Companion to the Hellenistic World*, 449–63, Malden, MA: Wiley-Blackwell.

Flemming, Rebecca (2005), 'Suicide, Euthanasia and Medicine: Reflections Ancient and Modern', *Economy and Society*, 34 (2): 295–321.

Fögen, Thorsten (2016), 'All Creatures Great and Small: On the Roles and Functions of Animals in Columella's *De Re Rustica*', *Hermes*, 144: 321–51.

Fögen, Thorsten and Thomas Edmunds, eds (2017), *Interactions between Animals and Humans in Graeco-Roman Antiquity*, Berlin: De Gruyter.

Forbes, Robert J. (1966), *Studies in Ancient Technology*, Leiden: Brill.

Foucault, Michel ([1984] 1990), *The History of Sexuality*. Vol. 3. *The Care of the Self*, transl. Robert Hurley, London: Penguin.

Fox, Sherry C. (2005), 'Health in Hellenistic and Roman Times: The Case Studies of Paphos, Cyprus and Corinth, Greece', in Helen King (ed.), *Health in Antiquity*, 59–82, London and New York: Routledge.

Foxhall, Lin (1998), 'Cargoes of the Heart's Desire: The Character of Trade in the Archaic Mediterranean World', in Nick Fisher and Hans van Wees (eds), *Archaic Greece: New Approaches and New Evidence*, 295–309, London: Duckworth.

Foxhall, Lin (2005), 'Village to City: Staples and Luxuries? Exchange Networks and Urbanization', in Robin Osborne and Barry Cunliffe (eds), *Mediterranean Urbanization 800–600 BC*, 233–48, Oxford: Oxford University Press.

Foxhall Lin and H. A. Forbes (1982), 'Sitometreia: The Role of Grain as a Staple Food in Classical Antiquity', *Chiron*, 12: 41–90.

Frede, Michael (1987), 'The Ancient Empiricists', in Michael Frede (ed.), *Essays in Ancient Philosophy*, 243–60, Minneapolis, MN: University of Minnesota Press.

Freisenbruch, Annelise (2007), 'Back to Fronto: Doctor and Patient in his Correspondence with an Emperor', in Ruth Morello and A. D. Morrison (eds), *Ancient Letters: Classical and Late Antique Epistolography*, 235–56, Oxford: Oxford University Press.

Frier, Bruce W. (2000), 'Demography', in Alan K. Bowman, Peter Garnsey and Dominic Rathbone (eds), *The Cambridge Ancient History: The High Empire, AD 70–192*. 2nd ed. Vol. 11, 787–816, Cambridge: Cambridge University Press.

Gagneux, Sebastien (2012), 'Host-Pathogen Coevolution in Human Tuberculosis', *Philosophical Transactions: Biological Sciences*, 367, no. 1590: 850–9.

Galagan, James E. (2014), 'Genomic Insights into Tuberculosis', *Nature Reviews. Genetics*, 15 (5): 307–20.

Gallant, Thomas W. (1991), *Risk and Survival in Ancient Greece: Reconstructing the Rural Domestic Economy,* Stanford, CA: Stanford University Press.

Garnsey, Peter D. A. (1988), *Famine and Food Supply in the Graeco-Roman World: Responses to Risk and Crisis*, Cambridge: Cambridge University Press.

Garnsey, Peter D. A. (1999), *Food and Society in Classical Antiquity,* Cambridge: Cambridge University Press.

Gazza, Vittorino (1956), 'Prescrizioni mediche nei papiri dell'Egitto Greco-Romano', *Aegyptus*, 36: 73–114.

Germain, Louis R. F. (1969), 'Aspects du droit d'exposition en Grèce', *Revue Historique de Droit Française*, 47: 177–97.

Gill, Christopher (2010), *Naturalistic Philosophy in Galen and Stoicism*, Oxford: Oxford University Press.

Ginouvès, René (1962), *Balaneutikè: Recherches sur le bain dans l'antiquité grecque*, Paris: de Boccard.

Ginouvès, René (1994), 'L'eau dans les sanctuaires médicaux', in René Ginouvès, A.-M. Guimier-Sorbets, Jacques Jouanna and Laurence Villard (eds), *L'eau, la santé et la maladie dans le monde grec*, 236–43, Paris: de Boccard.

Gitton-Ripoll, Valérie (2008), 'Chiron, le cheval-médecin ou pourquoi Hippocrate s'appelle Hippocrate', in Isabelle Boehm and Pascal Luccioni (eds), *Le médecin initié par l'animal*, 211–34, Lyon: Maison de l'Orient et de la Méditerranée – Jean Pouilloux.

Gleason, Maud W. (2009), 'Shock and Awe: The Performance Dimension of Galen's Anatomy Demonstrations', in Christopher Gill, Tim Whitmarsh and John Wilkins (eds), *Galen and the World of Knowledge*, 85–114, Cambridge: Cambridge University Press.

Goebel, V. and Peters, J. (2010), 'Veterinary Medicine', in G. L. Campbell (ed.), *Oxford Handbook of Animals in Classical Thought and Life*, 589–606, Oxford: Oxford University Press.

Gorrini, Maria Elena (2005), 'The Hippocratic Impact on Healing Cults: The Archaeological Evidence in Attica', in Philip J. van der Eijk (ed.), *Hippocrates in Context. Papers Read at the XIth International Hippocrates Colloquium, University of Newcastle-upon-Tyne, 27–31 August 2002*, 135–56, Leiden: Brill.

Gosselain, Olivier (1992), 'Technology and Style: Potters and Pottery among the Bafia of Cameroon', *Man New Series*, 27 (3): 559–86.

Gourevitch, Danielle (2000), 'Hicesius' Fish and Chips', in David Braund and John Wilkins (eds), *Athenaeus and His World*, 483–91, Exeter: Exeter University Press.

Gourevitch, Danielle (2001), 'Le nourrisson et sa nourrice: Étude de quelques cas pédiatriques chez Galien', *Revue de Philosophie Ancienne*, 19: 63–76.

Graham, Emma-Jayne (2013), 'The Making of Infants in Hellenistic and Early Roman Italy: A Votive Perspective', *World Archaeology*, 45 (2): 215–31.

Graham, Emma-Jayne (2016), 'Wombs and Tombs in the Roman World', *Material Religion*, 12 (1): 251–4.

Greenlaw, Cybelle (2011), *The Representation of Monkeys in the Art and Thought of Mediterranean Cultures*, Oxford: Oxford University Press.

Greene, Kevin (2008), 'Learning to Consume: Consumption and Consumerism in the Roman Empire', *Journal of Roman Archaeology*, 21: 64–82.

Griffin, Miriam ([1976] 1992), *Seneca: A Philosopher in Politics*, Oxford: Oxford University Press.

Grivell, Timothy, Helen Clegg and Elizabeth C. Roxburgh (2014), 'An Interpretative Phenomenological Analysis of Identity in the Therian Community', *Identity: An International Journal of Theory and Research*, 14 (2): 113–35.

Grmek, Mirko D. ([1983] 1989), *Diseases in the Ancient Greek World* [Les maladies à l'aube de la civilisation occidentale]. Translated by Mireille Muellner and Leonard Muellner, Baltimore, MD: Johns Hopkins University Press.

Grmek, Mirko D. (1996), *Il calderone di Medea: La sperimentazione sul vivente nell'antichità*, Rome: Editori Laterza.

Gruen, Erich S. (2011), *Rethinking the Other in Antiquity*, Princeton, NJ: Princeton University Press.

Hadot, Pierre (1984), 'Marc Aurèle était-il opiomane?' in E. Lucchesi and H. D. Saffron (eds), *Mémorial André-Jean Festugière: Antiquité païenne et chrétienne*, 35–50, Geneva: Cramer.

Hankinson, R. J. (1991a), 'Greek Medical Models of Mind', in S. Everson (ed.), *Psychology*. Companions to Ancient Thought, vol. 2, Cambridge: Cambridge University Press.

Hankinson, R. J. (1991b), 'Galen's Anatomy of the Soul', *Phronesis*, 36: 197–233.

Hankinson, R. J., ed. (2008), *The Cambridge Companion to Galen*, Cambridge: Cambridge University Press.

Hanson, Ann Ellis (1987), 'The Eight-Months Child and the Etiquette of Birth: *obsit omen!*', *Bulletin of the History of Medicine*, 61: 589–602.

Hanson, Ann Ellis (1990), 'The Medical Writers' Woman', in David M. Halperin, John J. Winkler and Froma I. Zeitlin (eds), *Before Sexuality: The Construction of Erotic Experience in the Ancient Greek World*, 309–38, Princeton, NJ: Princeton University Press.

Hanson, Ann Ellis (2010), 'Doctors' Literacy and Papyri of Medical Content', in Herman F. J. Horstmanshoff and Cornelis van Tilburg (eds), *Hippocrates and Medical Education. Selected Papers read at the XIIth International Hippocrates Colloquium, Universiteit Leiden, 24–26 August 2005*, 187–204, Leiden: Brill.

Hanson, Ann Ellis, and Monica Green (1994), 'Soranus of Ephesus: *Methodicorum princeps*', in Hildegard Temporini and Wolfgang Haase (eds), *Aufstieg und Niedergang der Romischen Welt*. Band II 37.2, 968–1075, Berlin: De Gruyter.

Hardy, Gavin and Laurence M. V. Totelin (2016), *Ancient Botany*, London: Routledge.

Harig, Georg (1977), 'Die antike Auffassung vom Gift und der Tod des Mithridates. (Le concept antique de poison et la mort de Mithridate)', *NTM. Schriftenreihe für Geschichte der Naturwissenschaften Technik und Medizin Leipzig*, 14(1): 104–12.

Harris, Charles R. S. (1973), *The Heart and the Vascular System in Ancient Greek Medicine*, Oxford: Clarendon Press.

Harris, William V., ed. (2013), *Mental Disorders in the Classical World,* Leiden: Brill.

Harris, William V. (2016), 'Popular Medicine in the Classical World', in William V. Harris (ed.), *Popular Medicine in the Greco-Roman World: Explorations*, 1–64, Leiden: Brill.

Harris, William V., ed. (2016), *Popular Medicine in Graeco-Roman Antiquity: Explorations*, Leiden: Brill.

Harris, William V. (2020), 'Scatological Asklepios: The Use of Excrement in Graeco-Roman Healthcare', *Journal of the History of Medicine and Allied Sciences*, 75 (1): 1–23.

Harrison, Adrian P., Ilenia Cattani and Jean M. Turfa (2010), 'Metallurgy, Environmental Pollution and the Decline of Etruscan Civilisation', *Environmental Science and Pollution Research*, 17: 165–80.

Heath, John (2005), *The Talking Greeks: Speech, Animals, and the Other in Homer, Aeschylus and Plato*, Cambridge: Cambridge University Press.

Heinimann, Felix (1945), *Nomos und Physis: Herkunft und Bedeutung einer Antithese im griechischen Denken des 5. Jahrhunderts,* Basel: F. Reinhardt.

Hillert, Andreas (1990), *Antike Ärztedarstellungen*, Frankfurt: Peter Lang.

Hin, Saskia (2013), *The Demography of Roman Italy: Population Dynamics in an Ancient Conquest Society (201 BCE–14 CE)*, Cambridge: Cambridge University Press.

Hingley, Richard (1997), 'Resistance and Domination: Social Change in Roman
    Britain', in David Mattingly (ed.), *Dialogues in Roman Imperialism*, 81–100, Ann
    Arbor, MI: *Journal of Roman Archaeology*.
Hodder, Ian (1982), *Symbols in Action*, Cambridge: Cambridge University Press.
Holford-Strevens, Leofranc ([1988] 2003), *Aulus Gellius: An Antonine Scholar and His
    Achievement*, Oxford: Oxford University Press.
Holmes, Brooke (2017), 'The Generous Text: Animal, Intuition, Human Knowledge
    and Written Tradition in Pliny's Books on Medicine', in Marco Formisano and
    Philip J. van der Eijk (eds), *Knowledge, Text and Practice in Ancient Greek Technical
    Writing*, 231–51, Cambridge: Cambridge University Press.
Horden, Peregrine and Nicholas Purcell (2000), *The Corrupting Sea: A Study of
    Mediterranean History*, Malden, MA: Blackwell.
Horky, Phillip S. (2017), 'The Spectrum of Animal Rationality in Plutarch', *Apeiron*,
    50 (1): 103–33.
Horstmanshoff, Herman F. J. (1976), 'The Ancient Physician: Craftsman or Scientist?',
    Bulletin of the History of Medicine, 31: 448–59.
Horstmanshoff, Herman F. J. (2004), 'Did the God Learn Medicine: Asclepius and
    Temple Medicine in Aelius Aristides' *Sacred Tales*', in Herman F. J. Horstmanshoff
    and Marten Stol (eds), *Magic and Rationality in Ancient Near Eastern and Graeco-
    Roman Medicine*, 325–42, Leiden: Brill.
Hughes, Jessica (2008), 'Fragmentation as Metaphor in the Classical Healing
    Sanctuary', *Social History of Medicine*, 21 (2): 217–36.
Hulttala, Anne (2007), *Le inscrizione sepulcrali latine nell'isola sacra*, Rome: Finnish
    Institute.
Ingold, T. (2001), 'Beyond Art and Technology: The Anthropology of Skill', in Michale
    B. Schiffer (ed.), *Anthropological Perspectives on Technology*, 17–32, Albuquerque,
    NM: University of New Mexico Press.
Isaac, Benjamin (2004), *The Invention of Racism in Classical Antiquity*, Princeton, NJ:
    Princeton University Press.
Israelowich, Ido (2012), *Society, Medicine and Religion in the* Sacred Tales *of Aelius
    Aristides*, Leiden: Brill.
Israelowich, Ido (2015), *Patients and Healers in the High Empire*, Baltimore, MD:
    Johns Hopkins University Press.
Israelowich, Ido (2016a), 'Medical Care in the Roman Army during the High Empire',
    in William V. Harris (ed.), *Perspectives on Popular Medicine in Classical Antiquity*,
    215–30, Leiden: Brill.
Israelowich, Ido (2016b), 'The Use and Abuse of Hippocratic Medicine in the *Apology*
    of Lucius Apuleius', *Classical Quarterly*, 67: 635–44.
Jackson, Ralph (1990a), 'Waters and Spas in the Classical World', in Roy Porter (ed.),
    The Medical History of Waters and Spas, 1–13, London: Wellcome Institute for the
    History of Medicine.
Jackson, Ralph (1990b), 'Roman Doctors and their Instruments: Recent Research into
    Ancient Practice', *Journal of Roman Archaeology*, 3: 5–27.
Jackson, Ralph (1993), 'Roman Medicine: Practitioners and their Practices', in
    Hildegard Temporini and Wolfgang Haase (eds), *Aufstieg und Niedergang der
    Romischen Welt*. Band II 37.1, 79–100, Berlin: De Gruyter.
Jackson, Ralph (1994a), 'The Surgical Instruments, Appliances and Equipment in
    Celsus' *De Medicina*', in Guy Sabbah and Philippe Mudry (eds), *La médecine de
    Celse: Aspects historiques, scientifiques et littéraires*, 167–209, Saint-Étienne:
    Publications de l'Université de Saint-Étienne.

Jackson, Ralph (1994b), '*Styphylagra, Staphylocaustes*, Uvulectomy and Haemorrhoidectomy: The Roman Instruments and Operations', in Antje Krug (ed.), *From Epidauros to Salerno. Symposium Held at the European University Centre for Cultural Heritage, Ravello, April 1990*, 167–85, Rixensart: Pact Belgium.

Jackson, Ralph (1995), 'The Composition of Roman Medical *Instrumentaria* as an Indicator of Medical Practice: A Provisional Assessment', in Philip J. van der Eijk, Herman F. J. Horstmanshoff and P. H. Schrijvers (eds), *Ancient Medicine in its Socio-Cultural Context. Papers Read at the Congress Held at Leiden University. 13–15 April 1992*, 189–208, Amsterdam: Rodopi Press.

Jackson, Ralph (1996), 'Eye Medicine in the Roman Empire', in Hildegard Temporini and Wolfgang Haase (eds), *Aufstieg und Niedergang der Romischen Welt*. Band II 37.3, 2228–51, Berlin: De Gruyter.

Jackson, Ralph (1999), 'Spas, Waters, and Hydrotherapy in the Roman World', in J. DeLaine and D. E. Johnston (eds), *Roman Baths and Bathing* (JRA Suppl.), 37: 107–16.

Jackson, Ralph (2007), 'The Surgical Instruments', in P. Crummy, S. Benfield, N. Crummy, V. Rigby and D. Shimmin (eds), *Stanway: An Élite Burial Site at Camulodunum*, 236–52, London: Society for the Promotion of Roman Studies.

Jacoby, Felix (1911), 'Zu Hippokrates' ΠΕΡΙ ΑΕΡΩΝ ΥΔΑΤΩΝ ΤΟΠΩΝ', *Hermes*, 46: 518–67.

Jacques, Jean-Marie (2008), 'L'animal et la médecine iologique: À propos de Nicandre de Colophon', in Isabelle Boehm and Pascal Luccioni (eds), *Le médecin initié par l'animal*, 49–61, Lyon: Maison de l'Orient et de la Méditerranée – Jean Pouilloux.

Jasny, Naum (1944), *The Wheats of Classical Antiquity*, Baltimore, MD: Johns Hopkins University Press.

Jenner, Mark S. R. and Patrick Wallis (2007), 'The Medical Market Place', in Mark S. R. Jenner and Patrick Wallis (eds), *Medicine and the Market in England and its Colonies, c. 1450–c. 1850*, 1–23, London: Macmillan Palgrave.

Jeong, Goun, Byung Chan Lim and Jong-Hee Chae (2015), 'Pediatric Stroke', *Journal of Korean Neurosurgical Society*, 57 (6): 396–400.

Johansen, T. K. (2012), *The Powers of Aristotle's Soul*, Oxford: Oxford University Press.

Johns, Timothy ([1990] 1996), *The Origins of Human Diet & Medicine: Chemical Ecology*, Tucson, AZ: University of Arizona Press.

Johnson, Matthew (1999), *Archaeological Theory: An Introduction*, Oxford: Blackwell Publishers.

Jones, Andrew (2002), *Archaeological Theory and Scientific Practice*, Cambridge: Cambridge University Press.

Jones, Christopher P. (1991), 'Aelius Aristides on the Water in Pergamon', *Archäologischer Anzeiger*, 111–7.

Jouanna, Jacques ([1990] 2012), 'Disease as Aggression in the Hippocratic Corpus and Greek Tragedy: Wild and Devouring Disease', in Philip J. van der Eijk (ed. and transl.), *Jacques Jouanna. Greek Medicine from Hippocrates to Galen. Selected Papers*, 81–96, Leiden: Brill.

Jouanna, Jacques ([1992] 1999), *Hippocrates*. Translated by M. B. DeBevoise, Baltimore, MD: Johns Hopkins University Press.

Jouanna, Jacques (2000), 'Maladies et médecine chez Aristophane', in Jean Leclant and Jacques Jouanna (eds), *Le théâtre grec antique: La comédie. Actes du 10ème colloque de la Villa Kérylos à Beaulieu-sur-Mer les 1er et 2 octobre 1999*, 171–95, Paris: Académie des Inscriptions et Belles-Lettres.

Jouanna, Jacques (2011), 'Médecine rationnelle et magie: Le statut des amulettes et des incantations chez Galien', *Revue des Études Grecques*, 124: 47–77.

Keyser, Paul T. and Georgia L. Irby-Massie, eds (2008), *The Encyclopaedia of Ancient Natural Scientists*, London: Routledge.

King, Helen (1998), *Hippocrates' Woman: Reading the Female Body in Ancient Greece*, London: Routledge.

Kleinman, Arthur (1980), *Patients and Healers in the Context of Culture*, Berkeley, CA: University of California Press.

Kokoszko, Maciej, Krzysztof Jagusiak and Zofia Rzeźnicka (2014), *Cereals of Antiquity and Early Byzantine Times*, Łódź: Łódź University Press.

Kollesch, Jutta (1997), 'Die anatomischen Untersuchungen des Aristoteles und ihr Stellenwert als Forschungsmethode in der aristotelischen Biologie', in Wolfgang Kullmann and Sabine Föllinger (eds), *Aristotelische Biologie: Intentionen, Methoden, Ergebnisse*, 367–74, Stuttgart: Franz Steiner Verlag.

Korpela, Jukka (1995), '*Aromatarii, pharmacopolae, thurarii et ceteri*: Zur Sozialgeschichte Roms', in Philip van der Eijk, Herman F. J. Horstmanshoff and Piet H. Schrijvers (eds), *Ancient Medicine in its Socio-Cultural Context. Papers Read at the Congress Held at Leiden University. 13–15 April 1992*, 101–18, Amsterdam: Rodopi.

Kron, Geoffrey (2012), 'Nutrition, Hygiene and Mortality: Setting Parameters for Roman Health and Life Expectancy Consistent with our Comparative Evidence', in Elio Lo Casco (ed.), *L'impatto della 'Peste Antonina'*, 193–252, Bari: Edipuglia.

Künzl, Ernst (1983), *Medizinische Instrumente aus Sepulkralfunden der römischen Kaiserzeit*, Cologne: Rheinland Verlag GmbH.

Künzl, Ernst (1996), 'Forschungsbericht zu den antiken medizinischen Instrumenten', in Hildgard Temporini and Wolfgang Haase (eds), *Aufstieg und Niedergang der Romischen Welt. Band II 37.3*, 2433–639, Berlin: De Gruyter.

Künzl, Ernst (2002), *Medizin in der Antike: Aus einer Welt ohne Narkose und Aspirin*, Stuttgart: Konrad Theiss Verlag GmBh.

Laes, Christian (2010), 'The Educated Midwife in the Roman Empire: An Example of Differential Equations', in Herman F. J. Horstmanshoff and Cornelis van Tilburg (eds), *Hippocrates and Medical Education. Selected Papers read at the XIIth International Hippocrates Colloquium, Universiteit Leiden, 24–26 August 2005*, 261–86, Leiden: Brill.

Lambert, Stephen and Laurence M. V. Totelin (2017), 'Funerary Monument of Phanostrate, Midwife and Doctor', *Attic Inscriptions Online*. Available online: www.atticinscriptions.com/inscription/CEG2/569 (accessed 5 October, 2020).

Lambrinoudakis, Vassilis (1994), 'L'eau médicale à Épidaure', in René Ginouvès, A.-M. Guimier-Sorbets, Jacques Jouanna and Laurence Villard (eds), *L'eau, la santé et la maladie dans le monde grec*, 225–36, Paris: de Boccard.

Langholf, Volker (2004), 'Structure and Genesis of Some Hippocratic Treatises', in Herman F. J. Horstmanshoff and Marten Stol (eds), *Magic and Rationality in Ancient Near Eastern and Graeco-Roman Medicine*, 219–75, Leiden: Brill.

Langslow, David R. (2000), *Medical Latin in the Roman Empire*, Oxford: Oxford University Press.

Lape, Susan (2010), *Race and Citizen Identity in the Classical Athenian Democracy*, Cambridge: Cambridge University Press.

Laskaris, Julie (2002), *The Art is Long:* On the Sacred Disease *and the Scientific Tradition*, Leiden: Brill.

Laskaris, Julie (2005), 'Error, Loss and Change in the Generation of Therapies', in Philip J. van der Eijk (ed.), *Hippocrates in Context. Papers read at the XI*

International Hippocrates Colloquium, University of Newcastle upon Tyne 27–31 August 2002, 173–89, Leiden: Brill.

Laskaris, Julie (2015), 'Treating Hemorrhage in Greek and Roman Militaries', in Geoff Lee, Helène Whittaker and Graham Wrightson (eds), *Ancient Warfare: Introducing Current Research, Volume I*, 273–90, Newcastle: Cambridge Scholars Press.

Laskaris, Julie (2016), 'Metals in Medicine: From Telephus to Galen', in William V. Harris (ed.), *Popular Medicine in Graeco-Roman Antiquity: Explorations*, 147–60, Leiden: Brill.

Laurence, Ray (2005), 'Health and the Life Course at Herculaneum and Pompeii', in Helen King (ed.), *Health in Antiquity*, 83–96, London: Routledge.

Leith, David (2009), 'The Qualitative Status of the *Onkoi* in Asclepiades' Theory of Matter', *Oxford Studies in Ancient Philosophy*, 36: 283–320.

Leith, David (2012), 'Pores and Void in Asclepiades' Physical Theory', *Phronesis*, 57: 164–91.

Leith, David (2015a), 'Elements and Uniform Parts in Early Alexandrian Medicine', *Phronesis*, 60: 462–91.

Leith, David (2015b), 'Erasistratus' *Triplokia* of Arteries, Veins and Nerves', *Apeiron*, 48: 251–62.

Leith, David (2016), 'How Popular Were the Medical Sects?', in William V. Harris (ed.), *Popular Medicine in Graeco-Roman Antiquity: Explorations*, 231–50, Leiden: Brill.

Leith, David (2020), 'Herophilus and Erasistratus on the Hēgemonikon', in Brad Inwood and James Warren (eds), *Body and Soul in Hellenistic Philosophy*, 30–61, Cambridge: Cambridge University Press.

Letts, Melinda (2015), 'Questioning the Patient, Questioning Hippocrates: Rufus of Ephesus and the Limits of Medical Authority', D.Phil. dissertation, University of Oxford.

Leven, Karl-Heinz (2004), '"At Times these Ancient Facts Seem to Lie before Me like a Patient on a Hospital Bed": Retrospective Diagnosis and Ancient Medical History', in Herman F. J. Horstmanshoff and Marten Stol (eds), *Magic and Rationality in Ancient Near Eastern and Graeco-Roman Medicine*, 369–86, Leiden: Brill.

Leven, Karl-Heinz (2005), 'Tierversuch', in Karl-Heinz Leven (ed.), *Antike Medizin: Ein Lexikon*, 866–7, München: C. H. Beck.

Leven, Karl-Heinz and U. Tröhler (2005), 'Vivisektion', in Karl-Heinz Leven (ed.), *Antike Medizin: Ein Lexikon*, 906–8, München: C. H. Beck.

Lévi-Strauss, Claude (1970), *The Raw and the Cooked*. trans. from *Le Cru et le cuit* 1964, London: Penguin.

Lewis, Gwyneth and Luc de Bernis, eds (2006), *Obstetric Fistula: Guiding Principles for Clinical Management and Programme Development*, Geneva: World Health Organization.

Liston, Maria A. and Susan I. Rostoff (2013), 'Babies in the Well: Archeological Evidence for Newborn Disposal in Hellenistic Greece', in Judith Evans Grubbs and Tim Parkin (eds), *The Oxford Handbook of Childhood and Education in the Classical World*, 62–82, Oxford: Oxford University Press.

Littman, Robert J. (2009), 'The Plague of Athens: Epidemiology and Paleopathology', *The Mount Sinai Journal of Medicine, New York*, 76 (5): 456–67.

Lloyd, Geoffrey E. R. (1983), *Science, Folklore and Ideology: Studies in the Ancient Life Sciences*, Cambridge: Cambridge University Press.

Lloyd, Geoffrey E. R. (1985), *Science and Morality in Greco-Roman Antiquity*: An inaugural lecture, Cambridge: Cambridge University Press. Reprinted in Lloyd,

Geoffrey E. R. (ed.) (1991), *Methods and Problems in Greek Science: Selected Papers*, Cambridge: Cambridge University Press.

Lloyd, Geoffrey E. R. (1991), 'Alcmaeon and the Early History of Dissection', in Geoffrey Lloyd (ed.)., *Methods and Problems in Greek Science*, 164–93, Cambridge: Cambridge University Press.

Lloyd, Geoffrey E. R. (1996), *Adversaries and Authorities: Investigations into Ancient Greek and Chinese Science*, Cambridge: Cambridge University Press.

Lloyd, Geoffrey E. R. (2003), *In the Grip of Disease: Studies in the Greek Imagination*, Oxford: Oxford University Press.

Lloyd, Geoffrey E. R. (2009), 'Galen's un-Hippocratic Case Studies', in Christopher Gill, Tim Whitmarsh and John Wilkins (eds), *Galen and the World of Knowledge*, 115–31, Oxford: Oxford University Press.

Long, Pamela O. (2001), *Openness, Secrecy, Authorship: Technical Arts and the Culture of Knowledge from Antiquity to the Renaissance*, Baltimore, MD: Johns Hopkins University Press.

Longrigg, James (2000), 'Epilepsy in Ancient Greek Medicine: The Vital Step', *Seizure: European Journal of Epilepsy* 9 (1): 12–21.

López Salvá, M. (1992), 'La leche como fármaco terapéutico en el *Corpus Hippocraticum*', in J. A. López Ferez (ed.), *Tratados Hipocráticos,* 251–62, Madrid: Editorial Gredos.

Lo Presti, Roberto (2008), *In forma di senso: L'encefalocentrismo del trattato ippocratico* Sulla malattia sacra *nel suo contesto epistemologico*, Rome: Carocci.

Lorenz, H. (2008), 'Plato on the Soul', in G. Fine (ed.), *The Oxford Handbook of Plato*, 244–66, Oxford: Oxford University Press.

Luce, Jean-Marc, ed. (2000), *Paysage et alimentation dans le monde grec,* Toulouse: Presses universitaires du Mirail.

Maehle A.-H. and U. Troehler (1987), 'Animal Experimentation from Antiquity to the End of the Eighteenth Century: Attitudes and Arguments', in Nicolaas A. Rupke (ed.), *Vivisection in Historical Perspective*, 14–47, London: Croom Helm.

Majno, Guido (1975), *The Healing Hand: Man and Wound in the Ancient World*, Cambridge, MA: Harvard University Press.

Malinas, Yves and Danielle Gourevitch (1982), 'Chronique anachronique, I: Suffocation subite chez la femme enceinte', *Revue Française de Gynécologie et d'Obstétrique*, 77: 753–55.

Männlein-Robert, Irmgard, (2014), 'Schmerz und Schrei: Sophokles' *Philoktet* als Grenzfall der Ästhetik in Antike und Moderne', *Antike und Abendland*, 60 (1): 90–112.

Mansfeld, Jaap (1989), 'Chrysippus and the "Placita"', *Phronesis*, 34: 311–42.

Mansfeld, Jaap (1990), 'Doxography and Dialectic: The *Sitz im Leben* of the "Placita"', *ANRW* II 36.4, 3056–229, Berlin: De Gruyter.

Martin, Roland and Henri Metzger (1976), *La religion grecque*, Paris: PUF.

Marganne, Marie-Hélène (1997), 'Les médicaments estampillés dans le corpus galénique', in Armelle Debru (ed.), *Galen on Pharmacology: Philosophy, History and Medicine. Proceedings of the Vth International Galen Colloquium, Lille, 16–18 March 1995*, 158–64, Leiden: Brill.

Massar, Natacha (2005), *Soigner et servir: Histoire sociale et culturelle de la médecine grecque à l'époque hellénistique*, Paris: De Boccard.

Massar, Natacha (2010), '"Choose Your Master Well": Medical Training, Testimonies and Claims to Authority', in Herman F. J. Horstmanshoff and Cornelis van Tilburg (eds), *Hippocrates and Medical Education. Selected Papers read at the XIIth International Hippocrates Colloquium, Universiteit Leiden, 24–26 August 2005*, 169–86, Leiden: Brill.

Mattern, Susan (2008), *Galen's Rhetoric of Healing*, Baltimore, MD: Johns Hopkins University Press.

Mattern, Susan (2013), *The Prince of Medicine: Galen in the Roman Empire*, Oxford: Oxford University Press.

Mattingly, David (2004), 'Being Roman: Expressing Identity in a Provincial Setting', *Journal of Roman Archaeology*, 17: 5–25.

Mattingly, David (2006), *An Imperial Possession: Britain in the Roman Empire 54 BC–AD 409*, London: Penguin Books.

Mauss, Marcel ([1934] 1979), 'Les techniques du corps', Reprinted in *Sociology and Psychology: Essays by Marcel Mauss Translated by Ben Brewster*, 95–135, London: Routledge.

Mayor, Adrienne (2010), *The Poison King: The Life and Legend of Mithradates, Rome's Deadliest Enemy*, Princeton, NJ: Princeton University Press.

McDermott, W. C. (1938), *The Ape in Antiquity*, Baltimore, MD: Johns Hopkins Press.

McGing, Brian C. (2012), 'Mithradates', in Simon Hornblower, Antony Spawforth and Esther Eidinow (eds), *The Oxford Classical Dictionary*, 4th edn, Oxford: Oxford University Press.

McNamara, Leanne (2003), '"Conjurers, Purifiers, Vagabonds and Quacks"? The Clinical Roles of the Folk and Hippocratic Healers of Classical Greece', *Iris: Journal of the Classical Association of Victoria*, 16–17: 2–25.

McQuaid, John (2015), *Tasty: The Art and Science of What We Eat,* New York: Scribner.

Mee, Christopher and Josette Renard, eds (2007), *Cooking Up the Past: Food and Culinary Practices in the Neolithic and Bronze Age Aegean*, Oxford: Oxbow Books.

Mee, Christopher, and Anthony Spawforth (2001), *Greece: An Oxford Archaeological Guide*, Oxford: Oxford University Press.

Metzger, Nadine (2015), 'Kynanthropy: Canine Madness in Byzantine Late Antiquity', *History of Psychiatry*, 3 (3): 318–31.

Miller, William I. (2009), *The Anatomy of Disgust*, Cambridge, MA: Harvard University Press.

Miles, Steven H. (2005), *The Hippocratic Oath and the Ethics of Medicine*, Oxford: Oxford University Press.

Millett, Martin (1990), *The Romanization of Britain: An Essay on Archaeological Interpretation*, Cambridge: Cambridge University Press.

Milne, Johns S. (1907), *Surgical Instruments in Greek and Roman Times*, Oxford: Clarendon Press.

Mitchell, Piers (2011), 'Retrospective Diagnosis and the Use of Historical Texts for Investigating Disease in the Past', *International Journal of Paleopathology*, 1: 81–8.

Mitchell, Stephen (2005), 'Olive Cultivation in the Economy of Roman Asia Minor', in Stephen Mitchell and Constantina Katsari (eds), *Patterns in the Economy of Roman Asia Minor*, 83–114, Swansea: Classical Press of Wales.

Molina, Monserrat (1981), 'Instrumental medico de epoca Romana en el Museo Arqueologico Nacional (Madrid)', *Archivo Español de Arqueologia*, 55: 255–62.

Moore, H. L. (1982), 'The Interpretation of Spatial Patterning in Settlement Residues', in Ian Hodder (ed.), *Symbolic and Structural Archaeology*, 74–9, Cambridge: Cambridge University Press.

Moritz, L. A. (1958), *Grain-Mills and Flour in Classical* Antiquity, Oxford: Clarendon Press.

Mudd, Shaun A. (2015), 'Constructive Drinking in the Roman Empire: The First to Third Centuries AD', PhD diss., University of Exeter.

Murray, Oswyn, ed. (1990), *Sympotica: The Papers of a Symposium on the Symposion*, Oxford: Clarendon Press.

Mylona, Dimitra (2008), *Fish-Eating in Greece from 500 BC to AD 700: A Story of Impoverished Fishermen or Lavish Fish Banquets?* Oxford: Archaeopress.

Mylona, Dimitra (2015), 'Fish', in John Wilkins and Robin Nadeau (eds), *A Companion to Food in the Ancient World*, 147–59, Malden, MA: Wiley Blackwell.

Naiden. F. S. (2012), 'Blessed Are the Parasites', in Christopher A. Faraone and F. S. Naiden (eds), *Greek and Roman Animal Sacrifice: Ancient Victims, Modern Observers*, 55–84, Cambridge: Cambridge University Press.

Naji, Myriem (2009), 'Gender and Materiality in-the-Making: The Manufacture of Sirwan Femininities through Weaving in Southern Morocco', *Journal of Material Culture*, 14 (1): 47–73.

Nash, Roderick (1972), 'American Environmental History: A New Teaching Frontier', *Pacific Historical Review*, 41 (3): 362–372.

Nutton, Vivian (1977), 'Archiatri and the Medical Profession', *Papers of the British School at Rome*, 32: 191–226.

Nutton, Vivian (1983), 'The Seeds of Disease: An Explanation of Contagion and Infection from the Greeks to the Renaissance', *Medical History*, 27: 1–24.

Nutton, Vivian (1985), 'The Drug Trade in Antiquity', *Journal of the Royal Society of Medicine*, 78: 138–45.

Nutton, Vivian (1986), 'Murders and Miracles: Lay Attitudes Towards Medicine in Classical Antiquity', in Roy Porter (ed.), *Patients and Practitioners: Lay Perceptions of Medicine in Pre-Industrial Society*, 25–53, Cambridge: Cambridge University Press.

Nutton, Vivian (1992), 'Healers in the Market Place: Towards a Social History of Graeco-Roman Medicine', in Andrew Wear (ed.), *Medicine in Society: Historical Essays*, 15–58, Cambridge: Cambridge University Press.

Nutton, Vivian (1993), 'Roman Medicine: Tradition, Confrontation, Assimilation', in Hildegard Temporini and Wolfgang Haase (eds), *Aufstieg und Niedergang der römischen Welt*. Band II 37.1, 49–78, Berlin: De Gruyter.

Nutton, Vivian (1995a), 'What's in an Oath?', *Journal of the Royal College of Physicians of London*, 29 (6): 518–24.

Nutton, Vivian (1995b), 'Medicine in the Greek World, 800–50 BC', in Lawrence Conrad, Michael Neve, Vivian Nutton, Roy Porter and Andrew Wear (eds), *The Western Medical Tradition: 800 BC to AD 1800,* Cambridge: Cambridge University Press.

Nutton, Vivian (1997), 'Galen on Theriac: Problems of Authenticity', in Armelle Debru (ed.), *Galen on Pharmacology: Philosophy, History and Medicine. Proceedings of the Vth International Galen Colloquium, Lille, 16–18 March 1995,* 133–52, Leiden: Brill.

Nutton, Vivian (2000), 'Medical Thoughts on Urban Pollution', in Valerie M. Hope and Eireann Marshall (eds), *Death and Disease in the Ancient City*, 65–73, London: Routledge.

Nutton, Vivian ([2004] 2013), *Ancient Medicine*, London: Routledge.

Osborne, Catherine (2007), *Dumb Beasts and Dead Philosophers*, Oxford: Oxford University Press.

Nutton, Vivian (2020), *Galen: A Thinking Doctor in Imperial Rome*, London: Routledge.

Overduin, Floris (2015), *Nicander of Colophon's Theriaca: A Literary Commentary*, Leiden: Brill.

Parker, Robert (1983), *Miasma: Pollution and Purification in Early Greek Religion*, Oxford: Oxford University Press.

Parkin, Tim (2013), 'The Demography of Infancy and Early Childhood in the Ancient World', in Judith Evans Grubbs and Tim Parkin (eds), *The Oxford Handbook of Childhood and Education in the Classical World*, 40–61, Oxford and New York: Oxford University Press.

Payne, Mark (2010), *The Animal Part: Human and Other Animals in the Poetic Imagination*, Chicago: University of Chicago Press.

Pérez Cañizares, Pilar (2010), 'The Importance of Having Medical Knowledge as a Layman: The Hippocratic Treatise *Affections* in the Context of the Hippocratic Corpus', in Herman F. J. Horstmanshoff and Cornelis van Tilburg (eds), *Hippocrates and Medical Education. Selected Papers Presented at the XIIth International Hippocrates Colloquium, Universeit Leiden, 24–26 August 2005*, 87–99, Leiden: Brill.

Perkins, Judith (1995), *The Suffering Self: Pain and Narrative Representation in the Early Christian Era*, London: Routledge.

Petit, Caroline (2017), 'Galen, Pharmacology and the Boundaries of Medicine: A Reassessment', in Lennart Lehmhaus and Matteo Martelli (eds), *Collecting Recipes: Byzantine and Jewish Pharmacology in Dialogue*, 51–80, Berlin: De Gruyter.

Petridou, Georgia (2015), 'Aelius Aristides as Informed Patient and Physician', in Georgia Petridou and Chiara Thumiger (eds), *Homo Patiens: Approaches to the Patient in the Ancient World*, 451–70, Leiden: Brill.

Petridou, Georgia (2016), 'Becoming a Doctor, Becoming a God: Religion and Medicine in Aelius Aristides' *Hieroi Logoi*', in Annette Weissenrieder and Gregor Etzelmuller (eds), *Religion and Illness*, 306–35, Eugene, OR: Cascade Books.

Petridou, Georgia and Chiara Thumiger, eds (2015), *Homo Patiens: Approaches to the Patient in the Ancient World*, Leiden: Brill.

Petrone, Pierpaolo, Massimo Niola, Pierpaolo Di Lorenzo, Mariano Paternoster, Vincenzo Graziano, Giuseppe Quaremba and Claudio Buccelli (2015), 'Early Medical Skull Surgery for Treatment of Post-Traumatic Osteomyelitis 5,000 Years Ago', *PloS One*, 10 (5).

Petsalis-Diomidis, Alexia (2005), 'The Body in Space: Visual Dynamics in Graeco-Roman Healing Pilgrimage', in Jas Elsner and Ian Rutherford (eds), *Seeing the Gods: Pilgrimage in Graeco-Roman and Early Christian Antiquity*, 183–218, Oxford: Oxford University Press.

Petsalis-Diomidis, Alexia (2010), *Truly Beyond Wonders: Aelius Aristides and the Cult of Asclepius*, Oxford: Oxford University Press.

Phillips, E. D. (1973), *Greek Medicine*, London: Thames and Hudson.

Pleket, H. W. (1995), 'The Social Status of Physicians in the Graeco-Roman World', in Philip J. van der Eijk, Herman F. J. Horstmanshoff and P. H. Schrijvers (eds), *Ancient Medicine in its Socio-Cultural Context. Papers Read at the Congress Held at Leiden University. 13–15 April 1992*, 27–34, Amsterdam: Rodopi Press.

Podolak, P. (2010), *Soranos von Ephesos: Peri psyches, Sammlung der Testimonien, Kommentar und Einleitung*, Berlin: De Gruyter.

Pohl, Rudolfus (1905), *De graecorum medicis publicis*, Berlin: Georg Reimer.

Pohlenz, Max (1938), *Hippokrates und die Begründung der wissenschaftlichen Medizin*, Berlin: De Gruyter.

Polito, Roberto (2006), 'Matter, Medicine, and the Mind: Asclepiades vs. Epicurus', *Oxford Studies in Ancient Philosophy*, 30: 285–335.

Pormann, Peter, ed. (2018), *The Cambridge Companion to Hippocrates*, Cambridge: Cambridge University Press.

Porter, Roy (1985), 'The Patient's View: Doing Medical History from Below', *Theory and Society*, 14: 175–98.

Porter, Roy ed. (1986), 'Introduction', in Roy Porter (ed.), *Patients and Practitioners: Lay Perceptions of Medicine in Pre-Industrial Society*, 1–22, Cambridge: Cambridge University Press.

Porter, Roy ed. (1986), *Patients and Practitioners: Lay Perceptions of Medicine in Pre-Industrial Society*, Cambridge: Cambridge University Press.

Purcell, Nicholas (1995), 'Eating Fish: The Paradoxes of Seafood', in John Wilkins, David Harvey and Michael Dobson (eds), *Food in Antiquity*, 132–49, Exeter: University of Exeter Press.

Rickman, Geoffrey E. (1971), *Roman Granaries and Store Buildings*, Cambridge: Cambridge University Press.

Riddle, John M. (1994), *Contraception and Abortion from the Ancient World to the Renaissance*, Cambridge, MA: Harvard University Press.

Roberts, Charlotte A. (2015), 'Old World Tuberculosis: Evidence from Human Remains with a Review of Current Research and Future Prospects', *Tuberculosis*, 95: S117–S121.

Roberts, Charlotte A. and Jane E. Buikstra (2003), *The Bioarchaeology of Tuberculosis*, Gainesville, FL: University Press of Florida.

Rocca, Julius (2003), *Galen on the Brain: Anatomical Knowledge and Physiological Speculation in the Second Century* AD, Leiden: Brill.

Rossignol, Benoît (2012), 'Le climat, les famines et la guerre: Éléments du contexte de la Peste Antonine', in Elio Lo Cascio (ed.), *L'impatto della "Peste Antonina"*, 87–122, Bari: Edipuglia.

Rowan, Erica (2014), 'Roman Diet and Nutrition in the Vesuvian Region: A Study of the Bioarchaeological Remains from the Cardo V Sewer at Herculaneum', D.Phil. diss., University of Oxford.

Rowlandson, Jane, ed. (1998), *Women and Society in Greek and Roman Egypt*, Cambridge: Cambridge University Press.

Rumor, Maddalena (2015), 'Babylonian Pharmacology in Graeco-Roman Dreckapotheke. With an Edition of Uruanna III 1–143 (138)', Diss. Berlin.

Rütten, Thomas (1996), 'Zootomieren im hippokratischen Briefroman: Motivgeschichtliche Untersuchungen zur Verhältnisbestimmung von Medizin und Philosophie', in Renate Wittern and Pierre Pellegrin (eds), *Hippokratische Medizin und antike Philosophie. Verhandlungen des VIII. Internationalen Hippokrates-Kolloquiums in Kloster Banz-Staffelstein vom 23. bis 28. September 1993*, 561–82, Hildesheim, Zürich, New York: Olms.

Rütten, Thomas and Leonie von Reppert-Bismarck (1996), 'Receptions of the Hippocratic Oath in the Renaissance: The Prohibition of Abortion as a Case Study in Reception', *Journal of the History of Medicine and Allied Sciences*, 51 (4): 456–83.

Saillant, Francine and Serge Genest, eds (2007), *Medical Anthropology: Regional Perspectives and Shared Concerns*, Oxford: Blackwell.

Salazar, Christine F. (2000), *The Treatment of War Wounds in Graeco-Roman Antiquity*, Leiden: Brill.

Salazar, Christine F. (forthcoming), 'Paul of Aegina on Venomous Animals', in Debby Banham (ed.), *The Missing Link: Studies in Early Medicine*, Oxford: Archaeopress.

Sallares, Robert (1991), *The Ecology of the Ancient Greek World*, Ithaca, NY: Cornell University Press.

Sallares, Robert (2002), *Malaria and Rome: A History of Malaria in Ancient Italy*, Oxford: Oxford University Press.

Sallares, Robert (2005), 'Pathocoenoses Ancient and Modern', *History and Philosophy of the Life Sciences*, 27 (2): 201–20.

Sallares, Robert (2006), 'Role of Environmental Changes in the Spread of Malaria in Europe during the Holocene', *Quaternary International*, 150 (1): 21–7.

Salles, Catherine (1985), 'Les cachets d'oculistes', in André Pelletier (ed.), *La médecine en Gaule: Villes d'eaux, sanctuaires des eaux*, 89–102, Paris: Picard.

Samama, Évelyne (2002), 'Empoisonné ou guéri? Remarques lexicologiques sur les *pharmaka* et *venena*', in Évelyne Samama and Frank Collard (eds), *Le corps à l'épreuve. Poisons, remèdes et chirurgie: Aspects des pratiques médicales dans l'Antiquité et au Moyen-Âge*, 13–27, Langres: Dominique Guéniot.

Samama, Évelyne (2003), *Les médecins dans le monde grec: Sources épigraphiques sur la naissance d'un corps médical*, Geneva: Droz.

Samama, Évelyne (2006), '*Thaumatopoioi pharmakopôlai*: La singulière image des préparateurs et vendeurs de remèdes dans les textes grecs', in Franck Collard and Évelyne Samama (eds), *Pharmacopoles et apothicaires: Les « pharmaciens » de l'Antiquité au Grand Siècle*, 7–27, Paris: l'Harmattan.

Say, Lale, Doris Chou, Alison Gemmill, Özge Tunçalp, Ann-Beth Moller, Jane Daniels, A. Metin Gülmezoglu, Marleen Temmerman and Leontine Alkema (2014), 'Global Causes of Maternal Death: A WHO Systematic Analysis', *The Lancet. Global Health*, 2 (6): 323–33.

Scarborough, John (1995), 'The Opium Poppy in Hellenistic and Roman Medicine', in Roy Porter and Mikulás Teich (eds), *Drugs and Narcotics in History*, 4–23, Cambridge: Cambridge University Press.

Scarborough, John and Vivian Nutton (1982), 'The Preface of Dioscorides' *De materia medica*: Introduction, Translation and Commentary', *Transactions of the College of Physicians of Philadelphia*, 5 (4): 187–227.

Scheidel, Walter (2007), 'A Model of Real Income Growth in Roman Italy', *Historia*, 56 (3): 322–46.

Scheidel, Walter (2012), 'Roman Wellbeing and the Economic Consequences of the Antonine Plague', in Elio Lo Cascio (ed.), *L'impatto della 'Peste Antonina'*, 265–95, Bari: Edipuglia.

Scheidel, Walter (2013), 'Disease and Death', in Paul Erdkamp (ed.), *The Cambridge Companion to Ancient Rome*, 45–59, Cambridge: Cambridge University Press.

Scobie, Alex (1986), 'Slums, Sanitation and Mortality in the Roman World', *Klio*, 68: 399–433.

Shaw, Brent D. (1996), 'Seasons of Death: Aspects of Mortality in Imperial Rome', *Journal of Roman Studies*, 86: 100–38.

Silk, M. S. (1996), 'Plagiarism', in Simon Hornblower and Antony Spawforth (eds), *The Oxford Classical Dictionary*, 3rd edn, 1088, Oxford: Oxford University Press.

Singer, Peter N. (2017), 'The Essence of Rage: Galen on Emotional Disturbances and their Physical Correlates', in Richard Seaford, John Wilkins and Matthew Wright (eds), *Selfhood and the Soul: Essays on Ancient Thought and Literature in Honour of Christopher Gill*, 161–96, Oxford: Oxford University Press.

Smith, Wesley D. (1979), *The Hippocratic Tradition*, Ithaca, NY: Cornell University Press.

Solmsen, F. (1961), 'Greek Philosophy and the Discovery of the Nerves', *Museum Helveticum*, 18: 150–97.

Soren, David (2003), 'Can Archaeologists Excavate Evidence of Malaria?', *World Archaeology*, 35 (2): 193–209.

Sparkes, B. (1995), 'A Pretty Kettle of Fish', in John Wilkins, David Harvey and Michael Dobson (eds), *Food in Antiquity*, 150–61, Exeter: University of Exeter Press.

Spatafora, Giuseppe (2007), 'Il sistema terapeutico nei poemi di Nicandro', *Giornale Italiano di Filologia*, 59 (1): 31–63.

Stafford, Emma (2004), '"Without You No One is Happy": The Cult of Health in Ancient Greece', in Helen King (ed.), *Health in Antiquity*, 142–57, London: Routledge.

Stathakopoulos, Dionysios C. (2004), *Famine and Pestilence in the Late Roman and Early Byzantine Empire: A Systematic Survey of Subsistence Crises and Epidemics*, Aldershot: Ashgate.

Stein, Michael (1997), 'La thériaque chez Galien: Sa préparation et son usage thérapeutique', in Armelle Debru (ed.), *Galen on Pharmacology: Philosophy, History and Medicine. Proceedings of the Vth International Galen Colloquium, Lille, 16–18 March 1995*, 199–209, Leiden: Brill.

Stivala, Joan (2015), 'Malaria and Miscarriage in Ancient Rome', *Canadian Bulletin of Medical History*, 32 (1): 143–61.

Stolberg, Michael (2015), 'Approaches to the History of Patients: From the Ancient World to Early Modern Europe', in Georgia Petridou and Chiara Thumiger (eds), *Homo Patiens: Approaches to the Patient in the Ancient World*, 499–518, Leiden: Brill.

Taborelli, Luigi and Silvia M. Marengo (1998), 'Il medicamento λύκιον e i suoi contenitori', *Archeologia Classica*, 50: 213–72.

Taborelli, Luigi and Silvia M. Marengo (2010), 'Microcontenitori per *medicamenta* di epoca ellenistica e romana', *Archeologia Classica*, 61: 211–42.

Tecusan, Manuela (2004), *The Fragments of the Methodists. Volume One: Methodism outside Soranus*, Leiden: Brill.

Temkin, Oswei ([1945] 1971), *The Falling Sickness: A History of Epilepsy from the Greeks to the Beginnings of Modern Neurology*, Baltimore, MD: Johns Hopkins University Press.

Thomas, Julian (1996), *Time Culture and Identity: An Interpretative Archaeology*, London: Routledge.

Thomas, Rosalind (1992), *Literacy and Orality in Ancient Greece*, Cambridge: Cambridge University Press.

Thomas, Rosalind (2000), *Herodotus in Context: Ethnography, Science and the Art of Persuasion*, Cambridge: Cambridge University Press.

Thumiger, Chiara (2014), 'Animals in Tragedy', in Gordon L. Campbell (ed.), *Oxford Handbook of Animals*, 84–98, Oxford: Oxford University Press.

Thumiger, Chiara (2017), *A History of the Mind and Mental Health in Classical Greek Medical Thought*, Cambridge: Cambridge University Press.

Thumiger, Chiara (2019), 'Animality, Illness and Dehumanisation: The Phenomenology of Illness In Sophocles' *Philoctetes*', in Giulia Maria Chesi and Francesca Spiegel (eds), *Undoing the Human: Classical Literature and the Post-Human*, 95–102, London, Bloomsbury.

Tieleman, Teun (1996), *Galen and Chrysippus on the Soul: Argument and Refutation in the* De Placitis *Books II–III*, Leiden: Brill.

Trancas, Bruno, Nuno Borja Santos and Luís D. Patrício (2008), 'O uso do ópio na sociedade romana e a dependência do princeps Marco Aurélio', *Acta Médica Portuguesa*, 21 (6): 581–90.

Totelin, Laurence M. V. (2004), 'Mithradates' Antidote: A Pharmacological Ghost', *Early Science and Medicine*, 9: 1–19.

Totelin, Laurence M. V. (2009), *Hippocratic Recipes: Oral and Written Transmission of Pharmacological Knowledge in Fifth- and Fourth-Century Greece*, Leiden: Brill.

Totelin, Laurence M. V. (2012a), 'Botanizing Rulers and their Herbal Subjects: Plants and Political Power in Greek and Roman Literature', *Phoenix*, 66 (1–2): 122–44.

Totelin, Laurence M. V. (2012b), 'And to End on a Poetic Note: Galen's Authorial Strategies in the Pharmacological Books', *Studies in History and Philosophy of Science Part A*, 43 (2): 307–15.

Totelin, Laurence M. V. (2016a), 'From *Technē* to *Kakotechnia:* Use and Abuse of Ancient Cosmetic Texts', in Marco Formisano and Philip J. van der Eijk (eds), *Knowledge, Text and Practice in Ancient Technical Writing*, 138–62, Cambridge: Cambridge University Press.

Totelin, Laurence M. V. (2016b), 'The World in a Pill: Local Specialties and Global Remedies in the Graeco-Roman World', in Rebecca Futo Kennedy and Molly Jones-Lewis (eds), *The Routledge Handbook of Identity and the Environment in the Classical and Medieval World*, 151–70, London: Routledge.

Totelin, Laurence M. V. (2016c), '*Pharmakopōlai*: A Re-Evaluation of the Sources', in William V. Harris (ed.), *Popular Medicine in Graeco-Roman Antiquity: Explorations*, 65–85, Leiden: Brill.

Totelin, Laurence M. V. (2020), 'Healing Correspondence', in Laurence M. V. Totelin and Rebecca Flemming (eds), *Medicine and Markets in the Graeco-Roman World and Beyond: Essays on Ancient Medicine in Honour of Vivian Nutton*, 17–36, Swansea: Classical Press of Wales.

Touwaide, Alain (2002), 'Veterinärmedizin. II. Klassische Antike', *Der Neue Pauly*, 12 (2), 146–7.

Trapp, Michael (2016), 'Introduction', in Donald A. Russell, Michael Trapp and Heinz-Günther Nesselrath (eds), *In Praise of Asclepius: Aelius Aristides Selected Prose Hymns*, 3–16, Tübingen: Mohr Siebeck.

Valamoti, Soultana M. (2009), 'Plant Food Ingredients and "Recipes" from Prehistoric Greece: The Archaeobotanical Evidence', in J. P. Morel and A. M. Mercuri (eds), *Plants and Culture: Seeds of the Cultural Heritage of Europe*, 25–38, Bari: Centro Europea per I Beni Culturali Ravello.

Vallance, John T. (1990), *The Lost Theory of Asclepiades of Bithynia*, Oxford: Oxford University Press.

van der Eijk, Philip J. (1997), 'Galen's Use of the Concept of "Qualified Experience" in His Dietetic and Pharmacological Works', in Armelle Debru (ed.), *Galen on Pharmacology: Philosophy, History and Medicine. Proceedings of the Vth International Galen Colloquium, Lille, 16–18 March 1995*, 35–57, Leiden: Brill.

van der Eijk, Philip J. (1999), 'The Anonymus Parisinus and the Doctrines of "the Ancients"', in Philip J. van der Eijk (ed.), *Ancient Histories of Medicine*, 295–331, Leiden: Bristol.

van der Eijk, Philip J. (2005a), 'The Methodism of Caelius Aurelianus: Some Epistemological Issues', in Philip J. van der Eijk (ed.), *Medicine and Philosophy in Classical Antiquity*, 299–327, Cambridge: Cambridge University Press.

van der Eijk, Philip J. (2005b), 'The Heart, the Brain, the Blood and the Pneuma: Hippocrates, Diocles and Aristotle on the Location of Cognitive Processes', in Philip J. van der Eijk, *Medicine and Philosophy in Classical Antiquity*, 119–35, Cambridge: Cambridge University Press.

van der Eijk, Philip J. (2015), 'Galen on the Assessment of Bodily Mixtures', in Brooke Holmes and Klaus-Dietrich Fischer, *The Frontiers of Ancient Science: Essays in Honor of Heinrich von Staden*, 675–98, Berlin: De Gruyter.

van Hooff, Anton J. L. (1990), *From Autothanasia to Suicide: Self-Killing in Classical Antiquity*, London: Routledge.

Vespa, Marco (2017), 'Why Avoid a Monkey: The Refusal of Interaction in
     Galen's *Epideixis*', in Thorsten Fögen and Edmund Thomas (eds), *Interactions
     between Animals and Humans in Graeco-Roman Antiquity*, 409–34, Berlin:
     De Gruyter.
von Staden, Heinrich (1975), 'Experiment and Experience in Hellenistic Medicine',
     Bulletin of the Institute of Classical Studies, 22: 178–99.
von Staden, Heinrich (1989), *Herophilus: The Art of Medicine in Early Alexandria*.
     Cambridge: Cambridge University Press.
von Staden, Heinrich (1991), 'Matière et signification: Rituel, sexe et pharmacologie
     dans le Corpus Hippocratique', *L'Antiquité Classique*, 60: 42–61.
von Staden, Heinrich (1992a), 'The Discovery of the Body: Human Dissection and its
     Cultural Contexts in Ancient Greece', *Yale Journal of Biology and Medicine*, 65 (3):
     223–41.
von Staden, Heinrich (1992b), 'Women and Dirt', *Helios*, 19: 7–30.
von Staden, Heinrich (1995), 'Anatomy as Rhetoric: Galen on Dissection and
     Persuasion', *Journal of the History of Medicine and Allied Sciences*, 50: 48–67.
von Staden, Heinrich (1996a), '"In a Pure and Holy Way": Personal and Professional
     Conduct in the Hippocratic Oath?', *Journal of the History of Medicine and Allied
     Sciences*, 51: 404–37.
von Staden, Heinrich (1996b), 'Liminal Perils: Early Roman Receptions of Greek
     Medicine', in F. Jamil Ragep and Sally P. Ragep (eds), *Tradition, Transmission,
     Transformation: Proceedings of two Conferences on Pre-Modern Science*, 369–418,
     Leiden: Brill.
von Staden, Heinrich (2000), 'Body, Soul, and Nerves: Epicurus, Herophilus,
     Erasistratus, the Stoics, and Galen', in J. P. Wright and P. Potter (eds), *Psyche and
     Soma: Physicians and Metaphysicians on the Mind–Body Problem from Antiquity to
     Enlightenment*, 79–116, Oxford: Oxford University Press.
von Staden, Heinrich (2012), 'The Living Environment: Animals and Humans in
     Celsus' *Medicina*', in Nicoletta Palmieri (ed.), *Conserver la santé ou la rétablir: Le
     rôle de l'environnement dans la médecine antique et médiévale*, 69–94, Saint-
     Étienne: Publications de l' Université de Saint-Étienne.
von Staden, Heinrich (2013), 'Writing the Animal: Aristotle, Pliny the Elder, Galen', in
     Markus Asper (ed.), *Writing Science: Medical and Mathematical Authorship in
     Ancient Greece*, 111–44, Berlin: De Gruyter.
Wallace-Hadrill, Andrew (2008), *Rome's Cultural Revolution*, Cambridge: Cambridge
     University Press.
Watson, Gilbert (1966), *Theriac and Mithridatium: A Study in Therapeutics*, London:
     Wellcome Historical Medical Library.
Wazer, Caroline (2016), 'Between Public Health and Popular Medicine: Senatorial and
     Popular Responses to Epidemic Disease in the Roman Republic', in William V.
     Harris (ed.), *Popular Medicine in Graeco-Roman Antiquity: Explorations*, 126–46,
     Leiden: Brill.
Webster, Jane (1997a), 'Necessary Comparisons: A Post-Colonial Approach to
     Religious Syncretism in the Roman Provinces', *World Archaeology*, 28 (3):
     324–38.
Webster, Jane (1997b), 'A Negotiated Syncretism: Readings on the Development of
     Romano-Celtic Religion', in David Mattingly (ed.), *Dialogues in Roman
     Imperialism*, 165–84, Portsmouth, RI: Journal of Roman Archaeology.
White, Kenneth D. (1970), *Roman Farming*, Ithaca, NY: Cornell University Press.

Wickkiser, Bronwen L. (2008), *Asklepios, Medicine, and the Politics of Healing in Fifth-Century Greece: Between Craft and Cult*, Baltimore, MD: Johns Hopkins University Press.

Wilkins, John (2012), 'Food and Drink in the Ancient World', in Kyri W. Clafin and Peter Scholliers (eds), *Writing Food History: A Global Perspective*, 11–23, London: Bloomsbury.

Wilkins, John (2015), 'Medical Literature, Diet and Health', in John Wilkins and Robin Nadeau (eds), *A Companion to Food in the Ancient World*, 59–66, Malden, MA: Wiley-Blackwell.

Wilkins, J. (1995), 'Introduction to Part II', in John Wilkins, David Harvey and Michael Dobson (eds), *Food in Antiquity*, 102–6, Exeter: University of Exeter Press.

Wilkins, John and Shaun Hill (2006), *Food in the Ancient World*, Oxford: Blackwell.

Wilkins, John (2015), 'Medical Literature, Diet, and Health', in John Wilkins and Robin Nadeau (eds), *A Companion to Food in the Ancient World*, 59–66, Malden, MA: Wiley Blackwell.

Wilkins, John (2017), 'Galen on the Relationship between Human Beings and Fish', in Thorsten Fögen and Edmund Thomas (eds), *Interactions between Animals and Humans in Graeco-Roman Antiquity*, 389–408, Berlin: De Gruyter.

Wilkins, John and Robin Nadeau, eds (2015), *A Companion to Food in the Ancient World*, Malden, MA: Wiley Blackwell.

Whitehorne, J. E. G. (1977), 'Was Marcus Aurelius a Hypochondriac?', *Latomus*, 36: 413–21.

Winder, Stephanie (2017), '"The Hands of Gods": Poison in the Hellenistic Court', in Andrew Erskin, Lloyd Llewellyn-Jones and Shane Wallace (eds), *The Hellenistic Court: Monarchic Power and Elite Society from Alexander to Cleopatra*, 373–408, Swansea: Classical Press of Wales.

Wöhrle, Georg (1990), *Studien zur Theorie der antiken Gesundheitslehre*, Stuttgart: Franz Steiner Verlag.

Woods, Robert (2007), 'Ancient and Early Modern Mortality: Experience and Understanding', *Economic History Review*, 60: 373–90.

Woolf, Greg (1998), *Becoming Roman: The Origins of Provincial Civilization in Gaul*, Cambridge: Cambridge University Press.

Woolf, Greg (2015), 'Ancient Illiteracy?', *Bulletin of the Institute of Classical Studies*, 58 (2): 31–42.

Wootton, David (2006), *Bad Medicine: Doctors Doing Harm since Hippocrates*, Oxford: Oxford University Press.

Worman, Nancy (2000), 'Infection in the Sentence: Discourse of Disease in *Philoctetes*', *Arethusa*, 33: 1–36.

Worster, Donald, ed. (1988), *The Ends of the Earth: Perspectives on Modern Environmental History*, Cambridge: Cambridge University Press.

Yegül, Fikret (2010), *Bathing in the Roman World*, Cambridge: Cambridge University Press.

Young, Gary K. (2001), *Rome's Eastern Trade: International Commerce and Imperial Policy 31 BC–AD 305*, Cambridge: Cambridge University Press.

Zelener, Yan (2012), 'Genetic Evidence, Density Dependence and Epidemiological Models of the "Antonine Plague"', in Elio Lo Cascio (ed.), *L'impatto della 'Peste Antonina'*, 167–77, Bari: Edipuglia.

Zucker, Arnaud (2008), 'Homme et animal: Pathologies communes et thérapies partagées', in Isabelle Boehm and Pascal Luccioni (eds), *Le médecin initié par l'animal*, 63–78, Lyon: Maison de l'Orient et de la Méditerranée – Jean Pouilloux.

CONTRIBUTORS

Patricia Baker is a Senior Lecturer in Classical and Archaeological Studies at the University of Kent, UK. Her areas of interest include the archaeology of ancient medicine and ancient conceptions of salubrious spaces. She is the author of *The Archaeology of Medicine in the Greco-Roman World* (Cambridge University Press, 2013) and has a recent paper in *World Archaeology*, 'Identifying the Connection between Roman Conceptions of "Pure Air" and Physical and Mental Health in Pompeian Gardens (*c.* 150BC–AD79): a multi-sensory approach to ancient medicine'.

Rebecca Flemming is Senior Lecturer in ancient history in the Classics Faculty of the University of Cambridge, and a Fellow of Jesus College. Her book *Medicine and the Making of Roman Women: Gender, Nature and Authority from Celsus to Galen* came out from Oxford University Press in 2000, and the volume she co-edited with Nick Hopwood and Lauren Kassell, *Reproduction: Antiquity to the Present Day* was published by Cambridge University Press in 2018. She is currently writing a book on medicine and empire in the Roman world.

Ido Israelowich is a Senior Lecturer in the Department of Classics, at Tel Aviv University. His research focuses on ancient medicine and Roman law. He is particularly interested in the social, economic and legal frameworks in which medicine was practised and in the influence of various disciplines and professions on the evolution of Roman law, and the way it has been administered.

Julie Laskaris received her doctorate in Classics from the University of California, Los Angeles, 1999. Before that, she was a modern dancer in New York. She is an Associate Professor in the Department of Classical Studies at the University of Richmond, Virginia. Her research interests centre on ancient Greek medicine. She is a past president of the Society for Ancient Medicine and Pharmacy.

David Leith is Lecturer in Classics at the University of Exeter. His research focuses on Graeco-Roman medicine, especially its interactions with philosophy. He has published on the Hellenistic and Roman medical sects and their theories, especially Herophilus, Erasistratus, Asclepiades and the Methodists, and has edited fragments of medical papyri for *The Oxyrhynchus Papyri* series. He is currently preparing an edition, with essays and commentary, of the testimonia on Asclepiades of Bithynia.

Chiara Thumiger is a classicist and historian of ancient science, currently holding a Kiel University Research Fellowship in the Cluster of Excellence Roots. Her interests lie in the area of history of psychiatry and of the representations of mental health, and more generally in the history of medicine. She has also researched and published on ancient emotions, tragedy and ancient animals. Recent publications are *A History of the Mind and Mental Health in Classical Greek Medical Thought* (Cambridge University Press, 2017), *Mental Illness in Ancient Medicine* (co-edited with P. Singer, Brill, 2018) and the edited volume *Holism in Ancient Medicine and Its Reception* (Brill, 2020). Her monograph about the ancient disease *phrenitis* and its afterlife in the Western medical tradition is forthcoming.

Laurence Totelin is Reader in Ancient History at Cardiff University. She specializes in the history of ancient pharmacology, gynaecology and botany. Her key works include *Hippocratic Recipes: Oral and Written Transmission of Pharmacological Knowledge in Fifth- and Fourth-Century Greece* (Brill, 2009), and with the botanist Gavin Hardy, *Ancient Botany* (Routledge, 2016).

John Wilkins is Professor Emeritus of Greek Culture at Exeter University. He works on Greek and Roman drama, food and medicine. Books include *Euripides: Heraclidae* (Oxford, 1993), *The Boastful Chef* (Oxford, 2000), *Food in the Ancient World* (with Shaun Hill, Malden MA, 2006), *Galien: Sur les facultés des aliments* (Paris, 2013). He co-edited *Food in Antiquity* (Exeter, 1995), *Athenaeus and his World* (Exeter, 2000), *The Rivals of Aristophanes* (London, 2000), *Galen and the World of Knowledge* (Cambridge, 2009), *A Companion to Food in the Ancient World* (Malden MA, 2016), *Selfhood and the Soul* (Oxford, 2017).

INDEX

abdomen 75, 157, 166, 171, 184
abortion
  and ethics and law 191, 198
  means to procure 15, 206
  safe and unsafe 87, 210 n.26
  spontaneous 69, 79; *see also* miscarriage
abscesses 75
Achilles (mythological hero) 109
acidity 60, 66 n.22
Acragas (river) 33
Actium (battle) 3, 7
acute pain 57, 108, 148–53, 155, 202
adolescents 76
adulteration 5, 10
advertisement 8
Aegean Sea 43
Aelius Aristides (Publius Aelius Aristides,
  orator) 22, 32–3, 147, 154–8, 161,
  162
Aeschylus (tragic poet) 93
Aesculapius (god) 135
Aetius (doxographer) 177, 179, 186
Aetius (of Amida, physician) 3, 43, 99,
  105
Africa
  North 29, 53, 72–3, 84, 147, 155
  Roman province of 29
  West 82
afterbirth 14
agency 143, 145, 157
Agricola (Gnaeus Julius Agricola, general) 25

agriculture 52, 69, 78, 109
  see also Cato, Columella, *Geoponica*,
    Palladius, Varro
Agrippa (Marcus Vispanius Agrippa,
  general) 37
Agrippina the Younger (Roman empress)
  17
air
  as an element 66, 146, 168, 172–3
  influence on health 26–7, 31, 36, 38–9,
    64, 79
  spreading diseases 126
  in the uterus 102
  see also pneuma, under Hippocratic
    treatises
Alcmaeon (of Croton, philosopher) 172,
  186 n.7
alcohol 64
Alexander (of Aphrodisias, philosopher)
  177
Alexander the Great (king) 3, 9, 52
Alexandria
  as centre of medical learning 113, 168,
    174, 179, 182
  sanctuaries of 154
  as urban centre 9, 32, 36, 208
  see also Zopyrus
Allianoi 36
alphabet 194
aluminium 138
Amasis Painter 74

Anacharsis (Scythian philosopher) 30
anaemia 72, 79, 86, 87
anaesthesia 119
analgesics 15
Anatolia 53
anatomical demonstrations 5, 175, 182
    see also epideixeis
anatomists 113, 182
anatomy
    Diocles and 106
    Galen and 107, 182–5; see also Galenic
        treatises
    Herophilus and 174–5
    and physiology 65, 105, 168, 185
    and vivisection 107
    see also physiology
Anaxagoras (of Clazomenae, philosopher)
    106
Andreas (of Carystus, physician) 4, 52
Andromachus the Elder (physician) 1
Andromachus the Younger (physician) 7
anger 64, 180
anima 165
animalization 110–11, 113
animals 93–117
    see also individual names of animals,
        Aristotle, bones, physiology
anise 17
ankles 39 n.1, 149
Annia Faustina (Roman princess) 154
Anonymus Londinensis 65 n.11, 168
Anonymus Parisinus 150, 173–4, 179–80
anthropologists 16, 17, 49
anthropology 25, 57
anthropotherapia 104–5
antidotes 1–18, 100–1, 153
    see also Mithradatium, under Galenic
        treatises
antimony 137
Antioch 39
Antiochus (of Ascalon, philosopher) 170
Antipater (medical author) 7
antipathy 115
Antonine Plague 73, 84
Antoninus Pius (Roman emperor) 148–50,
    152
Antonius Musa (physician) 37
Antyllus (physician) 38
anxiety 64
apes 107–8

Aphrodisias 52
    see also Alexander
Apollo (god) 38, 192
Apollonius Mys (physician) 4
Apollonius (of Tyana, philosopher) 205–6
apotropaic function 104
appetite 46, 58, 146, 165, 180, 184
apprenticeship 189–90, 193–4, 200
Apuleius (Lucius Apuleius Madaurensis,
        Latin rhetorician) 29–31
aqueducts 37–8, 90 n.5
Arabia 9–10
Arcadia 201
archaeologists 11, 32–3, 71, 121–2, 125,
    129–32, 135, 141
archaeology 11–12, 26, 36, 44, 52, 79–80,
    119–41
    see also bioarchaeology
Archagathus (physician) 207–8
Archaic period 10, 12, 32, 33
archiatroi 153
Archigenes (physician) 1, 18 n.2
architects 22, 24–7, 38, 207
architecture 22, 26, 27, 39
    see also buildings, Vitruvius
Arctic Ocean 77
aristocracy 75, 146
Aristophanes (comic poet) 195
Aristotle (philosopher) 24, 56, 113, 172
    Dissections 106
    History of Animals 106
    Nicomachean Ethics 194
    On Marvellous Things Heard 114 n.9
    On the Soul 61
    Parva Naturalia 106
armies 26–7, 29, 39, 73, 153
    see also soldiers
ars 209
arsenic 73–4, 137
art 23, 70, 129
Artemidorus (of Daldis, diviner) 154
Artemis (goddess) 10, 79, 94
arterial system 175–6, 184
arteries 145–6, 174, 176, 184
arthritis 150, 154
artisans 26, 40 n.4, 194
Asclepeia 32–4, 44, 157
Asclepiades (of Bithynia, physician) 3, 46,
    52, 170, 177–8
Asclepiads 193

Asclepius
   and Aelius Aristides 22, 147, 155–8,
     163
   association with animals 110–11, 190
   cult of 32–3
   dedications to 193
   healing by 164, 204
   as a hero 109
   invocations to 192
   see also Aesculapius, caduceus, Galen,
     temples and sanctuaries of Asclepius
Asia 9, 25, 29, 72, 150, 155
Asia Minor 3, 32, 43, 53, 147
asses 95
astringents 54, 57, 60–1, 64, 99, 196
astrologers 146
Athenaeus (of Attaleia, physician) 38, 178
Athenaeus (of Naucratis, rhetorician) 46,
     52, 63, 174
Athens 33, 145, 208
   see also Plague of Athens
athletes 62, 116 n.30
athletics 75
atoms 137, 178, 180
Attalus III (of Pergamum, king) 9
audiences 22–3, 108, 146, 155, 163 n.4
Augustus (Roman emperor) 8, 12, 17, 27,
     37
Aulus Gellius (Roman author) 5, 145, 148,
     158, 162
authenticity 10
authority 2–8, 185–6, 189–201
authorship 2, 8, 191, 197–200
autochthony 25
autonomy 158, 206
autumn 47, 76

Babylonia 111, 115 n.24
back 149
bacteria 81, 86, 89 n.2, 90 n.5, 126
Baiae 34, 36–7
Barbarians 25, 30, 40 n.18, 104
barley 44, 49, 57
barrenness 36
   see also under Hippocratic treatises
bathing 34–5, 53, 64, 66 n.26, 132, 151–2,
     157
baths 34–7, 64, 116 n.30, 151–2, 156,
     169, 205
battlefields 46

battles 32, 73
   see also Actium
beans 16, 49, 61–2, 66 n.16
bears 94, 107
beavers 10, 100
   see also castoreum
beef 54, 95
bees 101, 110, 114 n.9, 154, 178
beet 51, 54
bile 99, 100, 115 n.26, 164 n.12, 180
   black 15, 53, 54, 66 n.20
   yellow 53, 66 n.20
   see also melancholy
bioarchaeology 71, 90 n.9
biomedicine 45–6
birds 95, 102, 108, 135–6
birth
   canal 88
   giving 86, 110, 159–6
   of humble 157
   life expectancy at 76, 91 n.16
   live 87
   multiple 86
   as polluting 102, 203
   see also childbirth
birthing chair 160, 203
birthplace 30, 31, 32
Bistocus (friend of Mithradates) 6
bites 5, 14, 101, 104–5, 112, 115 n.19
bitterness 60–1
Black Death 82
Black Sea 3
bladder 47, 50, 87, 155
bladder stones 36, 72, 88
bleeding 113, 128, 195
blindness 72
blister beetles 102
blood
   and digestion 53–4, 56, 95
   excessive 47; see also bloodletting
   as a humour 66 n.20
   as an ingredient 99–100, 103–4,
     115 n.20
   nature of 58
   and pneuma 146, 176
   as a poison 112
   pressure of 86
   purges of 155–7
   quantity in the body 31–2
   spitting of 80, 154

on surgical instruments 134
transfusion of 87
see also anaemia, menstrual blood,
    women
blood making 53, 54, 56
    see also liver
blood vessels 146, 183
bloodletting 47–8, 50, 65 n.12, 110, 156–7
bloodstream 77, 86
boars 94–5
bones
    of animals 82, 94
    consuming of human 103
    cranial 125, 180
    diseases of 72, 75, 80
    of foetus 87–8
    and malnutrition 91 n.17
    as material 132
    remains of 71–2, 80
    setting of 75
    see also surgery
books
    cookery 58
    medical 145–6, 189–90, 194–5, 200,
        203
    see also notebooks, textbooks
botanists 66 n.18
    see also ethnobotanists
botany 9, 52
bowels 47, 48, 58, 145
boys 91 n.16, 205
bracelets 133
brain 47, 61, 75, 105, 107–8, 125, 165–87
    see also meninges, ventricles
brass 140
bread 43, 52, 57, 58
breath 146, 151, 155, 173
    see also pneuma
breathing 46, 64, 108, 156
Britain 25, 130
bronze 124–5, 130, 132, 137, 139–40,
    148
Bronze Age 73
brucellosis 72
Bubonic Plague 83
buckles 133
buildings 21, 38, 81, 131
burials 79, 84, 90 n.10, 130, 131–2, 134–5
butchers 73, 119, 147, 207
butter 96, 97, 99

Byzantine Empire 44, 83
Byzantium 43, 203

caduceus 135–6
Caelius Aurelianus (medical author) 169
Caerleon 35
cakes 57
Calcidius (philosopher) 178
calories 46
Campania 34, 36
cancer 71, 72
cannabis 53
cantharis 100
Caracalla (Roman emperor) 3, 11
cardamon 9, 17
cardiocentrism 170, 173
Carians 40 n.18
caries 75
Carthaginians 30
    see also Mago
cassia 9
castoreum 10, 100–1
castration 110
cataplasms 104
cataracts 104, 128, 133
catarrhs 151, 156, 161
caterpillars 99
catheters 88, 129, 202
Cato (Marcus Porcius Cato, agricultural
    writer) 109
cattle 82, 109
cautery 3, 123, 125, 207
cedar 53
cellulitis 86
Celsus (medical author) 7, 28, 35–6, 45,
    52, 89, 92 n.32, 125, 128, 130
cereals 43–4, 48–9, 58
cerebellum 174
character 25, 29–32, 39, 40 n.7
Charmis (physician) 37
cheese 95–7, 99, 82
chefs 46
chemotherapy 46
chest 75, 99, 152–3, 157, 161, 166
chickpeas 58–9
childbirth 70, 72, 79, 84–9, 196, 203
    see also afterbirth, chorion, fistulas
children
    bearing of 73, 104
    caring for 208

death of 17, 70, 80, 90 n.10
diseases of 77–8, 82, 97, 99, 152
eighth-month 161
feeding of 96, 98
and games 26
and the Hippocratic *Oath* 193
loss of 153
risks faced by 76, 79, 85
on steles 203
voices of 3
see also adolescents, boys, girls, infant,
    infant and child mortality, labour,
    lactation, newborns, *under*
    Hippocratic treatises
chills 14, 156
Chiron (centaur) 109–11
cholera 72, 151, 164 n.12
chorion 100, 104
chronic pain 147, 151, 161
Chrysippus (of Soli, philosopher) 176,
    178
Chthonic deities 133
cicadas 95
Cicero (philosopher) 158–9
cinnamon 9–10
circus games 5, 26
cities 23, 37–9, 44, 72, 79, 83, 145
citron 52
city planning 26
city walls 27
civic environment 34, 37–8
Claudius (Roman emperor) 17, 37, 103
cleansing 32, 104
Cleopatra (queen) 7, 16
Cleophantus (medical author) 7
cleverness 30
climates 23–9, 36, 39, 43, 56, 72–3
    see also microclimates
clitorises 89
cocks 5
coffee 61–2
cognition 78, 166, 177
coinage 148
coins 120, 140
collyrium stamps 133, 135–6
Cologne 134–5
colonies 31
colonization 129
Colophon 125, 157
    see also Nicander

Columella (Lucius Junius Moderatus
    Columella, agricultural writer) 44,
    109
comedy 100
    see also Aristophanes
commanders 25–7
Commodus (Roman emperor) 3, 10, 11,
    153–4
Competition 144, 146, 162, 200, 208
competitive consumption 10–12
complexion 47
conception 14, 100
conquests 9, 72
Constantinople 83
constipation 47, 51, 61
consumerism 11–12
consumption (disease) 157
convalescence 22, 32, 35
cookers 11
cooking 45, 53, 67 n.27, 81
copper 137–40
copper alloy 122–3, 127–8, 130–1, 136–7,
    139–41
Corinth 33, 182
corpses 84, 116 n.30
Corpus Hippiatricorum Graecorum 109
Cortes 61
Cos 32
    see also Hippocrates, Philinus, Praxagoras
cosmetics 102–3
coughs 14, 80, 97, 157
countryside 49, 83
courtiers 3, 17
courts (royal) 3, 9, 16, 103, 148, 154, 179,
    210 n.29
courts (of law) 29, 31, 198
Coventina (Romano-British goddess) 133
crabs 96, 104
cramps 100
cranioclasts 88
Crateuas (physician) 3, 4, 52, 201, 210 n.23
cremation 71, 130
criminals 3, 5, 74
crocodiles 10, 115 n.15, 178
Cumae 34
cupping 128
cupping vessels 144, 155, 189
curator aquarum 37–8
cursus honorum 148
Cyprus 104

dairy 94, 96–7
Damocrates (medical author) 2, 7, 8
Danube 152
death rates 74, 76, 78
deer 94–5, 101, 103, 115 n.20
  see also stag
deforestation 69, 78
delirium 47
Delos 33
Democritus (philosopher) 106, 179–81, 201
demography 44, 49, 75–7, 89
depression 46, 49
desires 11–12, 46, 77, 184, 207
despondency 48
detoxification 63, 66 n.26
diabetes 45, 46, 49
diagnosis 48, 50, 53, 61, 153, 196
  see also retrospective diagnosis
diarrhoea 114 n.9
dietetics 17, 50, 52, 56, 63, 94, 97, 110
dieticians 50
Digest 37
digestion
  issues with 17, 95, 99
  process of 15, 53–4, 58, 63–4, 176
  see also blood, liver, stomach
Dio Cassius (historian) 17, 37, 84, 153
Diocles (of Carystus, physician)
  and dissection 106
  and food 46, 51–2, 56–7
  and the heart 173–4
  and hygiene 34
Diodorus Siculus (historian) 202
Diogenes (of Apollonia, philosopher) 172
Dionysopolos 132
Dioscorides (of Anazarbus, medical author)
  4, 10, 52, 99, 101, 105, 154
Dioskuroi 111
Diphilus (of Siphnus, physician) 52, 63
diphtheria 72
disability 77–8, 85
diseases 69–92
  *see also individual names of diseases and
    affected parts of the body*, endemic
    diseases, epidemics, fevers, sacred
    disease, symptoms, women, *under*
    Hippocratic treatises
disgust 97, 99, 102, 103, 115
dissection105–8, 113, 128, 174, 175
  see also Aristotle, vivisection

dissectors 123
diuretics 60, 63, 64
dizziness 154
dogs 95, 98, 103, 104, 110–12
domestication 69, 82, 89
Domitian (Roman emperor) 37
donkeys 94, 98
drains 37, 52
dreams 154–8, 162, 164 n.26, 193, 195
Dreckapotheke 97, 99, 101–5
drills 129
drug sellers 191, 202–3
drugs
  compound 7, 15, 73, 202
  Egyptian 46, 104
  Hippocratic 58, 100
  poisoning 17
  polypharmaceutical 9, 16
  prophylactic 1, 14, 16
  psychotropic 97
  simple *see under* Galenic treatises
  see also individual names of drugs,
    antidotes, plants
dunameis 51, 53, 60–1
dung 99, 102–4, 115 n.26
  see also excrement
dyes 11
dysentery 50, 77, 99
dyspepsia *see* indigestion

Early Modern period 46, 147
ears 51, 116 n.30, 124–6, 172–3
earth
  as an element 56, 66 n.19, 168
  fruits of 30, 51, 57
  from Lemnos 10
ebola 83
eclampsia 86, 91 n.26
economy 11, 109
Edelstein, Ludwig 45, 198
efficacy 14–16, 101, 109, 136, 168
effluvia 27
eggs 95, 99, 100, 102, 106
Egypt 10, 115 n.26, 144, 159–60, 162,
  192
Egyptians 30
einkorn 43
elbows 149, 156, 161
elderly 80
electuaries 17

elements 28, 53, 66, 137–8, 168, 178
    see also air, earth, fire, water
elephants 99, 108, 115 n.15
elites
    educated 30, 145, 147
    local 155
    male 144
    Roman 11, 152
    senatorial 154
    social 3, 10, 14, 163
    see also patients
embryotomies 88
emesis 16
emetics 69
emmer 43
emollients 99
emotions 165, 172, 173, 177, 184
    see also anger, disgust, fear, grief
empeiria 3
Empiricists 3, 9, 168–9, 193
    see also Heraclides, Mantias, Zopyrus
encephalocentrism 170, 182
endemic diseases 72–3, 77–82
energy 46, 48, 53, 66 n.13, 75, 137
enslaved people 3, 14. 73, 76, 206
environment 5, 11, 21–41, 64, 95, 108,
    162
    see also civic environment
environmental determinism 31
Epicureanism 166, 177–8
Epicurus (philosopher) 153
Epidaurus 32, 33, 34, 202
epideixeis 108
epidemics 24, 72–3, 77, 82–4, 89, 90 n.12
    see also under Hippocratic treatises
epigrams 203
epigraphical record 12
epilepsy 70, 90 n.9, 104, 105, 172–4
Erasistrateans 64, 182
Erasistratus (of Ceos, physician) 47, 106,
    146, 168, 175–8, 182–5
Ethiopia 84
ethnobotanists 69
ethnographers 5, 26
ethnography 31, 32
Euphrates 39
Euripides (tragic poet) 112
Europe 9, 10, 25, 45, 72, 77, 82
euthanasia 191
excrement 99, 102–3, 105, 116 n.30

exercise 26, 28, 46, 60, 64–5, 152, 157, 195
experience 2–3, 56, 143–64
experimental method 106
experimentation 51
experiments 4, 5, 18, 60, 106, 184
expertise 170, 185, 199, 200
eyes
    black 47
    and the brain 173
    bright 113
    green 136
    issues with 14, 70, 159, 161
    medicines for 133
    and suffering 112

faeces 103
    see also dung, excrement
familia 12
family
    of birth 87
    imperial 149, 154
    nuclear 12
    of patients 143–4, 147–52, 158, 161–2
    and teaching of medicine 193–4, 197,
        198, 203
famine 21, 49, 58, 66 n.23, 71, 73, 82–3,
    89
Far East 52
farmers 44, 48, 73
farming 44, 73, 194
fashion 7, 10–12, 36
fasting 7, 47, 64, 158
fat 51, 94, 99–100, 115 n.26
fatigue 64
favism 72
Favorinus (of Arles, orator) 146
Fayum 160
fear 17, 50, 112–13, 151, 159, 172
feet 112, 149–50, 163 n.9, 173
Female Genital Cutting 87–8
fertility 30, 104, 206
festivals 94
fevers
    consuming 145
    as a disease 14, 50, 64–5, 70, 86,
        152–3, 155–6, 158–9, 161, 196
    enteric 47
    fits of 47
    malarial 162
    quartan 77

rheumatic 72
semitertian 77
as a symptom 16
tertian 77
yellow 73
figs 1, 7, 8, 17
filariasis 73
files (instrument) 129
fingers 127, 132, 149
fire 66 n.19, 81, 168
firewood 27
fish 44, 46, 54, 66 n.13, 78, 94–6
fishermen 73
fishing 46, 73
fistulas
    anal 88, 91 n.29
    obstetric 86–9, 91 n.29
    see also under Hippocratic treatises
floods 21, 78
flowers 1, 10, 114 n.9, 135
fluxes 145, 151, 152, 161, 204
fodder 27, 53, 95
foetus 14, 79, 87–8, 98, 102, 191
    see also under Hippocratic treatises
fogs 27
folk medicine *see* popular medicine
fomentation 150
food 1–2, 43–67, 93–7, 146, 152, 195,
    197
    see also individual names of foods,
        Diocles, digestion, dietetics, famine,
        hunger, malnutrition, nutrition,
        plants, recipes, women
food abstinence 157, 205
food chain 100, 113
food preparation 57–9, 122
food–medicine continuum 16–18
food shortages 45, 48–9, 82–4
Food Studies 43
foodstuffs 52, 56–7
    see also under Galenic treatises
food supply 43–4, 49, 58, 73
food tasters 17
forceps 88, 126–7, 130, 133, 135
forum 26
foxes 95
frankincense 9
fraud 15, 103
freedpeople 5, 12, 203
friendship 149–50

Frontinus (Sextus Julius Frontinus,
    engineer) 37–8
Fronto (Marcus Cornelius Fronto,
    grammarian) 147–52, 154–8,
    163 n.11
frugality 46
fruits 1, 49, 50, 57, 62, 66 n.13
fumigations 102

Galen (of Pergamum, physician)
    and his competitors 197, 204
    devotion to Asclepius of 153, 193
    imitators of 200
    as imperial physician 3, 5, 152–4, 158,
        162, 196
    as the new Hippocrates 198–9
    representations of 4, 107
    as source about Hellenistic authors 3
    teachers of 157; *see also* Satyrus
    as wondermarker 204
Galenic and pseudo-Galenic treatises
    Avoiding Distress 10, 134, 194
    Causes of Pulses 38
    *Commentary to Hippocrates' Epidemics
        VI* 100, 115 n.19
    Introduction or 'the Doctor' 179
    On Anatomical Procedures 107, 108,
        137, 182
    On Antidotes 1, 3, 5–12, 14, 16, 153
    On Good and Bad Juices 49–50
    On Mixtures 17, 53, 66
    On My Own Books 153, 182, 183, 200
    On Prognosis 108, 152–4, 196, 204
    On Recognizing the Best Physician 207
    On Synectic Causes 178
    *On the Composition of Drugs according
        to Kind* 8, 9, 15, 154
    *On the Composition of Drugs according
        to Places* 9, 123, 198–200
    *On the Opinions of Hippocrates and
        Plato* 178, 183, 186 n.10, 187 n.19
    On the Order of My Own Books 193
    On the Powers of Simple Drugs 5, 48,
        42–4, 60, 65, 66 n.18, 99, 103
    On the Preservation of Health 38, 53,
        62, 64, 132
    On the Properties of Foodstuffs 43, 45,
        48, 51–4, 56, 58–61, 63–6, 96
    On the Therapeutic Method 190
    On the Use of Respiration 186 n.10

On the Usefulness of Parts of the Body
    108
On Theriac to Pamphilianus 2
On Theriac to Piso 1, 5–6, 10–12, 15, 17
*The Capacities of the Soul Depend on
    the Mixtures of the Body* 170, 185
Thrasybulus 164 n.21
gall 100, 104
gaming boards 130
gangrene 112
garlic 60–1
garum 44
Gaul 25, 20, 135
Gauls 30
gender 14, 56, 98, 102–3, 114 n.4,
    115 n.26, 145, 193
generals 3, 6, 10, 27, 28, 32
    see also Agricola, Agrippa, Germanicus,
        Pompey the Great
genitals 87–8, 100, 129, 202–3
    see also Female Genital Cutting, penis,
        vagina
genomics 82, 89
Geoponica 44, 109
Germanicus Caesar (Germanicus Julius
    Caesar, general) 21–2, 26
Germans 25, 30
Germany 21, 135
ginger 9, 60
girls 73, 84–5, 87, 91 n.16
gladiators 104
glass 129, 132
goats 94–5, 98, 105, 107, 109
gold 84, 132, 137, 189
gourds 54–5
gout 14, 72, 150, 163 n.9
grains 44, 48, 49
grass 49, 57, 62, 103
Great Fire of Rome 10, 192
grief 64, 172
groin 149–50
growth 64, 76, 85, 87, 91 n.17, 165
gums 39 n.1, 99
gymnastic trainers 146, 156–7, 162,
    164 n.21
gynaecological treatises 88, 97, 102, 113,
    191, 194
    see also under Hippocratic treatises
gynaecological treatments 14, 96–8, 100,
    102, 104, 206

Hadrian (Roman emperor) 10
Hadrian's Wall 133
haemorrhage 47, 75, 86, 91 n.27
haemorrhoids 127
hair 47, 104, 113, 116 n.30
hand
    ailments of 70, 149, 159, 205
    and the brain 173
    holding of 203
    of the physician 134–5, 185
    washing of 105
    writing by 7, 149, 194
Hardknott Pass 28
hares 94, 95, 205–6
Harris stripes 76, 91 n.17
headaches 58
healthcare 21–3, 26, 33, 35–6, 110, 130
healthcare providers 22, 23, 25, 146
hearing 172
heart
    as central organ 170–1, 173–8, 182,
        184
    motion of 146
    as 'nurse of anger' 180
    see also hēgemonikon, ventricles, *under*
        Hippocratic treatises
heart disease 45, 46, 49
heatstroke 64
hedgehogs 95
hēgemonikon 166, 176–9
Helen (mythological character) 46
hellebore 70, 100, 106, 201
Hellenistic kingdoms 9
hemlock 201
hepatitis 72
Heracles (Greek god) 33, 112, 135–6
    see also Hercules
Heraclides (of Tarentum, Empiricist
    physician) 52
herbalists 201, 208
herbs 106, 110
Herculaneum 8, 52, 75, 76, 131
Hercules (god) 135
Herodian (historian) 39
Herodotus (historian) 25, 40 n.18
heroes 46, 109, 112–13
    see also Achilles, Asclepius
Herophilus (of Chalcedon, physician) 106,
    168, 174–80, 182–5
Hesiod (poet) 103

hills 28
Hippocrates (of Cos, physician)
   and Democritus 180–1, 201
   conferring authority on the Hippocratic
      Corpus 2, 191, 198–9
   name of 111
   students of 193
Hippocratic Corpus (history and
   constitution of) 2, 179, 183, 190,
   199
Hippocratic medicine 33, 46, 47, 145
Hippocratic physicians 45, 47, 58
Hippocratic question 198
Hippocratic treatises
   Aphorisms 90 n.6
   Epidemics 1 18, 47, 195–6
   Epidemics 2 184, 187 n.19
   Epidemics 3 95
   Epidemics 5 86, 147
   Epidemics 7 86, 147
   Law 186
   Letters 180–1, 201
   Oath 190–9, 201–3, 206, 208
   On Airs, Waters and Places 23–4, 27,
      29–30, 34, 36, 38, 43, 87
   On Ancient Medicine 57, 197
   On Barrenness 87, 100, 104
   On Decorum 189
   On Diseases 1 86
   On Diseases of Women 85, 91 n.27,
      100, 102, 104, 113, 115 n.16, 196
   On Fistulas 91 n.29
   On Joints 80, 196
   On Regimen 51, 56, 60, 95, 98, 178
   On Regimen in Acute Diseases 60, 63,
      97
   On the Art 207
   On the Heart 106
   On the Nature of Man 66 n.20
   On the Nature of the Child 85, 106,
      191
   On the Nature of Woman 98, 102, 104,
      206
   On the Sacred Disease 70, 90 n.9,
      105–6, 172–4, 179, 181, 183–4,
      205
   Prognostic 90 n.6, 196
   Prorrhetic 196
Hippocratic triangle 18
historiography 21, 25

Homer (poet) 43, 46, 63
Homo erectus 69
honey 10, 17, 94–5, 97, 100, 114 n.9,
   152
hooks 88, 130, 132, 135
Horace (poet) 37
horns 101, 104, 107, 115 n.20, 129
horses 57, 94–5, 98, 109, 111
hotels 36
household gods 149
households 7, 151, 158, 159, 208
hudrophobia 110, 112
humoural balance 14, 26, 46, 53, 128
humoural system 26, 66 n.20, 110
humours 15, 18, 46–66, 110
   see also bile, blood, phlegm
hunchbacks 70, 80, 197
hunger 45, 50, 113
hunter-gatherers 82
hunters 73
hunting 46, 94, 112, 205
husbandry 108
hybridization 110, 130
hydromel 97
hydrotherapy 33–4
Hygieia (goddess) 192
hygiene 34, 37, 86, 125
hymens 89
hypochondriacs 50, 147
Hypsas (river) 33

iamata 156
Iambic poetry 100
ibis 136
illiteracy 12, 189
Illyrium 39
immigrants 29, 76
immigration 72, 76, 83
immortality 6, 180, 185
incantations 205
incense 12
incontinence 87, 89
India 9, 10, 201
indigestion 14, 58, 196
infant and child mortality 162
infant exposure 91 n.16
infanticide 91 n.16
infants 78, 80, 85, 90 n.10, 99, 116 n.30,
   203
   see also newborns

infections
    bacterial 46, 72, 86
    causes of 27, 69, 72, 73
    cutaneous 73
    malarial 78–9, 82
    post-partum 86
    pyogenic 72
    seasonal 75
    treatment of 75
    viral 46
infertility 15
influenza 90 n.3
innkeepers 29
insanity 36
inscriptions 12, 32, 111, 144, 203
insects 79, 99–100, 108
insomnia 47
instruments *see* surgical instruments
intellectual property 8, 200
invasions 129
iology 99–100
Iphigenia (mythological character) 132
iris 10
iron 72, 127, 129–32, 137–40
irrigation 69
Isidore (of Seville, scholar) 109
Islam 46
Italy 7, 36, 71, 75–6, 78–80

jaundice 14
Jesus (of Nazareth, religious leader) 205
Jews 30, 82
joints 74, 148–51, 161
    see also under Hippocratic treatises
juices
    good and bad 49–51, 53–4, 64
    of plants 16, 60, 201
    raw and cooked 51, 56
    in the soil 36
    and tastes 60–1
    see also under Galenic treatises
Julia Domna (Roman empress) 210 n.29
juniper 53, 61
Juturna (deity) 38
Juvenal (poet) 1, 3, 18 n.2

keys 132
kidney stones 88
kidneys 14, 100
knees 22, 39 n.1, 149, 151

knives 88, 132, 189
kyphosis 70, 80–1

labour 73, 85–7, 89, 203, 205
lactation 15
ladders 197
lambs 94–5
lameness 39 n.1
lamps 131, 132
lancets 189
lard 100
laughter 7, 172, 181, 201
laws 40 n.18, 158, 198, 206
    see also under Hippocratic treatises
laxatives 15, 51, 69, 97, 98
laypeople 21, 24, 33, 101, 109, 208
lead 72, 137, 139–40
    see also poisoning
Lebedus 157
Lebena 33
leeks 61
legumes 44, 49
leishmaniasis 72
Lemnos 10, 112
Lenaeus (freedman) 5
lentils 49
leprosy 72, 77
letters 144, 149–52, 155, 158–9, 161,
        163
    see also under Hippocratic treatises
lettuce 53–4
life expectancy 75–6, 78, 90 n.15, 91 n.16
ligaments 150, 166
ligulae 123–4, 126
lions 94, 99, 104, 115 n.15, 205
literacy 12, 194–5, 197, 203, 208
liver
    as cause of appetite 180, 184
    diseases of 14
    as an ingredient 99
    mauling of 110
    nature of 176
    role in blood-making 54, 56, 183–4
Livia (Roman empress) 8, 17
Livy (historian) 83
lizards 8
locusts 178
loins 149
London Pharmacopoeia 2
Lucian (of Samosata, satirist) 135, 189, 192

Lucius Verus (Roman emperor) 84, 148, 152
Lucretius (philosopher) 74, 103
lukion 11
lungs 80, 176, 184
lussa 110, 112
luxury 46, 95, 189
Lysimachus (Hellenistic king) 52

madness 112, 165, 172, 201
  see also insanity
magia 29–30
magic 80, 97–8, 100–4, 113, 136, 206
magical papyri 102, 115 n.22, 136
magical rituals 80, 201
magicians 146, 205
Mago (the Carthaginian, agricultural
  writer) 109
make-up 123
malaria 72–3, 75–9, 83, 89, 90 n.11
malnutrition 48, 73, 76, 82, 85, 91 n.17
Mantias (Empiricist physician) 9, 52
manufacturing 119, 130–1, 134, 136, 140
manuscripts 4, 167, 192, 194
Marc Antony (Roman politician) 16
Marcus Aurelius (Roman emperor)
  and antidotes 10–11, 15–17
  correspondence of 148–50, 155, 156,
   158
  and Galen 3, 196
  Meditations 153
mares 58
market sellers 3
marriage 72, 87
marrow 100, 166
marshes 24, 26–8, 79
Martial (poet) 35, 36
Martialis (physician) 182
Masinissa (king) 31
massages 50, 53, 63–4, 66 n.26, 150
masseurs 64, 191
Massilia 37
materia medica 25, 45
maternal mortality 70, 86, 89
Mauretania 10
Measles 83, 90 n.3
meat 54, 82, 94–6, 114 n.4
meconium 116 n.30
Medea (mythological character) 112
medical marketplace 23, 146, 158, 200–1,
  207, 208

Mediterranean cultures 97
Mediterranean region 43, 52, 73, 77, 102,
  130–1
melancholy 15
melicrat *see* hydromel
memory 184, 194
menarche 84–5
meninges 176–7, 182, 184, 186 n.10
menses 14
menstrual blood 104, 113, 116 n.30
menstruation 15, 102
  see also menarche
mental disorders 15, 112, 165, 169, 172,
  174
mental health 64–5
merchants 10, 18
mercury 137
Messene 33
metallurgy 73
metalworkers 73
Methodists 64, 169, 193, 251
  see also Soranus, Themison
Mexico 61
mice 102
microbes 73, 89
microbiome 89
microclimates 24, 43
midwives 146, 160–1, 191, 201, 203–4, 208
  see also Phanostrate
migrations 21, 82
military campaigns 84, 152, 153
military camps 27–8, 32, 38–9, 79
military experts 24
milk
  animal 58, 61, 82, 94–100
  human 104–5, 116 n.30
  kourotrophic 104
  see also lactation
mills 44
mind 2, 14–15, 18, 30–1, 64–5, 165–87
minerals 9–10, 25, 33, 39, 45, 201
miners 74
mirror 125, 132, 140
miscarriage 69
mists 27
Mithradates VI (of Pontus, king) 1, 3–9,
  12, 14, 18, 153, 210 n.23
Mithradatium 1–18
mixtures (*kraseis*) 53, 56, 61–2, 66
  see also under Galenic treatises

Mnesitheus (physician) 46, 51–2, 60, 63–4
Moesia 132
monkeys 104
moon 135
morality 5
morals 82
mortality rates 72, 75–6, 78–9
  see also infant and child mortality, maternal mortality
mortars 136
mosquitoes 77–9
mothers 7, 79, 85–8, 98–9, 104, 159–60, 203
mountains 30, 78, 113
mouth of the stomach 54, 154
mouths 70, 75, 97, 113
mules 102, 106
Mulomedicina Chironis 116 n.42
murder 31, 191
Muscio (medical writer) 89
muscles 36, 53, 75, 100
mushrooms 17
music 194
mustard 10
myrrh 9, 10
myrtle 61–2
Mysia 43

Naples 36, 52
nard 9, 10, 154
nausea 47, 48
Near East 10, 84, 101
neck 70, 149
necrosis 87–8
needles 128, 130, 133, 134
Neolithic 43, 69–70, 82
Nero (Roman emperor) 1, 34
Nerva (Roman emperor) 37
nerves 14, 150, 175 8, 182, 184
nervous system 174–6, 178–9, 182–5
newborns 79
Nicander (of Colophon, poet) 4, 100–1
Nicostratus (medical author) 8
Noricum 137
nostrils 47, 172, 184
notebooks 7
nutrition 44–50
nutritionists 47
nuts *see* walnuts

octopus 96
Oea (North African city) 30
ointments 123, 125, 126, 154
olive oil 53
Onasander (military writer) 27
onions 56, 60, 61, 66 n.13, 67 n.27
opisthotonos 14
opium 15–16, 201
oral transmission of knowledge 194
orators 144, 147, 150, 154–5, 158
oratory 149, 155
Oribasius (of Pergamum, physician) 3, 38, 43, 52, 99
osteoarthritis 72, 74, 75
osteomalacia 72
osteoporosis 72
Ostia 195, 203–4
otters 100, 115 n.16
oxen 57, 107
oxymel 97
Oxyrhynchus 161, 192

Paccius (Lucius Lutatius Paccius, incense seller) 12
Paccius (medical authority) 12, 14
Paget's disease 72
paideia 31
pains
  bodily 94
  chronic 147, 151, 161
  cries of 112–13
  feeling of 66 n.20, 162, 172, 203
  relief from 189
  see also acute pain, analgesics, chronic pain
painting 160 199
  see also Amasis Painter
paints 123
Palladius (Rutilius Taurus Aemilianus Palladius, agricultural writer) 44, 109
Panacea (goddess) 192
panic attacks 112
panthers 99
paralysis 36, 205
parasites 69–71, 73, 77–9, 89, 90
Park Collection 120–5, 129–31, 134, 137–8, 141
Parthians 30
pater familias 208
pathocoenosis 77

pathogens 72, 83
patienthood 93, 111, 112
patients
    disobedient 207
    elite 147–59, 162
    female 159–61
    Galenic 153
    wealthy 207
    see also Aelius Aristides, Fronto, Marcus
        Aurelius
Paul (of Aegina, medical writer) 3, 89, 99,
        101, 124
Pausanias (geographer) 32
peaches 11
peasants 44, 48, 49, 208
peddlers 12
pelvis 85–6
penis 100, 202
pepper 44, 48, 49, 208
Pergamum 32, 36, 154–7, 159, 162
    see also Attalus, Galen
Pericles (statesman) 83
peripneumonia 14
peritonitis 86
Persia 179
perspiration 99
pertussis 72, 90 n.3
pessaries 104, 191–2, 201
pestilences 28, 37, 72
Phanostrate (midwife) 203, 210 n.26
pharmacists 13
pharmacology 3, 17, 45, 52, 56, 94,
        97–105, 108, 110, 115 n.15
    see also antidotes, Dreckapotheke,
        drugs
pharmaka 17
pharmakeia 103
Philadelphia 159
Philinus (of Cos, physician) 168
Philoctetes (mythological character) 112
philosophers 26, 65, 145–6, 168, 170,
        175–7, 185, 193–4
    see also individual names of
        philosophers, Presocratic
        philosophers
Philostratus (sophist) 205
phlegm 53, 66 n.20, 173, 205
Phoenicians 30
phosphorus 139
phrenitis 47, 169, 179

phthisis 36, 80
Phylotimus (medical writer) 46
physiology
    and anatomy 65, 168, 185
    animal 106, 108
    causation in 51
    human 47, 95, 110, 113, 172–4, 177
physique 29, 30
pia mater 177, 180
pigs 90 n.3, 94, 104, 106–8
pilgrimages 22
pins 133
physicians
    amateur 3
    itinerant 23, 24
    literate 122, 145, 194–5, 197
    public 40 n.5, 207
placebo effect 16
placenta 86, 91 n.27, 104
plagiarism 200
Plague of Athens 82, 83–4, 91 n.23
plagues 21, 24, 69, 82, 112
    see also Antonine Plague, bubonic
        plague, Plague of Athens
plains 28, 45
plainsmen 30
plantain 154
plants
    as foods 44, 49, 51–2, 61, 66 n.23
    as drugs 45, 100–1, 106, 109, 201
    gathering of 201–2
    see also names of individual plants,
        domestication
plasters 157
Plato
    Gorgias 40 n.5, 46, 59
    Menexenus 25
    Phaedrus 181, 194
    Protagoras 181, 193
    Republic 45, 46, 195
    Timaeus 166, 171, 180
    see also psychology, *under* Galenic
        treatises
pleasure 46, 57, 59, 66
pleurisy 14, 72
Pliny the Elder (encyclopaedist)
    Natural History 8 115 n.20
    Natural History 21 17, 114 n.9
    Natural History 23 7
    Natural History 25 3, 5, 21–2

Natural History 28 99–100, 104–5, 115
Natural History 29 7, 37, 207–8
Natural History 31 35–6
Natural History 33 74
Natural History 36 136
Pliny the Younger (letter writer) 158
pluralism of ancient medicine 147, 162,
    191
Plutarch (philosopher) 3, 32, 63, 106,
    116 n.39
pneuma 146, 172–8, 184
  see also blood
Pneumatists 170, 193
pneumonia 72
podagra 150
poiotētes 53, 61
poisoning
  arsenic 74
  attempts at 16
  lead 72
  protection against 9, 66 n.18
  threat of 1, 4, 7, 17
  see also drugs
poisons
  administering of 17
  deadly 16, 100–1, 110
  experimenting with 5
  ingestion of 3, 6, 115 n.19, 178
  protection against 11, 14, 16, 153; *see*
    also antidotes, Mithradatium
  suicide with 6, 191
  see also blood, mushrooms, *pharmaka*,
    snakes, *venenum*
policy makers 26, 39
poliomyelitis 72
pollution 74, 202–3
Pompeii 11, 76, 127, 131
Pompey the Great (Gnaeus Pompeius
    Magnus, general) 3, 5–7
Pontus 97, 100
  see also Mithradates VI
popular medicine 3, 105, 114 n.3
pores 26, 36, 53, 64, 67 n.26
pork 66 n.13, 95
porridge 58
Posidonius (of Apamea, philosopher) 24,
    178
potency 201
Pott's disease 80, 81
pottery 129, 130, 132, 194

poultry 95, 110
poverty 71, 80
Praxagoras (of Cos, physician) 106, 173–4
predators 69
pre-eclempsia 86
pregnancy 15, 79, 84–5, 91 n.26, 159–61,
    206
Presocratic philosophers 106, 194
preventive medicine 45–6, 62, 64–5
priests 22, 81, 191
primum non nocere 195
probes 121–7, 130, 132–4, 139–40
professionalization of medicine 146,
    163 n.2
prognosis 23–4, 196–7
  see under Galenic treatises, Hippocratic
    treatises
Prometheus (titan) 93, 110, 112
proteins 86, 94
psuchē 65, 165
psychology
  and diet 51
  environmental 29
  of Galen 65, 185
  medical 110, 176, 178
  of Plato 51, 65, 66 n.14, 166, 179–86
public health 26, 29, 37, 39, 46
pulse 146, 151, 196
  see also under Galenic treatises
pulses (food) 49
pungency 54, 57, 60–1, 64, 66 n.22
purgatives 15, 69–70, 99
purges 36, 57, 64, 106, 155–7
purification 202, 205
purifiers 146, 205
pus 70, 90 n.6, 134
pustules 128
Pythagoras (philosopher) 198

quacks 14, 189, 205
quails 100
Quintus Serenus (medical author) 7

rabies 110, 205
racism 29–30
rains 27
rape 87
recipes
  of antidotes 5–6
  compilations of 200

and Dreckapotheke 99–100
exchange of 161
for food 58
in the Hippocratic Corpus 9, 58, 96,
    104, 191, 201
on papyri 97, 115 n.26
pharmacological 97, 101
in Theophrastus 97
verse 194
see also Mithradatium
rectum 87, 91 n.29
refugees 83
regimens 150, 195
    see also under Hippocratic treatises
religion 32, 62, 129, 158
    *see also names of individual gods and
        goddesses,* festivals, sacrifice, temple
        medicine, votive offerings,
        worshippers
reproduction 64, 79, 86, 102, 165, 176
respiration 172–3, 175–7
    see also under Galenic treatises
respiratory system 162
rest 64, 151, 152, 161
restaurants 36
retractors 130
retrospective diagnosis 14, 70, 83, 90 n.9
rhetors 29–31
rhododendrons 114 n.9
rickets 72
rings 130, 132, 133
rivers 22, 28, 33, 78, 156
    see also Acragas, Hypsas, Tiber
roads 36, 38
Roe v. Wade 198
Roman provinces 129–33, 137, 159
Romanization 129–30
root cutters 3, 191, 201
roots 5, 49, 51, 61
roses 1, 17
rubbish deposits 132
rue 7
Rufus (of Ephesus, medical writer) 4, 99
rust 128, 135, 136, 138, 189
rustics 58
rye 43

Sabinus (physician) 38
Sacred Disease 70, 90 n.9, 205 *see also*
    epilepsy, *under* Hippocratic treatises

sacrifice 62, 94–5, 157
sailors 73, 197
saliva 99
salivation 16
Sallust (historian) 163 n.9
salmonella 72
salt 7, 51, 58
salubriousness 27–8
salvation 156
sanitation 38, 69, 72, 73
Satyrus (Galen's teacher) 157
saws 107, 129, 130
scala naturae 117 n.48
scalpels 127–8, 130, 132, 134–5, 137
scapegoating 82
schist 136
schistosomiasis 73
sciatica 14
scorpions 101
Scribonia Attice (Roman midwife) 203–4
Scribonius Largus (medical writer) 7, 14,
    103, 150
scurvy 72
Scyfax (king) 30
Scythians 30, 58
seas 22, 36, 46, 197
    see also seawater
seasoning 58–9
seasons 24, 27–9, 56, 77
    see also autumn, diseases, infections,
        spring, summer, winter
seawater 36
sects 15, 169, 170, 190, 193
seizures 70–2
self-healing 103
self-medication 150, 162
Semonides (poet) 103
Seneca the Younger (philosopher) 25, 151
sensation 154, 162, 166, 171–2, 174–8,
    182, 184
senses 50, 62, 167, 171–3
    see also hearing, sight, smell, taste,
        touch
septicaemia 86
Septimius Severus (Roman emperor)
    3, 11
Serapis (god) 154
Sermoneta (Italian village) 78
Severus Alexander (Roman emperor) 39
sewers 38, 52

sex 46, 202, 206
  see also sexual intercourse
Sextus Empiricus (philosopher) 170
sexual abuse 206
sexual intercourse 1, 195, 202, 206
sexual violence 87, 89, 91 n.30
sexual symbolism 100
sexual violence 87, 89
sheep 94, 106, 107, 109, 154
shepherds 73
shoes 133
shopping 200
shops 20, 131
shoulders 74, 149
Sicily 33
sickness 27, 57, 73, 113, 154
sight 205
silicon 138, 139, 140
silver 135, 137, 140, 189, 202
sinews 36, 150, 155
skeletons 71
skin
  ailments of 50, 99
  observation of 47
  oiling of 53, 66 n.26
  rosy 156
  shedding of 110
  and surgery 127–8
  see also infections
skink 8, 10, 14
skulls 104
slavery 74, 77
slaves 151, 206–8
  see also enslaved people
sleep 46, 63, 64, 195
  see also dreams, insomnia
sleeping sickness 73
sleeplessness 48, 64, 172
smallpox 72, 73, 83, 84
smell
  bad 105, 112
  as cause of illness 27
  sense of 50, 61, 102, 172, 186 n.7
Smyrna 71, 156–7, 162, 182
snails 95
snakes
  associated with Asclepius 111, 190
  poisonous 100–1, 104–5, 112
  self-renewal of 11
  see also vipers

soap 11
social classes 48, 75
social climbers 3
Socrates (philosopher) 181
soil 29, 30, 36, 43, 53, 128
soldiers
  British 135
  healthy 62
  Roman 21–2, 26, 28, 39, 84
  sick 114 n.9, 73
  veteran 31
Sophists 31, 157, 205
Sophocles (tragic poet) 112
Soranus (of Ephesus, physician) 34, 48,
      85–7, 92 n.32, 169, 203
Sostratus (medical author) 99
soul 15, 51, 63–4, 66 n.14, 153, 165–87
  see also psuchē, under Galenic
      treatises
Spain 25, 61
Spartans 83, 144 n.4
spas 22, 36
spasms 112, 174
spatula probes 121, 123, 125–6, 130,
      139
spectacles 5
spectators 26, 108
sperm 103, 176
spices 17
spiders 101
spindle whorls 132
spittle 104, 116 n.30
spleen 14, 78, 176, 183
spoon probes 126–7, 134, 140
spoons 121–4, 132, 137–9
spring (season) 29, 49, 66 n.23
springs 22, 33–8, 133, 156–7
stags 100, 101
Stanway 130–2, 135
staphylococcus 72
stars 24, 135
starvation 73, 82
statuettes 71, 132
steatite 136
steel 128, 137
sterility 100, 102, 106
  see also barrenness
Stoicism 152, 166, 170, 176–8, 183
Stoics 176, 177, 185
  see also Chrysippus

stomach
    ailments of 14, 99, 151, 153–4, 156–7
    and digestion 51, 54, 58, 63–4
    see also mouth of the stomach
Strabo (geographer) 32, 35, 36, 74
strigils 132
strokes 70, 72, 90 n.9
stylus 121–3, 139
suet 100
Suetonius (historian) 35
suffering 87, 94, 108, 110–13, 143, 158
sugar 61
suicide 6, 7, 87, 191
summer 24, 27, 28, 49, 76
sun 27, 30, 31, 135, 178
surgery 45–6, 110
    bone 125, 127, 129
    dental 127
    specialization in 191–2
surgical instruments 11, 88, 105, 119–41,
        189, 195, 203–4
    see also individual names of
        instruments, blood
swamps 79
sweat 47, 103–5, 116 n.30, 134
swine 95
swords 6
sympathy 115 n.20, 161
symposium 46, 62–4, 145
    see also wine
symptoms
    of Aulus Gellius 145–6
    description of 161–2
    of dysentery 47–8
    of epidemic diseases 82–3
    of malaria 79
    of Marcus Aurelius 152, 156
    of phrenitis 169
    remission of 16
    role in identifying illnesses 70
    of tuberculosis 80
Syria 39, 124, 130
Syrians 30
syrups 17

Tacitus (historian) 17, 25, 35
tanners 73
taste
    aesthetic 11
    corrective of 97

and diagnosis 53
and humours 56, 60–1
and pleasure 46, 59–62, 66 n.17
sense of 50, 61, 102, 172
of substances 10, 24, 54, 62
Tatian (theologian) 103–4
tears 172
technē 93, 109, 110, 194, 196, 197,
        201–2, 209
    see also ars
technologies 89, 129–30, 135
teeth 22, 75, 91 n.16, 116 n.30, 123
    see also surgery
temple medicine 33, 39, 62
temples and sanctuaries of Asclepius 22,
        32–3, 154, 157, 162, 202
tendons 150, 166
Tertullian (theologian) 169, 174, 178
testicles 10, 100, 202
tetanus 14, 72
textbooks 22, 26
texture 15, 53–4, 56, 58
thalassemia 72, 79
theatre 26, 113
Themison (of Laodicea, physician) 169
Theophrastus (of Eresus, philosopher) 52,
        97, 106, 172, 201–2
therapeutics 97, 102, 110
theriac 1–2, 5, 9, 11, 14–17, 153, 156
    see also under Galenic treatises
Thessalus (Methodist physician) 190
Thessaly 100
thirst 47, 48
Thrace 43
throat 6, 106, 152, 161
Thucydides (historian) 25, 40 n.11, 82–4
Tiber 78, 79
Tiberius (Roman emperor) 14
tin 137, 139–40
Tivoli 35
toes 149
toilet items 125–7, 133
toilets 90 n.4
tongue 61, 123, 126, 154, 172–3
tonsils 127
topography 23, 25, 39
tortoises 178
torture 5, 18, 150
touch 53, 61, 66 n.26
tourism 32–4, 6

towns 8, 24, 39, 49
toxicology 97
toxins 75
trade 9–10, 12, 72, 82–3, 189
tragedy 112
Trajan (Roman emperor) 17, 25, 35
travels 72, 83, 99, 161
treacle 17
trees 28, 49
trepanation 75, 125
Tricca 32
Troezen 33
trotters 51
Troy 46
tuberculosis 71–3, 75–6, 80–2, 89
    see also Pott's disease
tumours 36
Tusculum 158
tweezers 127
typhoid 72, 76, 83
typhus 83

ulcers 99, 103, 152
Umbria 79
unguent sellers 12
unguents 11, 99, 100
urbanism 26
urbanization 21, 69
urinary tract 87, 129
urine
    diagnosis by 47, 48, 50, 86
    as a drug 99, 102–5, 116 n.30
    flow of 129
    retention of 14
    substances to promote 63
uterus 87, 102, 106
    see also womb
Utica 53
uvulae 127

vagina 87, 102, 104, 202
Varro (Marcus Terentius, agricultural
    writer) 24, 109
vegetable growers 29
vegetables
    as foods 51, 57, 65 n.13, 95
    growing of 29, 31, 49
    Phliasian 29
vegetarian diet 98, 158
vegetation 25, 26, 29, 39

Vegetius (Publius Flavius Vegetius Renatus,
    military writer) 22, 27–8, 31–2
veins 50, 54, 56, 145, 149, 176
venenum 17
venesection 152, 157
venoms 18, 101, 115 n.19
ventricles
    of the brain 174, 184
    of the heart 175
Vesuvius 8, 75–6, 86
veterinary art/medicine 94, 108–10,
    116 n.42
Vienna Dioscorides 4
Villa Vesuvio 11
Vindonissa 132
vinegar 51, 57, 97
vipers 1, 14, 100
virtues 30, 31, 99, 104, 153
viruses 71, 89 n.2
vision 58, 61, 136, 155, 172
vitamins 16, 72
Vitruvius (Marcus Vitruvius Pollio,
    engineer) 22, 26–8, 35–6, 38
vivisection 107–8, 116 n.41, 174–5
volcanoes 21
votive offerings 22, 23, 85, 98, 119, 131,
    133, 171

waking 64
walnuts 7, 11
warfare 22, 87, 91 n.30
wars 73, 87
    Mithradatic 3
    World War I 135
water
    boiling 51– 8
    curative 32–6, 64, 133
    drinking 22, 96, 150
    as an element 66 n.19, 168
    and malaria 78–9
    marshy 24
    to mix medicines in 16
    to mix with other drinks 63, 67, 152
    supply of, 24, 27–8, 31, 37–9, 69, 77,
        90 n.5
    taste of 54– 7
    to wash hands with 105
    see also aqueducts, curator aquarum,
        seawater, under Hippocratic
        treatises

wax 101, 116 n.30, 134
wealth 1, 9, 46, 62, 162, 208
weaving 74, 194
wellbeing 45
wells 38, 79, 133
wheats 43–4, 49, 57, 58
winds 24, 30, 39, 43, 58
wine
    Chian 10
    expensive 46
    making of 31
    to mix medicines in 7, 16, 17, 102
    as nourishment 63–4, 152
    red/black 50, 63–4
    tawny 64
    Thasian 29
winter 24, 28, 49
witches 191
womb 88, 115 n.16, 196, 205–6
women
    anatomy of 106, 129
    blood of 14–15, 113; *see also* menstrual
        blood, menses
    diseases of 3, 47, 72, 74, 86–9, 203
    as food makers 58
    infertile 36
    nursing 73
    pregnant 48, 69, 79, 86–7, 89, 191
    as victims of violence 87, 91 n.30, 206
    voices of 3, 114, 159
    and weaving 74
    see also birth, childbirth, hymens,
        midwives, mothers, patients,

regnancy, sexual organs, uterus,
    under Hippocratic treatises
wood 126, 135, 160, 175
woodworking 129
wool 74, 99, 100, 154, 159, 202
workers 62–3
workshops 13, 131, 207
World Health Organization 87
worms 89 n.2, 100
worshippers 22, 32, 33
wounds
    in the belly 100
    healers of 207
    treatment of 70, 111, 123, 126
    ulcerous 112
    of war 31–2, 73, 90 n.13
wrestlers 103
writing 150, 194–5
    see also literacy
writing tools 122
    see also stylus

Xenocrates (medical author) 7
xenophobia 30
Xenophon (philosopher) 114 n.9,
    194
xerophthalmia 72
X-Ray Florescence 136–7

Zeus (god) 157
zinc 137, 139–40
Zopyrus (of Alexandria, Empiricist
    physician) 3, 5